Computed
Tomography
of the Body

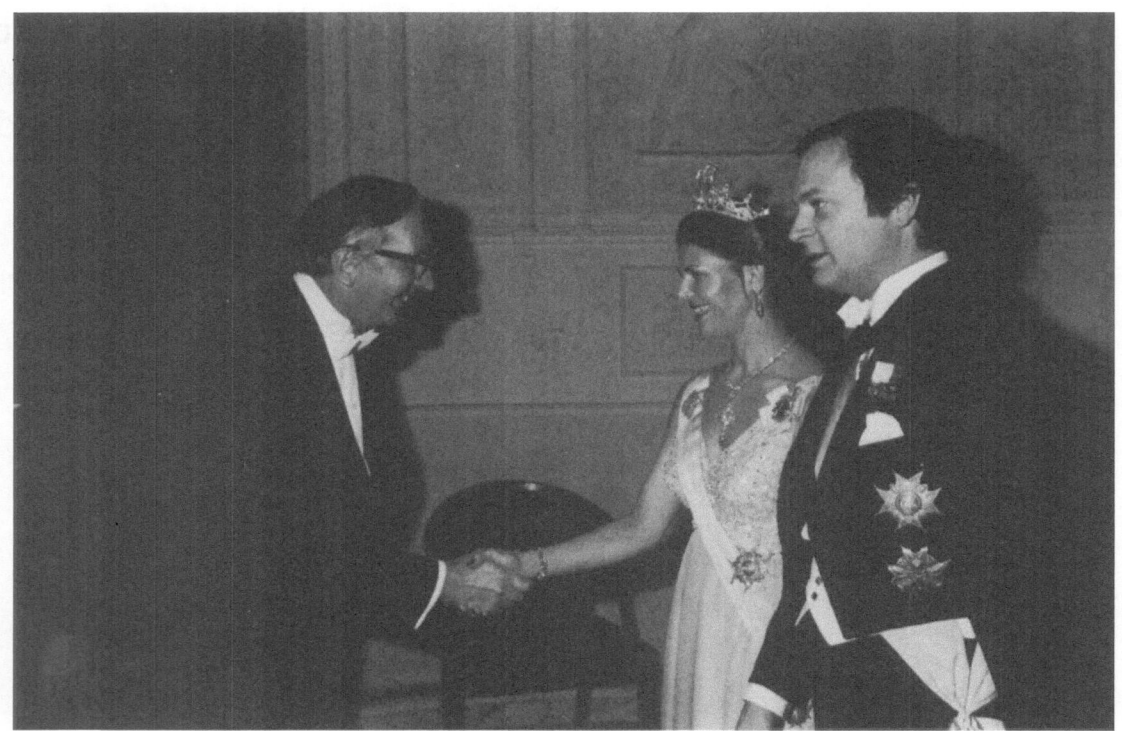

We would like to acknowledge the pioneer work of Sir Godfrey Hounsfield, CBE, FRS, in the development of computed tomography. He is seen here with King Carl Gustav and Queen Silvia after the award of the 1979 Nobel Prize in Medicine

Computed Tomography of the Body

A RADIOLOGICAL AND CLINICAL APPROACH

Janet E. Husband, MRCP, FRCR

*Consultant Radiologist and Honorary Senior Lecturer,
Institute of Cancer Research, Royal Marsden Hospital, Sutton; and
Consultant Radiologist, BUPA Medical Centre, London*

and

Ian Kelsey Fry, DM, FRCP, FRCR

*Consultant Radiologist, St Bartholomew's Hospital, London; and
Director, CT Scanning Unit, BUPA Medical Centre, London*

First edition 1981
Reprinted 1983, 1985

Published by
Scientific and Medical Division
MACMILLAN PUBLISHERS LTD
London and Basingstoke
Companies and representatives throughout the world

Typeset in Great Britain by
PINTAIL STUDIOS LTD
Ringwood, Hampshire

ISBN 978-0-333-25585-8   ISBN 978-1-349-04254-8 (eBook)
DOI 10.1007/978-1-349-04254-8

To our long-suffering families

Contents

The Contributors   vii

Preface   ix

1   Basic Principles *with R. Parker*   1
    The scanner   1
    The image   3
    Storage of data   6
    Resolution   6
    Slice width   6
    Partial volume effect   6
    Artefacts   7
    Radiation   7
    Resolution and its relationship to dose   8

2   General Considerations – Technical   9
    Outlining the bowel   10
    Reducing movement artefacts   11
    Bladder emptying   12
    Scanogram or scout view   13
    Enhancement   14
    Care of the patient   16
    Planning and supervision of the
      examination   16

3   General Considerations – Clinical   17
    The clinical value of computed
      tomography   19
    Relationship to other techniques   20
    Computed tomography and ultrasound   20
    How useful is computed tomography?   21

4   The Thorax – Mediastinum   23
    Technique of examination   23
    CT anatomy   23
    Mediastinal masses   27
    Heart   36

    Use and accuracy of computed
      tomography   36

5   The Thorax – Lungs, Pleura and Chest
    Wall   40
    Technique of examination   40
    CT anatomy   40
    Pulmonary nodules   44
    General lung disease   47
    Pleural disease   49
    Chest wall   51
    Use and accuracy of computed
      tomography   52

6   The Abdomen – Kidney   55
    Technique of examination   55
    CT anatomy   55
    Renal mass lesions   58
    Other renal and perirenal lesions   64
    Use of computed tomography and
      relationship to other techniques   68

7   The Abdomen – Adrenals   71
    Technique of examination   71
    CT anatomy   71
    Adrenal masses   73
    Other adrenal lesions   77
    Accuracy and relationship to other
      techniques   77

8   The Abdomen – Liver and Biliary Tract   81
    Technique of examination   81
    CT anatomy   82
    Focal liver disease   85
    Diffuse liver disease   89
    Gall-bladder disease   91
    Use and accuracy of computed
      tomography   93

9 The Abdomen – Pancreas   97
    Technique of examination   97
    CT anatomy   98
    Signs of pancreatic disease   102
    Differential diagnosis and the use of
       computed tomography in pancreatic
       disease   108
    Accuracy of computed tomography
       and relationship to other techniques   109

10 The Abdomen – Miscellaneous Topics   113
    The retroperitoneal and peritoneal
       spaces   113
    Ascites   123
    Aorta   123
    Inferior vena cava   124
    Use of computed tomography in
       assessment of intra-abdominal
       masses   125
    Spleen   126
    Gastrointestinal tract   127
    Aspiration techniques guided by
       computed tomography   128

11 Lymph Node Disease of the Abdomen
    and Pelvis   132
    Technique of examination   132
    CT anatomy and abnormal
       appearances   132
    Para-aortic and retrocrural nodes   134
    Nodes in other upper abdominal sites   137
    Accuracy of computed tomography   140
    Use of computed tomography in lymph
       node disease   142

12 The Pelvis   146
    Technique of examination   146
    CT anatomy   148
    Bladder   151
    Rectum   154
    Female genital tract   157
    Prostate   159
    Miscellaneous pelvic conditions   161
    Use of computed tomography   162

13 The Musculo-Skeletal System   165
    Technique of examination   166

    CT anatomy   166
    Tumours   171
    Use of computed tomography in
       tumours of bone and soft tissues   177
    Trauma   178
    Congenital and developmental lesions   181
    Vertebral column and spinal cord   181

14 The Spinal Cord   by P. Pullicino   184
    Technique of examination   184
    Intramedullary lesions   185
    Intradural extramedullary lesions   185
    Extradural lesions   187
    Metrizamide CT myelography   187

15 The Head and Neck   with C. A. Parsons   189
    Paranasal sinuses   189
       Technique of examination   189
       CT anatomy   189
       Tumours   191
    Pharynx   194
       Technique of examination   194
       CT anatomy   195
       Tumours   196
    Larynx   198
       Technique of examination   198
       CT anatomy   198
       Tumours   199
    Parotid gland   201
       Technique of examination   201
       CT anatomy   201
       Tumours   202

16 The Orbits   by G. A. S. Lloyd   204
    Technique of examination   204
    Abnormalities of the orbit   205
    Use of computed tomography in
       orbital diagnosis   208

17 Computed Tomography in Oncology   210
    Primary diagnosis   210
    Staging   211
    Monitoring response to treatment   213
    Radiotherapy treatment planning   215

Index   219

The Contributors

G. A. S. Lloyd, DM, FRCR

Consultant Radiologist, Royal National Throat, Nose and Ear Hospital, London

R. Parker, PhD, MSc

Senior Lecturer in Physics, Royal Marsden Hospital, Sutton

C. A. Parsons, FRCS, FRCR

Consultant Radiologist, Royal Marsden Hospital, Sutton

P. Pullicino, MD, MRCP

Research Fellow, National Hospital for Nervous Diseases, London

Preface

The effective use of a diagnostic imaging technique depends on both radiologist and clinician understanding what the technique can do and how to use it. We have, therefore, set out to provide an introduction to computed tomography of the body describing not only the technique and interpretation of scans but also the value of scanning in clinical practice. The essentially technical aspects of scanning have been kept to the minimum required to understand how the scans are done and how they are interpreted.

The resources available in a department of medical imaging are usually in excess of the ability to use them to best advantage. When a new technique is introduced it often continues to be used just because it is there. This is unlikely to happen with computed tomography (CT) scanning of the body because of the way in which its introduction has coincided with a time of diminishing resources and, in some quarters, of increasing disenchantment with high-technology medicine. Very proper questions are being asked about the justification for scans in terms of their effect on the management of the patient and on the outcome of the disease. Experience is too limited for definitive answers to be given to such questions at this time, but there is already considerable agreement about the main applications of the method and its relation to other imaging techniques.

Our personal experience is limited to the use of a second-generation scanner, the EMI 5005 General Purpose Scanner. Many of the reports in the literature refer to studies on this or some similar type of machine. The development of new faster scanners has already improved picture quality and there is little doubt that the number of clinical situations in which CT scanning is the investigation of choice will expand. In particular, the introduction of dynamic scanning is likely to have important clinical implications. Such developments are, however, unlikely to invalidate the general principles which have already been established.

One of us (JH) first gained experience of CT scanning with Dr Louis Kreel of Northwick Park Hospital. We are both happy to have this opportunity of putting on record our recognition of Dr Kreel's special contribution to the understanding of the principles of CT scanning of the body.

Between us we have experience of scanners in three other institutions – the Royal Marsden Hospital, the BUPA Medical Centre and St Bartholomew's Hospital – and we would like to acknowledge the immense help that we have had from numerous radiological and clinical colleagues in these institutions. It is a pleasure to recognise the part played by our radiological colleagues working with the scanners – Dr J. S. Macdonald, Dr Colin Parsons and Dr Stephen Golding at the Royal Marsden Hospital, Dr P. Travers, Dr D. G. Shaw, Dr P. Gishen, Dr M. Kellett and Dr R. Dick at the BUPA Medical Centre, and Dr Adrian Dixon and Dr Elizabeth White at St Bartholomew's Hospital.

We have been fortunate to work with skilled and dedicated radiographers who have handled their sometimes temperamental machines with great expertise and patience. The radiographers in charge of the departments – Mrs Dorothy Mears, Mrs Jacqueline Seckel, Miss Sandy Jewell and Miss Marion Hallett – have not only managed their departments with great competence but have also found time for the extra work involved in research and the documentation of results.

Having access to a new imaging technique capable of examining any part of the body soon exposes the radiologist's ignorance of many clinical conditions. Much of the content of this book is the result of discussion with surgeons and physicians and we are grateful for their stimulus and interest. In particular, Professor Michael Peckham and Dr Neil Hodson at the Royal Marsden Hospital have done a great deal towards helping to define the precise role of computed tomography in the management of malignant disease. Their advice has been invaluable but they should not be held responsible for any of the views that we have expressed.

We would like to record our appreciation of the contributions from the Cancer Research Campaign and the Department of Health and Social Security who have generously financed research at the Royal Marsden Hospital and from the Trustees of St Bartholomew's Hospital and the Research Fund of the BUPA Medical Centre, both of whom have supported research on the scanners of their institutions.

Also, we would like to thank Mrs Judy Grimes and Mr John Higgins for help with producing the illustrations and Mrs Julie Jessop and Mrs Janice O'Donnell for their enthusiastic and expert secretarial help with the manuscript.

Finally, we would like to thank the following for their kind permission to reproduce figures: the Cancer Research Campaign, Dr Foley (Milwaukee County Hospital, Milwaukee, Wisconsin), International General Electric (New York), Pitman Press, Dr Robinson (Leeds General Infirmary), *Radiology*, Siemens AG UB Med (Erlanger, West Germany), Dr T. P. Naidich (The Edward Mallinckrodt Institute of Radiology, St Louis, Missouri), Dr M. Sage (Department of Radiology, Flinders Medical Centre, Bedford Park, South Australia), Dr L. A. Gilula (The Edward Mallinckrodt Institute of Radiology, St Louis, Missouri), Dr Haughton (Milwaukee General Hospital, Milwaukee, Wisconsin), Dr Hoare and Dr Stanley.

London, 1981 J.E.H.
I.K.F.

1

Basic Principles

with Roy Parker

Computed tomography (CT) is an x-ray technique which uses a computer to reconstruct an image of a thin slice of the body. The main advantage of CT over conventional radiology is that very small differences of attenuation of x-rays can be recorded so that fine variations in tissue density can be detected. Images are usually obtained in the axial plane. A CT examination entails obtaining a series of scans through the part of the body to be examined, the slices usually being about 1 cm thick (figure 1.1).

The basic parts of the system are shown diagrammatically in figure 1.2. An x-ray source and an array of detectors are mounted on a scanning gantry which moves round the patient. These detectors record the number of x-ray photons emerging from the patient as the gantry rotates. The information recorded by the detectors is processed in a computer system and the reconstructed image is displayed on a video monitor as a grey-scale image.

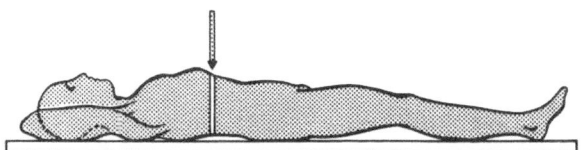

Figure 1.1 CT produces an image of a thin slice of the patient in cross section

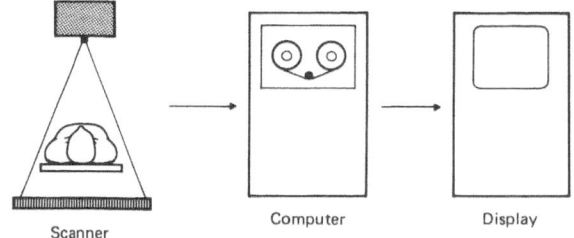

Figure 1.2   Basic CT system

THE SCANNER

Scans are obtained with the patient lying on an x-ray table with the part to be examined lying within the aperture of the gantry so that the x-ray tube rotates around the patient (figure 1.3).

The original scanning system developed by Hounsfield (1973) uses a translate–rotate movement in which the x-ray source traverses the patient and is then rotated through a small angle and a further traverse made. The whole process is repeated until the x-ray source has completed an arc around the patient of at least 180° (figure 1.4). For mechanical reasons, most machines using this type of system require scan times of between 15 and 20 s. The EMI (CT5005) General Purpose Scanner referred to in this book is such a scanner. The major advantage of this original scanning system is that

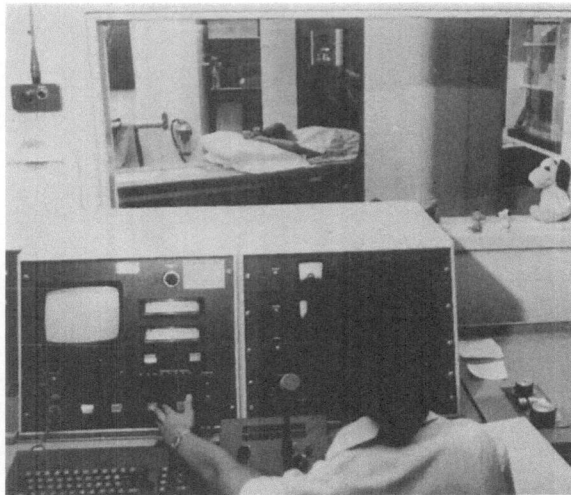

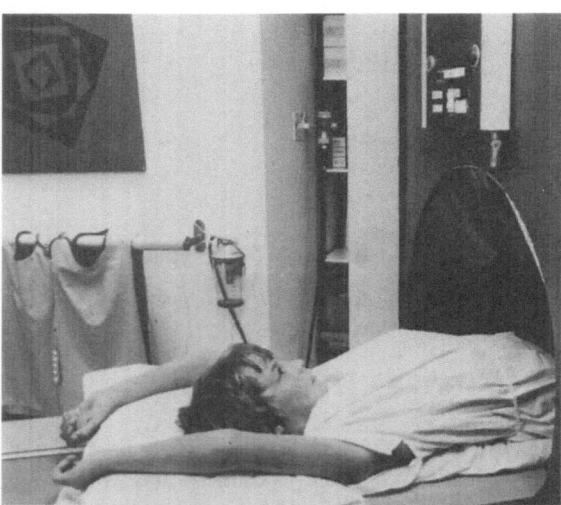

Figure 1.3 The EMI (CT5005) General Purpose Scanner. (Top) General view from operator's console. (Bottom) Patient prepared for abdominal scan. (Reproduced by kind permission of the Cancer Research Campaign)

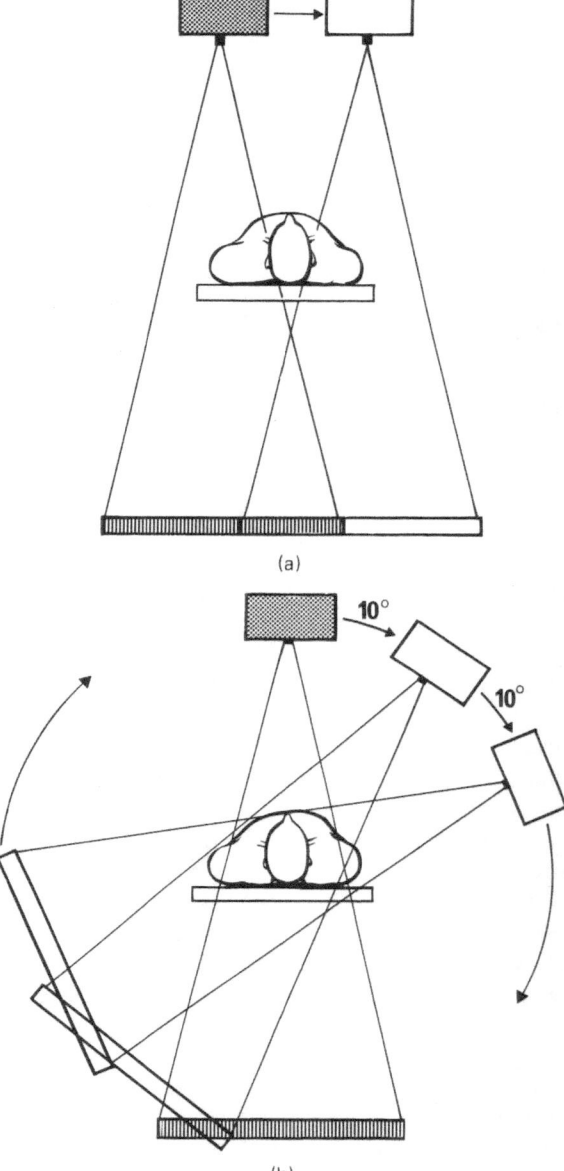

Figure 1.4 Translate–rotate system: (a) translate movement, (b) rotation

individual detectors scan across the patient and it is possible to calibrate them at each traverse. Since the image quality is highly dependent on the stability and reproducibility of the mechanical movements and of the electronic equipment, such calibrations are beneficial and account for the good picture quality obtained with this method even during its

early development. It is widely used for brain scanning and in the slower whole-body machines. From this original system, several different types of scanner have been developed to achieve short scan times of the order of 3 to 5 s.

Shorter scan times are most obviously achieved by using a rotate-only motion as shown in figure 1.5. The x-ray beam is wide enough to encompass the patient so that the traversing movement is no longer necessary although a greater number of detectors is required. The whole assembly (x-ray tube and detector array) rotates around the patient and scan times as short as 2 or 3 s have been achieved. Mechanically, the design is fairly simple, but stringent demands are placed on the stability of the system since each detector images a particular circular path around the centre of rotation, and it is not possible to calibrate the whole system with the patient in position. Great ingenuity has been shown in reducing these problems, but nevertheless this type of system (rotate–rotate) is prone to circular artefacts.

The disadvantage of circular artefacts is overcome if a stationary circular array of detectors is employed with a rotating x-ray tube (figure 1.6). Clearly the complexity and expense is increased, but calibration is possible continuously as each detector effectively moves across the patient. The time required for a scan is similar to that using the rotate–rotate method.

A drawback of both the rotate–rotate and stationary-detector methods is the diameter of the detector ring that is required. This must encompass both the patient and the x-ray tube (*see* figures 1.5

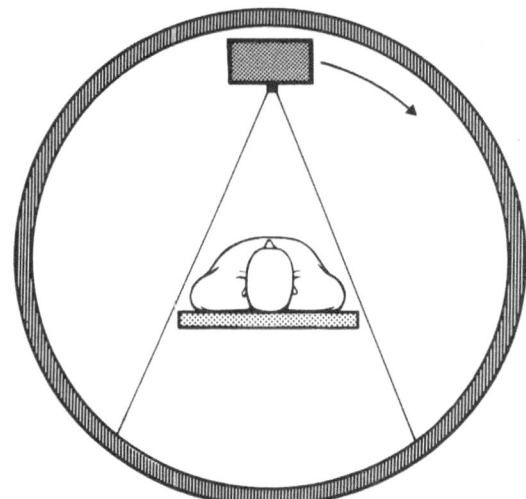

Figure 1.6   Stationary–rotate system

and 1.6), which means that a large number of detectors must be used to achieve good spatial resolution. It would be preferable for the x-ray tube to be situated outside the detector ring so that the detectors are close to the patient. Some manufacturers have achieved this either by tilting the plane of the detectors away from the x-ray beam or by some type of eccentric motion.

THE IMAGE

The image consists of a matrix of picture elements (*pixels*) each representing the degree of attenuation of x-rays at that point in the body. The pixel size depends on the number of pixels forming the image matrix. Thus, using the EMI CT5005 scanner with a matrix of 320×320, the pixel size is approximately 0.75 mm $\times$ 0.75 mm. Using the 160×160 matrix, the pixel size is approximately 1.5 mm $\times$ 1.5 mm.

Since each image represents a certain thickness of tissue, the attenuation value recorded at a point actually represents the mean value obtained from a volume of tissue (the *voxel*) (figure 1.7).

A scale of CT numbers has been introduced which relates the attenuation values of tissues to that of water, the CT number of which is designated zero. The CT numbers for different tissues using the

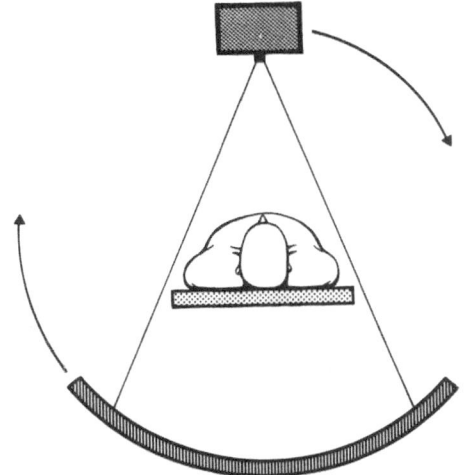

Figure 1.5   Rotate–rotate system

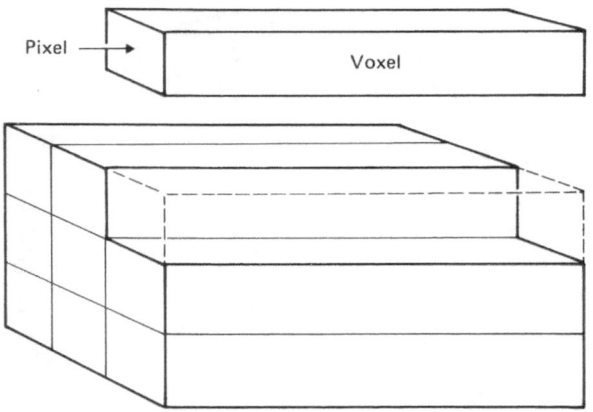

Figure 1.7   Schematic representation of part of a CT section

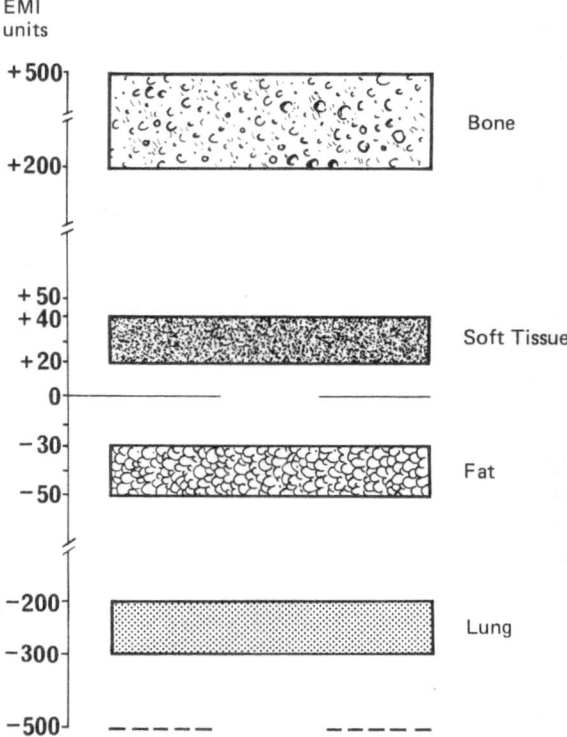

Figure 1.8   Scale of CT numbers (EMI units) showing values for body tissues (1 EMI unit equals 2 Hounsfield units)

EMI scale are shown in figure 1.8. The CT number for air is −500, for dense bone +200 to +500, for soft tissues +20 to +40 and for fat −30 to −50. CT numbers are closely related to the physical density of the tissue. For this reason, changes in CT number are often referred to as alterations in density. Many machines, including the EMI brain scanners, use the Hounsfield scale, in which two Hounsfield units correspond to one EMI unit. The EMI scale is used in the present text.

The different CT numbers are displayed on a video monitor as a grey-scale image. The great majority of body scans are viewed as if looking at the patient from the feet. Scans of the head and upper part of the neck are conventionally viewed as if looking down from above.

Since only a limited number of grey-scale steps can be appreciated by the human eye, only a limited range of values can be distinguished simultaneously. For this reason, the viewing console is provided with a set of controls which enable the observer to select a range of values for display appropriate to the tissue being examined. The centre of the range is known as the *window level* and the range of density values displayed on either side of the window level is known as the *window width*. The smaller the range of density values represented by each grey-scale step, the greater the contrast. For this reason, a narrow window width is used when examining structures such as the liver or brain, when small differences in density can be important. Relatively wider widths are more commonly used in body scanning, when the shape and contours of structures are the main criteria for diagnosis.

The effect of varying window level is illustrated in figure 1.9 which shows the appearance of a scan through the thorax at three different window levels whilst keeping the window width constant at 200. At a window level between −300 and −400 (figure 1.9a), the soft tissues of the mediastinum and chest wall appear white and the vessels of the lungs are seen as a network traversing the lung parenchyma. As the window level is increased to approximately +20 EMI units (figure 1.9b), the lungs become black, the vessels are no longer visible and the soft tissues of the mediastinum and chest wall can then be examined, but the bone still appears white. Increas-

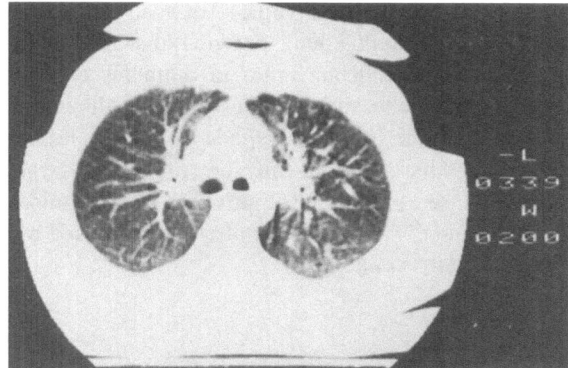

Figure 1.9(a)

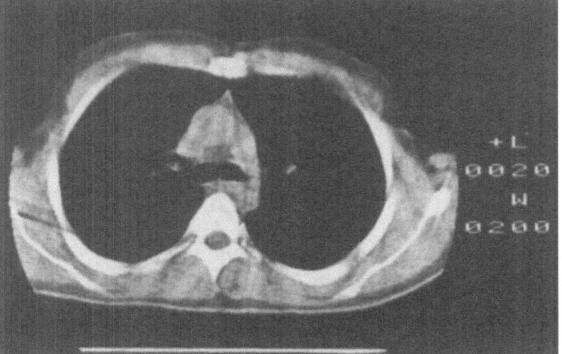

Figure 1.9(b)

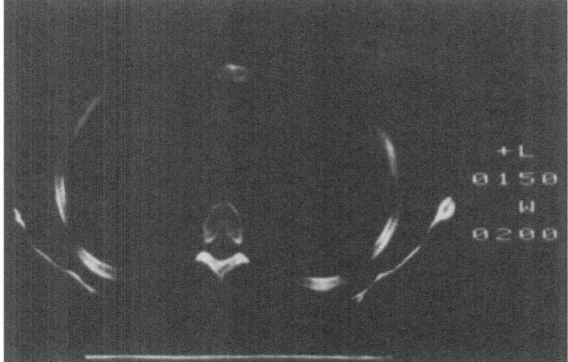

Figure 1.9(c)

Figure 1.9 CT scan taken at the level of the tracheal bifurcation to show the effect of changing window level ($\pm L$) with constant window width (W) of 200 EMI units. The image has been manipulated to show: (a) the lungs, window level −339 EMI units; (b) the soft tissues, window level +20 EMI units; and (c) the bone, window level +150 EMI units

ing the window level to between +100 and +200 EMI units demonstrates the architecture of bone, but in this range the soft tissues are not visible (figure 1.9c).

The effect of varying window width whilst keeping the window level constant is illustrated in figure 1.10. At a window width of 400, the step in the grey scale represents a wide range of CT numbers so that there is very little contrast and the liver appears homogeneous. The tissue outlines are, however, sharply defined (figure 1.10a). With a window width of 40, there is much more contrast and metastases are readily seen within the liver. Tissue outlines are, however, less clear (figure 1.10b).

Various other facilities are available on the viewing console, but the precise details depend on

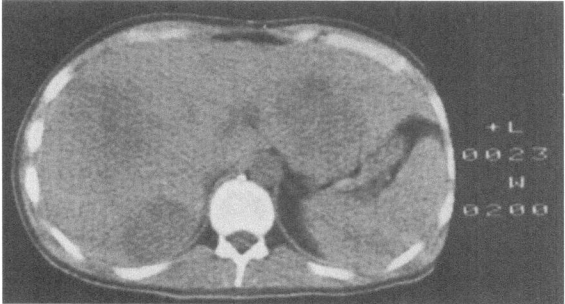

Figure 1.10(a)

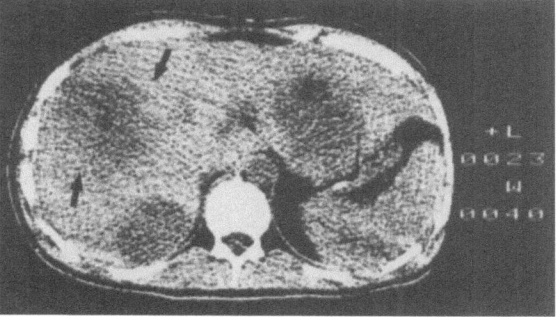

Figure 1.10(b)

Figure 1.10 CT scan through liver with multiple metastases showing effect of varying window width (W) with constant window level of +23 EMI units: (a) $W =$ 200 EMI units; (b) $W = 40$ EMI units. The metastases are best shown when viewed with a narrow window

the manufacturer. For example, it is possible to obtain a statistical calculation of the mean attenuation values and standard deviation within a region of interest which is outlined using a roller ball or light pen directly onto the CT image. Other facilities include measuring a direct line between two points, and enlargement of a quadrant for easier visualisation. A facility that is becoming increasingly important is the ability to combine contiguous slices to reconstruct images in other planes. This is only of value in scanners providing thin slices, approximately 5 mm, since the resolution of the reconstructed image with thicker slices is rarely helpful.

These unique facilities of CT enable the observer to manipulate the CT data so that the maximum information can be obtained from the scans. It is thus essential that all reporting is done directly from the viewing console rather than from hard copies, such as Polaroid prints or normal film. These hard copies are useful records for the clinician and the radiologist, but illustrate only the salient features of a complex examination.

STORAGE OF DATA

CT information can be stored using the normal computer media of magnetic tape and floppy discs. Magnetic tape is very suitable for long-term storage. Floppy discs, similar to small gramophone records, are more applicable to short-term storage. Large computer discs are used for image storage on the scanner itself, and on the latest scanners these can hold several hundred images. Many radiologists prefer to report scans without interfering with the routine operation of the scanner and this can be achieved by using a remote reporting station (independent viewing console) equipped with its own computer together with floppy-disc and magnetic-tape readers.

RESOLUTION

The size of a lesion that can be detected depends on the density difference between the lesion and the surrounding normal tissue. For example, in the lung the

difference in attenuation values between the mass and the air-containing lung parenchyma is so high that lesions as small as 3 mm in diameter can be identified. In a site such as the liver, in which the density difference between a space-occupying lesion and the liver parenchyma may be small, even large lesions can be difficult or impossible to recognise. Differences in CT number can often be increased by the use of contrast agents.

SLICE WIDTH

The thickness of tissue scanned is usually 5 to 13 mm but, because of the design of the collimator system, slices are not usually of constant width. Figure 1.11 illustrates the shape of the slice obtained with the EMI CT5005 General Purpose Scanners (P. A. Hobday and R. P. Parker, unpublished). It can be seen that partial volume effects are more likely at the surface than at the centre of the patient. This has a bearing on choosing the appropriate spacing between the scans. If the spacing is selected on the basis of the slice width at the centre, then tissues near the surface will be included on two contiguous slices and will be irradiated twice with the resultant increase in radiation exposure. However, if selection is based on the slice width at the surface, then there is a volume of tissue which will not be included in the images.

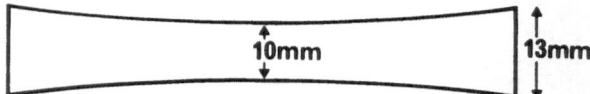

Figure 1.11 Shape of CT section (EMI CT5005 General Purpose Scanner)

PARTIAL VOLUME EFFECT

When interpreting CT scans, it is essential to remember that the EMI number of each voxel is the mean of the attenuation values of all the structures within it. A structure or lesion which only partially occupies the thickness of the slice is subject to partial volume averaging. This has two effects: first, normal structures only partially contained within a

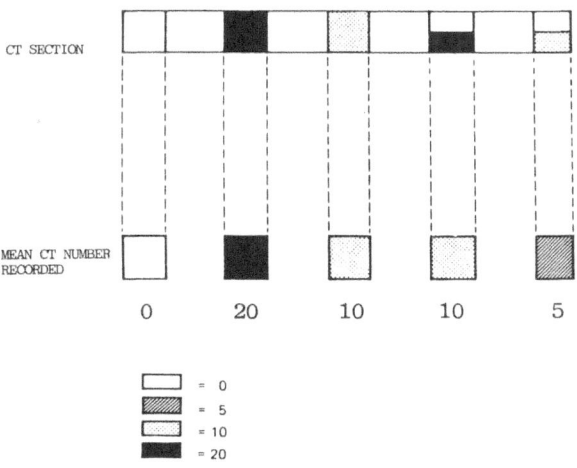

CT SECTION

MEAN CT NUMBER
RECORDED

0   20   10   10   5

☐ = 0
▨ = 5
☐ = 10
■ = 20

Figure 1.12   Partial volume effect

slice may give misleading anatomical appearances which can only be resolved by examination of contiguous slices; secondly, the composition of a lesion only partially included within the slice may be misinterpreted. A mean attenuation value recorded from such a lesion will be false, approximating towards that of the surrounding normal tissue (figure 1.12). For instance, a small cyst in the liver may return attenuation values which suggest a solid tumour rather than a fluid-containing cyst. Some small lesions may be missed altogether.

ARTEFACTS

Artefacts are produced by movement and by structures of very high density. They take the form of linear streaks and may so degrade the image that interpretation is impossible. They not only interfere with visualisation of structures but also invalidate density measurements.

The commonest artefacts are produced by respiratory, cardiac and bowel movements. They are frequently seen using 15 to 20 s scanners but are greatly reduced when 3 to 5 s scanners are used. Particularly dense artefacts can be produced when high-density material, such as metal clips, barium,

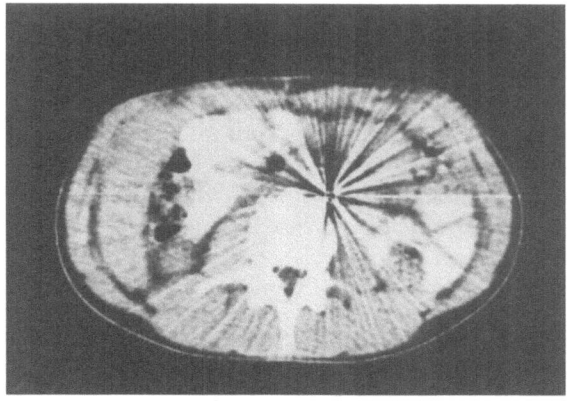

Figure 1.13   CT scan through the abdomen showing gross artefacts from a surgical metal clip

Myodil or hip prostheses, are included within the scan, even if there is no associated movement (figure 1.13).

Malfunction of the scanner and its related equipment can result in a variety of artefacts, but these are normally well characterised and disappear on correction of the fault.

RADIATION

The radiation dose to the patient during a CT scan is well within the range associated with other diagnostic x-ray investigations such as intravenous urography or barium studies. The skin dose for a single slice varies from approximately 1.0 to 2.5 R (röntgen) according to the type of equipment and technique used (McCullough and Payne, 1978; Hobday and Parker, 1978). For a series of contiguous non-overlapping slices at normal scan speeds, the exposure is higher due to side-scattered radiation but is usually within the range 3.0 to 5.0 R. However, the exposure is dependent on the type and design of machine and the latest CT scanners utilise x-ray photons more efficiently, thus reducing the radiation exposure required for a given contrast resolution.

Perhaps more important than the skin dose at any one point is the *integral dose*, which is the total amount of radiation absorbed by the body and which takes into account the area exposed. Even CT examinations involving numerous scans may not encompass areas as large as those exposed in conventional radiology and frequently the area is quite small.

It is clear that the exposure to a given patient is determined by many factors, including scan speed, slice width and slice interval. If slices overlap, there will be a significant increase in exposure.

RESOLUTION AND ITS RELATIONSHIP TO DOSE

The CT number corresponding to each pixel has associated with it an uncertainty or noise value due primarily to the statistical variations in the number of x-ray photons. This depends on the design of the machine, but most of all on the x-ray dose given to the patient. The amount of noise limits the ability to distinguish adjacent areas of differing density (*contrast resolution*). In order to appreciate small variations in density, a coarse image matrix is selected so that the noise is averaged over a larger area. Thus, spatial resolution is sacrificed to obtain better contrast resolution. For example, using the EMI General Purpose Scanner, brain scans are viewed with a 160×160 matrix, whilst those of the thorax or abdomen are displayed on a 320×320 matrix.

It has been shown that for a fixed slice width

$$\text{noise} \propto \sqrt{\left(\frac{1}{\text{dose} \times (\text{pixel width})^3} \right)}$$

Thus, to halve the noise the dose must be quadrupled and to decrease the pixel width by a factor of two increases the noise by a factor of 2.7 unless the dose is increased by a factor of 8. In addition, the noise is inversely proportional to slice thickness.

REFERENCES

Hobday, P. A. and Parker, R. P. (1978). Radiation exposure to the patient in computerized tomography. *British Journal of Radiology*, **51**, 925–926

Hounsfield, G. N. (1973). Computerised transverse axial scanning (tomography): Part I. Description of system. *British Journal of Radiology*, **46**, 1016–1022

McCullough, E. C. and Payne, J. T. (1978). Patient dosage in computed tomography. *Radiology*, **129**, 457–463

2

General Considerations – Technical

As with other x-ray examinations, the technique will be tailored to answer the clinical questions. Details of the technique used for different organs and different clinical problems are discussed in the appropriate chapters. Only principles of technique which are generally applicable are discussed here. Although the account refers to experience based on the use of the EMI CT5005 General Purpose Scanner, it applies to other scanners of the same type. Most of the text is equally applicable to faster scanners, although these can be expected to give sharper images and can, in some patients, provide more information (figure 2.1).

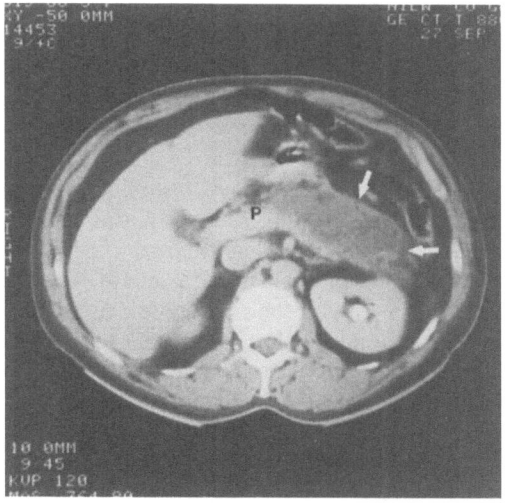

Figure 2.1(b)

Figure 2.1   CT scan of two patients with pseudocysts (arrowed) of the pancreas (P). (a) Scan taken using the EMI CT5005 General Purpose Scanner – scan time 18 s. (b) Scan taken using a faster machine. With both systems, the lesion is identified but more anatomical detail is provided in the image produced by the faster machine. (Scan (b) is reproduced by kind permission of Dr Foley)

INSTRUCTIONS TO PATIENT

Patients having abdominal scans should eat nothing for some hours before the examination. Apart from this, there are no special instructions.

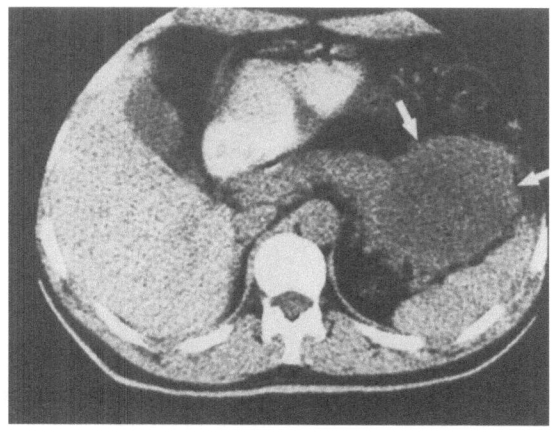

Figure 2.1(a)

OUTLINING THE BOWEL

The bowel usually has an attenuation value similar to that of other soft tissues unless it contains air (figure 2.2). It may, therefore, produce an appearance indistinguishable from a soft tissue mass unless outlined with contrast medium. The contrast medium is usually Gastrografin, which is a dilute mixture of one of the urographic contrast media (sodium meglumine diatrizoate) with some flavouring material and a wetting agent. We give patients having scans of the abdomen or pelvis 300 ml 5% Gastrografin on arrival in the department (not less than 30 min before the scan) and a further 300 ml just before the scan. Following the second dose, the patient lies on his/her right side to ensure that the contrast medium enters the duodenum and proximal small bowel (figure 2.3). When examining the lower abdomen and pelvis, it is important to ensure that the distal bowel is outlined with contrast medium; to save time, in-patients can be given Gastrografin in the ward.

The taste of Gastrografin has been likened to that of aniseed or Pernod. Unfortunately, this is not so. Some patients find it unpleasant and children may refuse to take it. In such circumstances, a urographic contrast medium such as sodium iothalamate (Conray 325) suitably diluted with orange juice is an acceptable, although more expensive, substitute.

Barium in the bowel produces gross streak

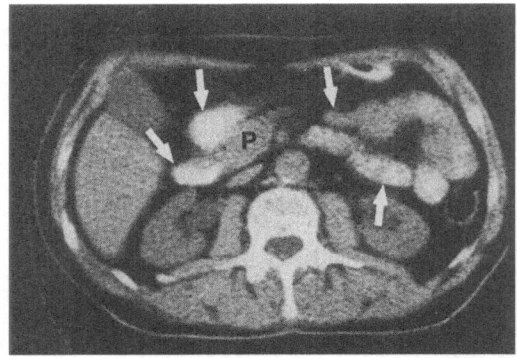

Figure 2.3 The duodenum and jejunum have been opacified with oral contrast medium (arrowed). The pancreatic head (P) is readily distinguished from the duodenum which lies lateral to it

artefacts (figure 2.4). For this reason, satisfactory CT scans cannot be obtained if there is a significant residue following barium examinations. This has to be borne in mind when planning the sequence of investigations.

Kreel (1979) recommends giving calcium phosphate orally, 1 g three times a day for two days before the examination, to outline the colon. In our experience, the colon is usually definable without contrast medium, except when examining the pelvis, in which case 5% Gastrografin should be instilled into the rectum to outline the rectum and sigmoid colon (figure 2.5).

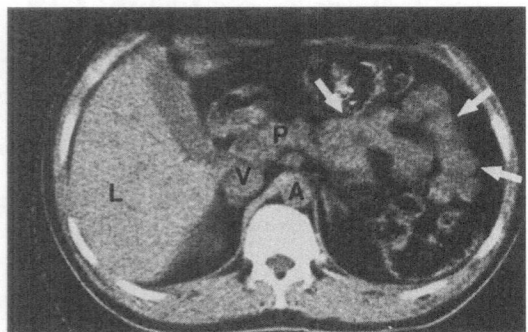

Figure 2.2 A normal CT scan. Loops of bowel (arrowed) have a similar density to the pancreas (P) and other soft-tissue structures within the abdomen. Liver (L), aorta (A), inferior vena cava (V)

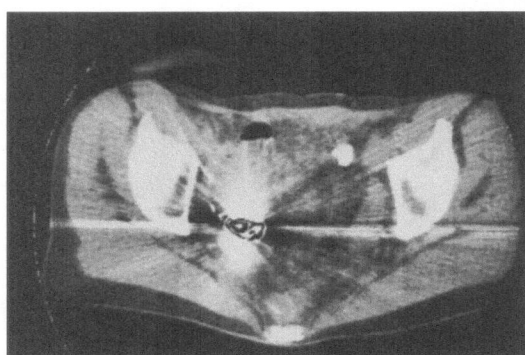

Figure 2.4 CT scan through the pelvis showing streak artefacts due to retained barium following a barium enema

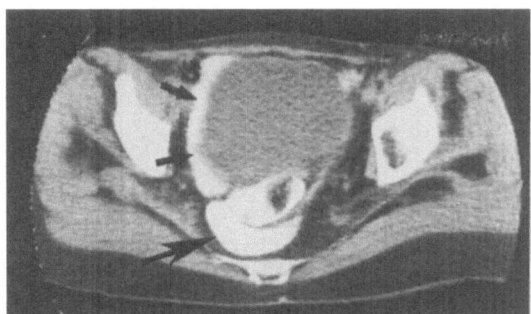

Figure 2.5   CT scan of pelvis, showing sigmoid colon outlined with rectal Gastrografin (large lower arrow). A loop of small bowel opacified with oral contrast medium (small upper arrows) is shown adjacent to the right wall of the bladder

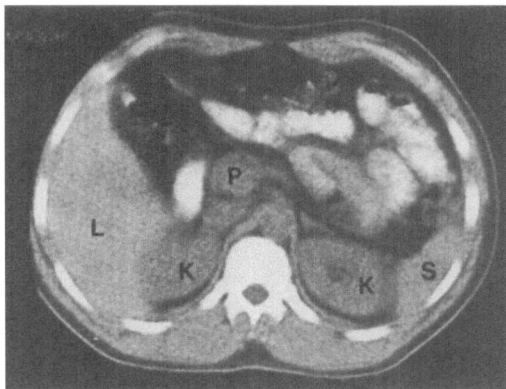

Figure 2.6(a)

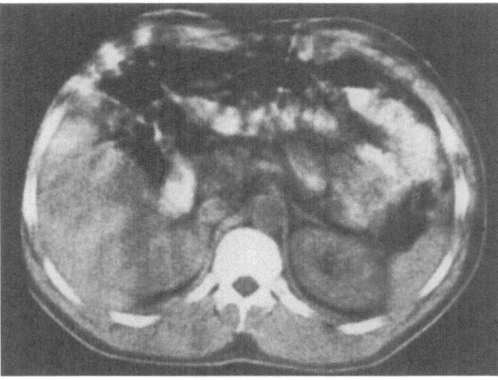

Figure 2.6(b)

Figure 2.6   CT scans taken at the level of the twelfth thoracic vertebra in the same patient. (a) Scan taken during suspended respiration and (b) scan taken with the patient breathing gently throughout. Liver (L), kidneys (K), spleen (S), pancreas (P)

REDUCING MOVEMENT ARTEFACTS

There are four causes of movement artefact:

- (a)   respiration,
- (b)   peristalsis,
- (c)   patient movement, and
- (d)   cardiac pulsation.

(a) Respiration

Using 18 to 20 s scanners, the patient has to stop breathing for this period if artefacts are to be avoided when the thorax or abdomen is being scanned (figure 2.6). Although most adult patients can achieve this, some find it difficult or impossible. In these, gentle steady respiration often results in a scan which, although it contains artefacts, provides all the diagnostic information that is required. Many patients find it easier to hold their breath in mid-inspiration rather than full inspiration.

When scanning structures which move with respiration, it is important to try to ensure that each scan is obtained at the same level of inspiration so that sequential scans accurately reflect the sequential internal anatomy.

(b) Peristalsis

Bowel movement produces streak artefacts, especially when the bowel contains air or dense contrast medium (figure 2.7). For this reason, patients having abdominal scans may need an antiperistaltic agent. We use Buscopan 20 mg intravenously (i.v.) or intramuscularly (i.m.) immediately before the scan, repeating the dose as necessary. When an atropine-like substance is contra-indicated, glucagon 0.25 mg i.v. can be given.

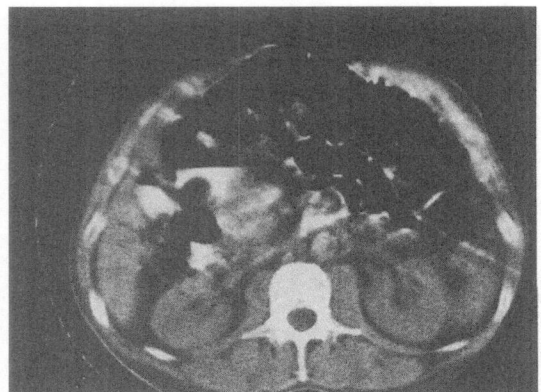

Figure 2.7   Streak artefacts produced by a large amount of air in the bowel

(c) Patient Movement

A restless patient may need some sedation but must still be able to cooperate. Occasionally, general anaesthesia is required; it is commonly needed if satisfactory scans are to be obtained in small children.

(d) Cardiac Pulsation

This produces some unavoidable streak artefacts which can lead to difficulties in interpretation (figure 2.8).

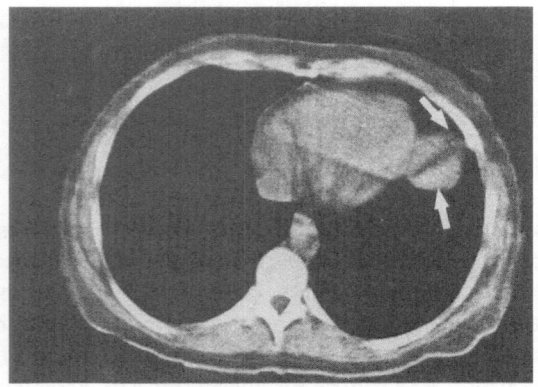

Figure 2.8   CT scan at the level of the heart showing a left parapericardial cyst (arrowed). Streaks across the image produce difficulty in interpretation of the density of this mass

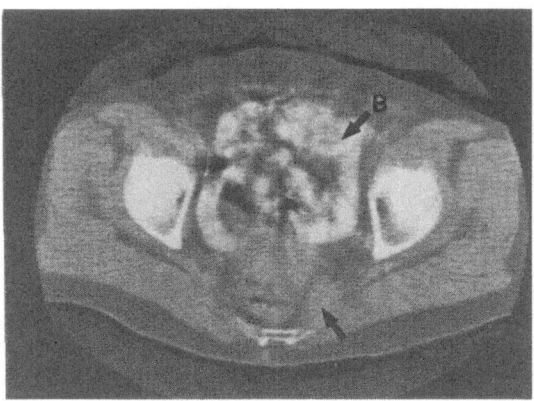

Figure 2.9(a)

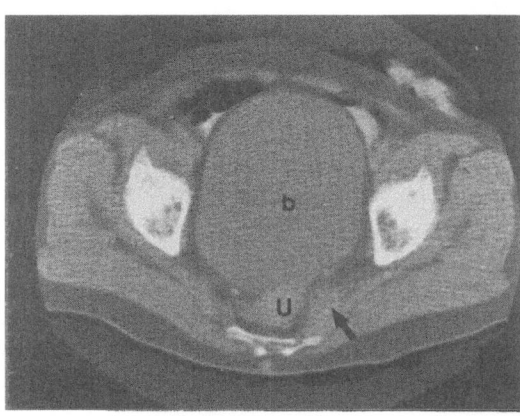

Figure 2.9(b)

Figure 2.9   Female patient with recurrent rectal carcinoma (arrowed). (a) With empty bladder showing bowel (B). (b) With full bladder (b) and uterus (U)

BLADDER EMPTYING

In general, patients should be asked to empty their bladder just before the scan to avoid discomfort during a prolonged examination, particularly when there is a diuresis following the use of intravenous contrast medium. When the pelvis is examined, however, the bladder must be full. This has the effect of pushing the small bowel out of the pelvis and simplifies interpretation of the scans (figure 2.9).

SCANOGRAM OR SCOUT VIEW

Some method is needed for defining the level at which a scan should be started and, more importantly, for localising and recording the precise levels at which scans are obtained. Newly developed scanners have the facility for projecting a conventional image of the part to be examined on the monitor – a so-called 'scout view' (figure 2.10). The appropriate starting level of the scan can be selected from this. The correct angle of gantry tilt can be judged from the lateral view. The levels at which the scans are actually obtained is readily recorded.

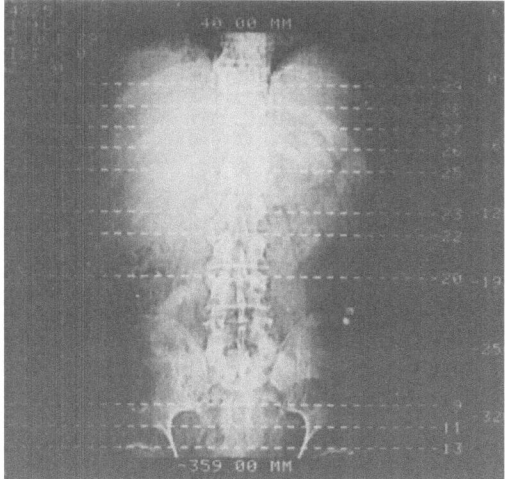

Figure 2.10(a)

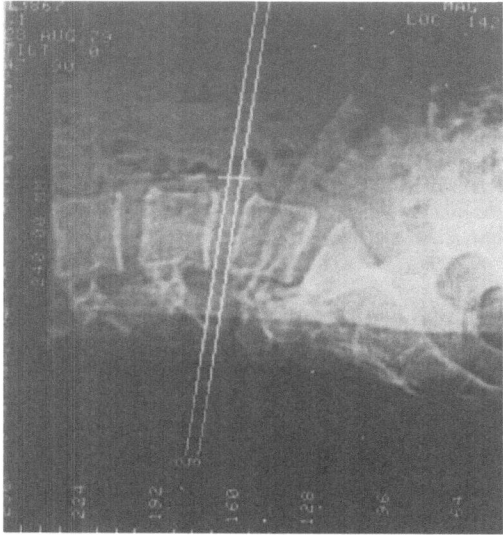

Figure 2.10(b)

Figure 2.10 Scout views obtained with the GE8800 Scanner. (a) Anteroposterior (AP) view, (b) lateral view. The level and angle of the slices are shown on the image. (Reproduced by kind permission of International General Electric)

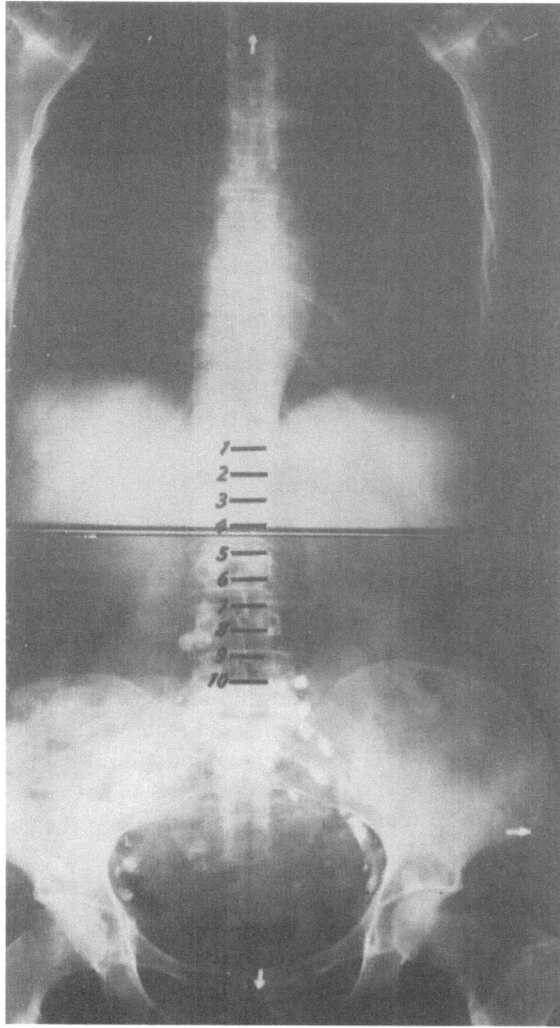

Figure 2.11 Scanogram film taken using a slit beam of x-rays. The level and number of slices is marked on the film at the time of the examination

When this facility is not available, as with older scanners, the same effect can be obtained by taking a slit beam radiograph of the area to be scanned with metal markers on the skin before the patient is placed on the scanner – a so-called 'scanogram' (figure 2.11). The position of the markers is recorded on the skin and used when positioning the patient in the scanner. The same film can be used for recording the levels of each scan and also for outlining the shape and size of a mass seen on the axial sections (*see* chapter 17). Quite apart from its use for localising the region to be scanned, a plain radiograph frequently provides important information and should always be available when interpreting a CT examination.

ENHANCEMENT

The term 'enhancement' is used during CT scanning to refer to the increase in density of the tissue after the injection of intravenous iodine-containing contrast medium. There are two types of enhancement as follows.

(a) General Opacification of the Tissues

This is produced partly by contrast medium in the vascular tree and partly by contrast medium in the extracellular space (except in the kidney where the contrast medium is also concentrated in the tubules). This type of opacification frequently improves the differentiation between normal and abnormal tissue by increasing the difference in contrast between them (figure 2.12). Most commonly, abnormal tissues enhance less than the surrounding tissues, but, occasionally, vascular lesions take up the contrast medium preferentially.

Because CT can readily detect smaller variations in tissue densities than is possible with conventional radiography, opacification of body tissues is readily detected after relatively small doses of contrast medium. For this reason, doses such as 50 ml sodium iothalamate containing 325 mg iodine/ml (Conray 325) are sufficient for general enhancement.

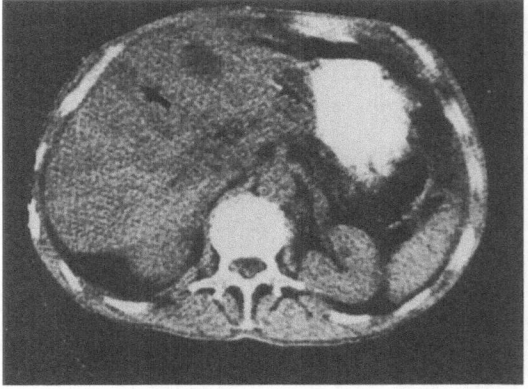

Figure 2.12(a)

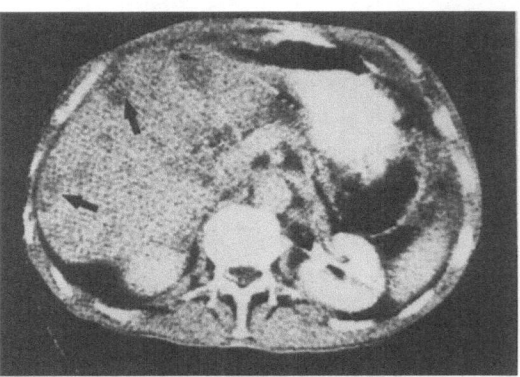

Figure 2.12(b)

Figure 2.12   CT scans of the liver: (a) pre-contrast, (b) post-contrast. Images are shown at the same window levels and window widths. The metastases shown in the precontrast scan are easier to identify after contrast enhancement (arrowed). Note general tissue opacification and concentration of contrast medium in the kidneys

(b) Opacification of Major Vessels

This is used to show vascular anatomy and pathology, and to distinguish vessels from other structures. To achieve this type of enhancement, the plasma level of contrast medium must be high and scans should be obtained during or immediately after injection, when the plasma level is at its peak. Some workers recommend a large dose of contrast medium such as that used for high-dose urography. Thus, Korobkin *et al.* (1978) recommend a dose of 100 ml Conray 325 a few minutes before the scan, followed by a bolus of a further 100 ml during the scan. Certainly this type of dose would give good visualisation of the major vessels. In our experience, much smaller doses are sufficient to enhance the vessels adequately for diagnostic purposes. A dose of 50 ml Conray 325 injected during the scan is usually adequate (figure 2.13).

The superior or inferior vena cava can be opacified using a smaller dose of contrast medium injected during the scan into the arm or leg as appropriate (figure 2.14).

It must always be remembered that urographic contrast media, especially in large doses, are

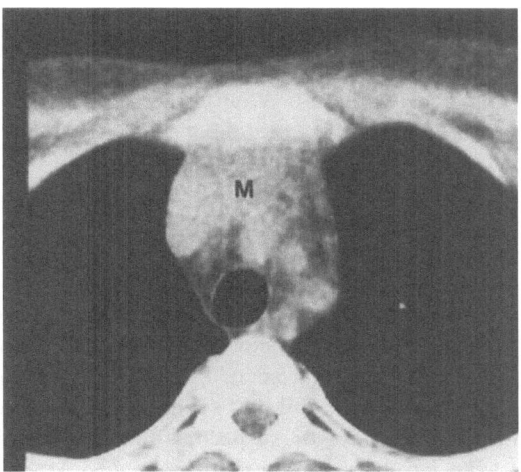

Figure 2.13(a)

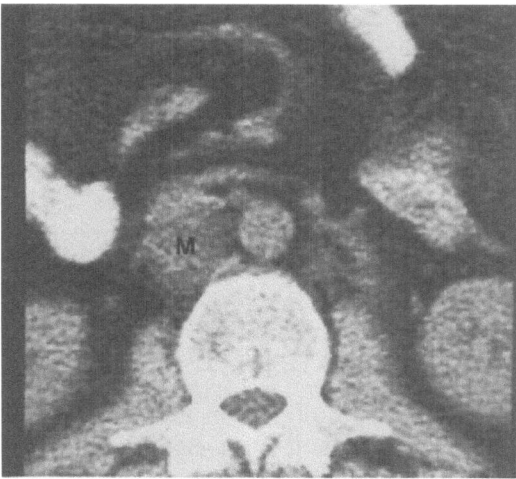

Figure 2.14(a)

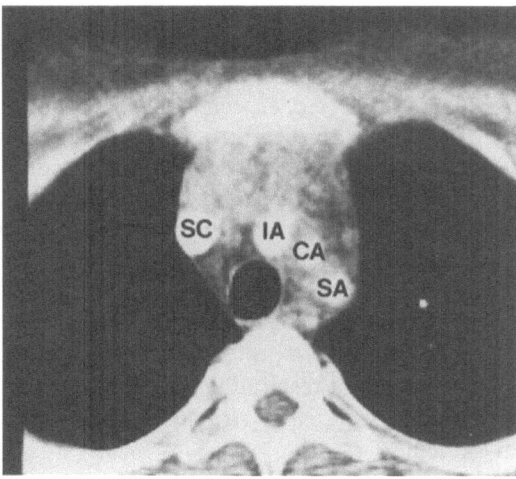

Figure 2.13(b)

Figure 2.13   CT scans through the upper mediastinum showing a lymph node mass anterior to the major vessels (M): (a) pre-contrast; (b) after the injection of 50 ml Conray 325. Superior vena cava (SC), innominate artery (IA), left common carotid artery (CA), left subclavian artery (SA)

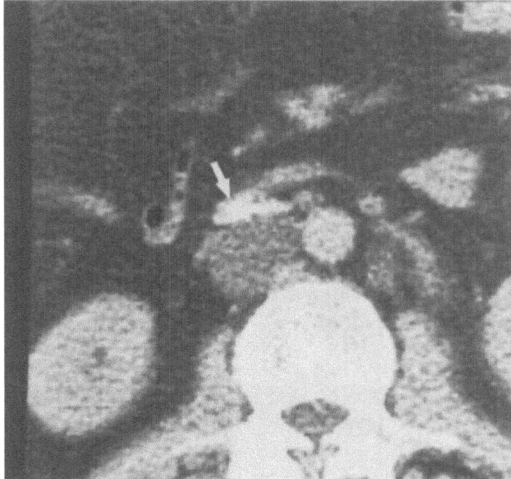

Figure 2.14(b)

Figure 2.14 Patient with abdominal nodal metastases from testicular teratoma. (a) In the pre-contrast scan, a mass (M) lies to the right of the aorta. The inferior vena cava is not easily distinguished from it. (b) After injection of contrast medium into a vein in the foot, the inferior vena cava is clearly identified and shown to be patent (arrowed)

potentially hazardous. Fortunately, unlike brain scans, a relatively small number of body scans require enhancement.

Dynamic Scanning

The development of 2 to 3 s scanners has enabled a rapid sequence of scans to be obtained, and this simplifies the technique of CT angiography by ensuring that scans are obtained at the most effective time. In addition, the pattern of sequential density changes in a tissue after the injection of intravenous contrast medium can be studied. The implications of this are not yet fully realised, but it seems to be one way in which CT might come to be used to study not only morphology but also pathophysiology.

CARE OF THE PATIENT

The great majority of patients are not disturbed by the examination. A few get claustrophobic in the scanners, especially when the scan is at the level of the upper thorax or higher. It is important that the radiologist and radiographer establish rapport with the patients, who often have strange ideas about what is going to happen to them and find the machine rather imposing and impersonal. In all but the oldest machines, scanning can take place without the radiographer entering the room between scans and it is easy for the patient to feel isolated, even though there is a microphone for communication with the radiographer. Rooms should be so designed that the patient can see the radiographer whilst scanning is taking place.

PLANNING AND SUPERVISION OF THE EXAMINATION

The radiologist has to decide what area should be scanned, how many scans are required, with what intervals between scans and with what slice thickness. What preparation is required? Is enhancement likely to be necessary?

The number of scans in an examination may vary from as many as 40, when a chest and abdomen are being scanned in a patient suspected of having metastatic disease, to as few as 4 or 5, when

monitoring the response of a known mass to therapy. The intervals between scans are also varied according to the size of the structure being scanned. Small structures, such as the adrenal glands, will require contiguous or even overlapping scans; large masses can be scanned at 2 or 3 cm intervals. The time taken for an examination will, therefore, vary widely according to the need for bowel opacification, the size of the area to be scanned and the need for enhancement. Patients having a CT scan of the body can expect to be in the department for between half an hour and two hours. When using a scanner such as the EMI CT5005, throughput will vary between about eight and ten patients in an eight-hour working day. Throughput may be higher using scanners with more rapid data processing.

Scanning of the body demands close supervision by the radiologist, and clinical examination of the area to be scanned is frequently important. Proven or unsuspected masses should be palpated before scanning to ensure that scans are obtained through the appropriate area and that scans can be precisely related to the mass or suspected mass. When the first scan has been obtained, this should be viewed on the operator's console to ensure that the examination is starting at the right level. When the initial set of scans has been obtained, the scans should be reviewed immediately. It is easy to be cursory about this step, especially as there is often a sense of urgency to proceed to the next patient. If a problem is not identified at this stage, the examination may prove to be inadequate and the patient may have to be recalled. The need for intervening or overlapping scans may be apparent, especially if there is suspicion that a partial volume effect is confusing the interpretation. When scanning the thorax and upper abdomen, it is important to check that variations in the depth of respiration have not led to parts of the mobile soft tissue structures being omitted from the scan.

REFERENCES

Korobkin, M., Kressel, H. Y., Moss, A. A. and Koehler, R. E. (1978). Computed tomographic angiography of the body. *Radiology*, **126**, 807–811

Kreel, L. (1979). *Medical Imaging: A Basic Course*, ed. L. Kreel, H M & M Publishers, Aylesbury

3

General Considerations – Clinical

CT scanning has revolutionised neurological and neurosurgical practice. The technique is ideally suited for the investigation of intracranial disease, not only for technical reasons but also because it replaces hazardous and expensive neuroradiological procedures (Thomson, 1979). Its impact on diagnosis elsewhere in the body has been less dramatic, mainly because the alternative methods of investigation are usually less hazardous than those used for intracranial disease. The technique is, however, available for investigating abnormalities in any part of the body, so that, even if only a small proportion of patients require a scan, the total demand for CT will be large. It is, therefore, important to try to define those situations in which CT is likely to be of most use. The technique and its value in each part of the body are discussed in the following chapters. Some general points about its use are discussed here.

WHAT TYPE OF PROBLEM?

CT scanning is potentially applicable to any diagnostic problem where there might be:

(a) a lesion large enough to distort the normal tissue outline (figure 3.1);
(b) a lesion whose density (attenuation value) differs significantly from that of the surrounding tissue (figure 3.2) – the detection of such a lesion will depend on its size and the degree of difference

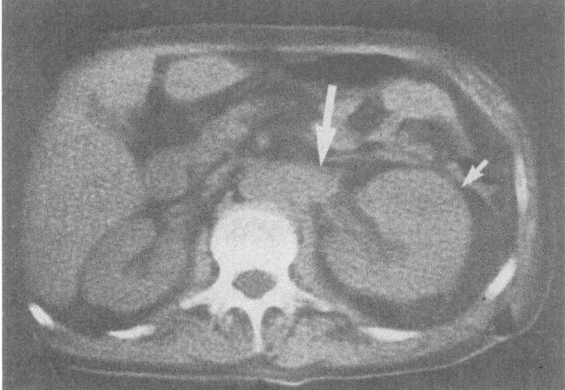

Figure 3.1 CT scan showing a carcinoma of the left kidney. The lesion is recognised because the kidney is enlarged and there is gross distortion of the renal outline (arrowed). Note lymph node enlargement of the left para-aortic nodes (large arrow)

in density between the lesion and the surrounding tissues (*see* p. 6); or
(c) a pathological change in the texture of a normal structure leading to detectable abnormality of density – for instance, fatty change in the liver (figure 3.3).

The capacity to determine tissue density means that CT not only shows the presence of an abnormality but may also determine its nature. Attenuation values in body scanning are, however, less precise than those in brain scans and only major differences, such as those between fat, fluid or soft

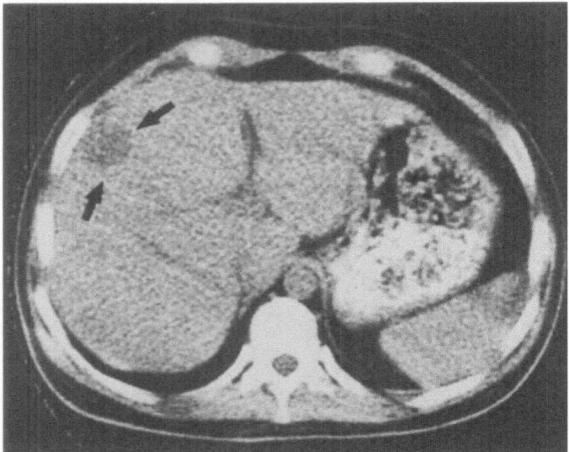

Figure 3.2 **Liver metastasis (arrowed). The lesion is identified because there is a significant difference between the attenuation values of normal liver parenchyma and tumour**

tissue, can be relied upon for diagnosis. The CT characteristics of different types of mass with attenuation values corresponding to soft tissue are not usually sufficiently distinctive to allow diagnosis of the nature of the mass. Thus, a tumour cannot be distinguished from an inflammatory mass by CT number alone, while benign and malignant tumours can have identical appearances.

PRIMARY DIAGNOSIS OR STAGING AND EXTENT OF KNOWN DISEASE?

The main value of CT of the body is its ability to define and detect masses. For this reason, it has rapidly found a place as a method of determining the stage and extent of malignant disease. Because the images can be obtained in the axial plane, the technique has a unique role in radiotherapy planning. The technique is, however, seriously undervalued if it is thought of only or mainly as a tool for the oncologist and radiotherapist. It is a powerful diagnostic tool for primary diagnosis. The indications for CT of the body have been reviewed in 1000 consecutive patients scanned at St Bartholomew's Hospital (Fry, 1981). The hospital has large departments of medical oncology and radiotherapy. About half the patients were scanned to determine the extent of known malignant disease or for radiotherapy treatment planning. Approximately 40% were scanned to resolve a diagnostic problem; the remaining 10% being scanned to assess or follow up known benign lesions.

WHAT TYPE OF PATIENT?

The quality of scans in most parts of the body, excluding the lungs and bones, depends on the way

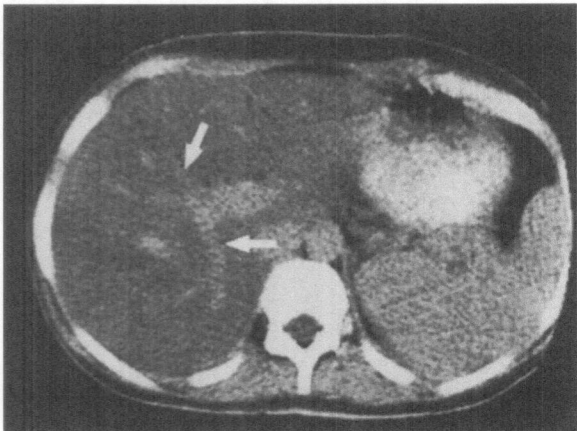

Figure 3.3 **Gross fatty infiltration of the liver. The density of the liver is less than that of other soft tissues so that the portal vessels are seen as relatively dense structures within it (arrowed)**

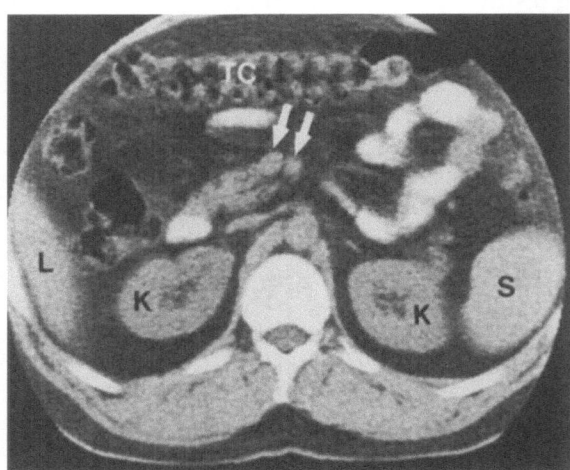

Figure 3.4 **Normal CT scan in a patient with abundant fat. Kidneys (K), spleen (S), tip of the right lobe of the liver (L), transverse colon (TC). The mesenteric vessels are arrowed**

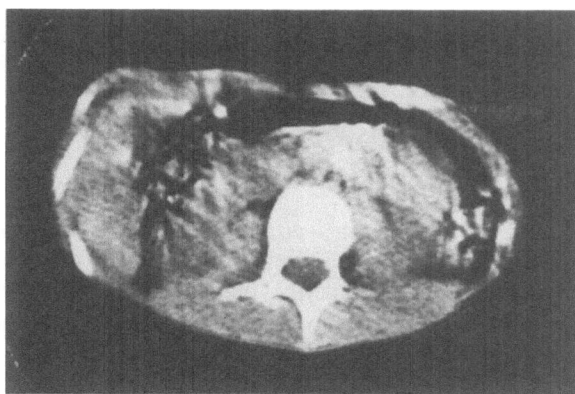

Figure 3.5   Poor-quality scan at the level of the third lumbar vertebra in a child with little intra-abdominal fat. This investigation was carried out because enlargement of the retroperitoneal nodes was suspected. No conclusive diagnosis could be made

in which the soft tissues are outlined by fat (figure 3.4). The fatter the patient the better the scan (only very rarely is a patient too fat to enter the scanner). It is worth noting that obese men have relatively greater amounts of intra-abdominal fat than obese women. In the latter, a much greater proportion of the fat lies in the superficial soft tissues. In very thin patients, the absence of fat may result in a scan that is uninterpretable. Children often have very little fat and this creates special problems, especially when they cannot hold their breath (figure 3.5).

THE CLINICAL VALUE OF COMPUTED TOMOGRAPHY

Assuming that the clinical question is valid, the effect of a technique on management depends on its appropriateness, its accuracy and its credibility. The range of conditions to which CT is applicable is very wide, but its use is limited by the general lack of availability and the relatively high cost. It is only appropriate for those problems which cannot be resolved so effectively by other techniques or which can only be resolved by techniques which are more hazardous, more unpleasant or more expensive.

An important factor when considering the appropriateness of CT is that the technique is not organ-specific. Many imaging techniques examine only one organ or system at a time. Should the referring clinician choose an inappropriate investigation, an abnormality may go undetected. With CT, all the tissues in the whole of each body slice are examined. For example, an examination directed at the liver includes all the upper abdominal structures, the lung bases, the bones and the superficial tissues. CT can therefore be helpful when symptoms and signs suggest the general site of a lesion without pointing to a specific organ.

Estimates of the accuracy of imaging techniques are difficult to interpret, particularly when the technology is changing rapidly. The figures do, however, have some value as a rough guide and as such are quoted in the following chapters. When interpreting statistics that compare the accuracy of one technique with another, there is the additional difficulty of ensuring that the techniques being compared have been carried out with the same degree of technical and interpretative skill. All too often, a highly sophisticated version of one technique is compared with an already aging version of another, or the results obtained by a dedicated expert using one technique are compared with those of another technique used by a routine clinical department. In this context, it is worth noting that one of the strengths of CT is that it is only minimally dependent on the skill of the operator. Good-quality examinations can be obtained as soon as the machine is installed.

Even though an imaging technique is capable of producing correct answers to clinically relevant questions, it does not always have the effect on management that might be expected. There are many reasons for this, including caution and conservatism; an important additional influence is the credibility of the information presented to the clinician. For an investigation to be useful, the result must be believed by the clinician with sufficient confidence for it to influence the management decision. Credibility will depend partly on previous experience of the method and partly on the reputation of the radiologist. An additional important element, however, is the way in which the information is presented. If the images are easily understood and abnormalities are clearly seen, then the report will not only be accepted but can also be acted upon.

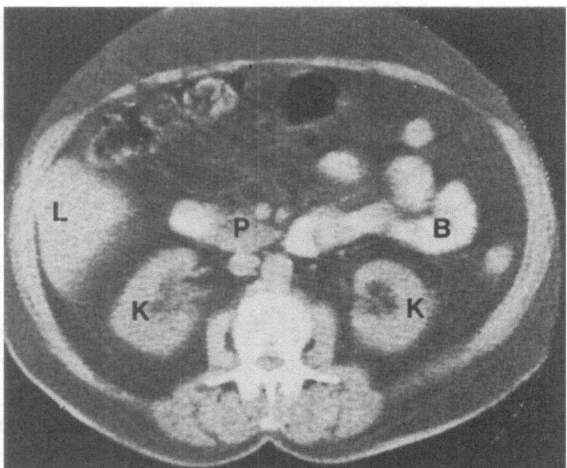

Figure 3.6   Scan through suspected abdominal mass in an obese patient. The scan shows only an excessive amount of fat and there is no evidence of an abnormal soft-tissue mass. Kidney (K), pancreas (P), liver (L), bowel (B)

One of the great advantages of CT as a diagnostic technique is that, in the majority of patients, the anatomy and pathology are clearly displayed and easily understood, and for this reason are accepted as the basis for decisions on management. Because of the credibility of CT and the fact that it is not organ-specific, a negative examination has more diagnostic impact than is usual with imaging techniques. This is especially so when a mass is suspected (figure 3.6).

RELATIONSHIP TO OTHER TECHNIQUES

In general, less hazardous, cheaper, more available and less painful and time-consuming investigations will be preferred, assuming that one can obtain comparable degrees of accuracy and credibility. Until now, CT of the body has not often been used as the investigation of first choice because a great many of the problems for which it might be applicable can be resolved without the need for hazardous investigations. For this reason, most CT scans of the body have been done when other techniques have failed to resolve the clinical problem. It seems likely as scanning time becomes more available, and the type and amount of information provided by CT is better

appreciated, that CT will be used earlier in the diagnostic sequence.

COMPUTED TOMOGRAPHY AND ULTRASOUND

These two techniques are often considered to be competitive but there is much less overlap between them than is commonly thought. They are, in general, complementary. The techniques are compared in table 3.1.

CT depends on the differential absorption of x-rays, whereas ultrasound depends on variations in acoustic impedance. It is hardly surprising, therefore, that the techniques vary widely in their applications and limitations. Ultrasound has no known ill-effects; CT is associated with the same risks due to low doses of radiation as other diagnostic x-ray examinations and should not be

Table 3.1   Comparison of ultrasound and CT

	Ultrasound	CT
Best use	Obstetric	Brain
Principal other uses	Abdomen Cardiac	Abdomen Thorax Any part of the body
Area examined	Localised	Whole-body slice
Plane of section	Infinitely variable	Limited
Physical constraints (fat, air, bone)	Frequent	Fewer
Operator dependence	Great	Minimal
Interpretation	Difficult	Easier
Credibility (acceptance by clinicians)	Limited (excluding obstetric and cardiac)	High
Acceptance by patient	Very high	Lower
Hazard	None	X-radiation
Cost	Low	Higher

used for the examination of pregnant women. Bony structures, air and excessive fat interfere with ultrasound but not with CT. Ultrasound images can be obtained in any plane that appears appropriate to the structure under examination. CT in general is limited to the axial plane. The facility for reconstructing images in different planes which is available on the newer machines has overcome this limitation to a certain extent.

Where one or other technique is at its most effective, there is no overlap. Thus, the best use of CT is for brain scanning and the best use for ultrasound is for the study of pregnancy. CT has little place, at present, in the management of heart disease, whereas echocardiography is a well established technique. CT is capable of examining any part of the body. This includes the head and neck, mediastinum, lungs and thoracic cage, and any bony structure; these areas can only be examined to a limited extent with ultrasound.

The only area of significant overlap is in the abdomen. Here an important consideration is that ultrasound is hindered by bone, air and excessive fat; 10 to 15% of abdominal ultrasound examinations fail because of interference from bony structures or because of excess bowel gas or fat. In general, fat patients are better examined with CT, thin patients and children with ultrasound.

The great advantages of ultrasound are that it is quicker and much more pleasant for the patient than CT, it carries no radiation hazard and is less expensive.

The two disadvantages of ultrasound compared with CT are that it is very operator-dependent and that the images are not readily understood by clinicians. Considerable training and experience are required if reliable abdominal ultrasound examinations are to be obtained. Even with good-quality grey-scale examination of the abdomen, the images are less acceptable than CT to the untrained observer. Many clinicians find ultrasound images difficult to understand and are frequently reluctant to base management decisions on ultrasound findings alone.

Apart from these general considerations, the relative advantages of the two techniques vary with the clinical problem. When both techniques are equally applicable, ultrasound will be used before CT, but the two techniques should be regarded as one diagnostic package, CT being used if the ultrasound examination is unsuccessful or equivocal, or the results are at variance with other evidence.

HOW USEFUL IS COMPUTED TOMOGRAPHY?

In order to justify the introduction of a new diagnostic technique, the technique should be shown to alter management so as to improve the outcome of disease. This is not easy to do and there are very few studies into the effect of any diagnostic test on the outcome of disease. Effect on management is a little easier to determine and reports relating to specific situations are discussed in the following chapters. Robbins *et al.* (1978) and Wittenberg *et al.* (1978) have attempted an overall view of the effect of CT on diagnostic understanding and choice of treatment in large groups of patients with clinical problems appropriate for CT scanning. The study by Robbins *et al.* (1978) was retrospective. They studied 687 patients and found that CT provided information that was not otherwise available and which changed diagnosis, prognosis or therapy in 23% of abdominal scans and 9% of scans of the thorax (93% of the abdominal scans had already had an ultrasound examination). Major surgery was avoided in 34 patients.

Wittenberg *et al.* (1978) carried out a prospective study in 184 patients. CT provided unique diagnostic information not available from other non-surgical procedures in 7% and significantly improved diagnostic understanding in an additional 34%. CT was very important compared with other factors in leading to a beneficial change in therapy in 7%, contributed to a change in therapy in a further 11% and reassured the physician about previously planned therapy in 43%. It improved the precision of previously planned treatment in 10%. Angiography was planned in 36 patients but only required in 14 after CT. Endoscopic retrograde pancreatography was contemplated in 37 patients but after CT was only carried out in 10. In 19% of patients, disease was excluded in the area scanned.

Both these studies were carried out when experience with CT was limited and some groups of patients were included in whom experience would suggest that CT is relatively ineffective. This is balanced by the fact that both groups included patients who were scanned to determine the extent of known malignant disease, a purpose for which CT is particularly well suited.

More sophisticated methods are required for studying the effect of diagnostic techniques on management and outcome of disease but these studies suggest that CT of the body when properly used can be an effective diagnostic tool with a significant impact on management in a very substantial proportion of patients.

REFERENCES

Fry, I. K. (1981). The role of CT in primary diagnosis – an overview. In *Computerised Axial Tomography in Oncology*, eds. J. E. Husband and P. A. Hobday, Churchill Livingstone, Edinburgh, pp. 14–19

Robbins, A. H., Pugatch, R. D., Gerzof, S. G., Faling, L. J., Johnson, W. C. and Sewell, D. H. (1978). Observations on the medical efficacy of computed tomography of the chest and abdomen. *American Journal of Roentgenology*, **131**, 15–19

Thomson, J. L. G. (1979). Cost effectiveness of an EMI brain scanner: an updated review 1977–78. *Health Trends*, **11**, 46–48

Wittenberg, J., Fineberg, H. V., Black, E. B., Kirkpatrick, R. H., Schaffer, D. L., Ikeda, M. K. and Ferrucci, J. T. (1978). Clinical efficacy of computed body tomography. *American Journal of Roentgenology*, **131**, 5–14

4

The Thorax – Mediastinum

On standard radiography, the mediastinal structures are packed closely together and on the frontal projection are largely obscured by bony structures. Even with tomography, it may not be possible to determine the origin and nature of lesions seen on the chest radiograph. In addition, some lesions are obscured by neighbouring structures and may not be detectable by any of the standard methods. For these reasons, the diagnosis of mediastinal abnormalities is one of the most rewarding uses for CT.

TECHNIQUE OF EXAMINATION

No preparation is required. Scans should be carried out with the breath held in full inspiration; scan intervals will vary with the nature of the problem. Vascular enhancement is frequently required.

Cardiac pulsation has prevented effective scanning of the heart using 20 s scanners but this is becoming practicable with the development of faster scanners and of electrocardiogram (ECG) gating techniques.

CT ANATOMY

If there is enough fat, the individual major vessels in the upper mediastinum can be seen surrounding the trachea from the level of the heart into the neck.

Through sequential scans it is possible to trace the innominate veins to the point where they unite to form the superior vena cava and to follow the course of the arteries arising from the aortic arch (figure 4.1a–c). Lower CT sections show the aortic arch and the superior vena cava. The arch passes posteriorly to the left and is closely related to the trachea and oesophagus (figure 4.1d). The oesophagus is easily identified; it frequently contains air.

Below the aortic arch the main pulmonary artery is seen on the left of and slightly anterior to the ascending aorta. The right pulmonary artery (figure 4.2) enters the hilum passing behind the superior vena cava and in front of the intermediate bronchus. The left pulmonary artery has a different course, passing over the left main bronchus. At a slightly lower level it is shown behind the left main bronchus (figure 4.2c). The pulmonary veins entering the left atrium form the lower part of the hilar shadows. The azygos vein is commonly seen as it enters the superior vena cava just above the tracheal bifurcation (figure 4.3).

In patients with abundant mediastinal fat, other normal structures can be recognised; for example, normal lymph nodes, nerves and remnants of the thymus. In adults, the amounts of mediastinal fat and residual thymic tissue vary considerably from patient to patient. The thymic tissue most commonly appears as small fragments of soft-tissue density within the mediastinal fat, but sometimes it is sufficiently well preserved to be seen as a defined

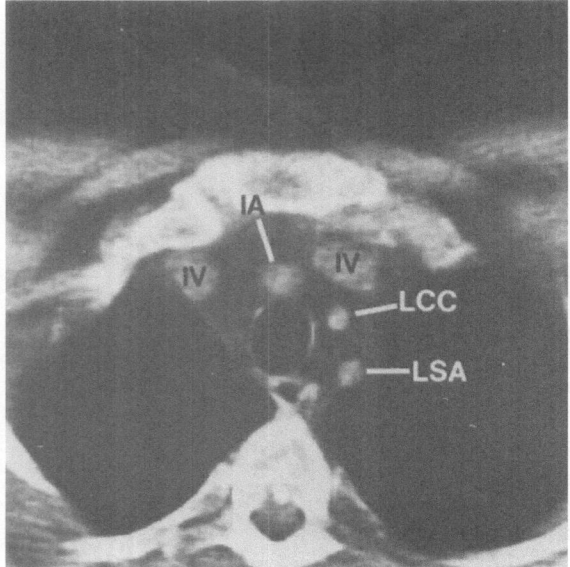

Figure 4.1(a)

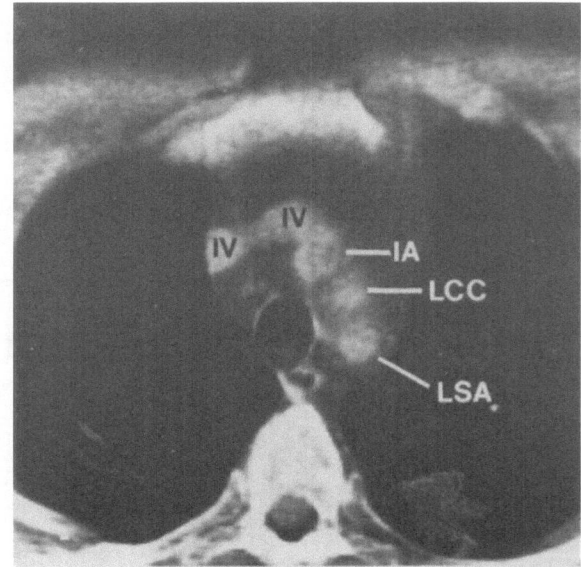

Figure 4.1(b)

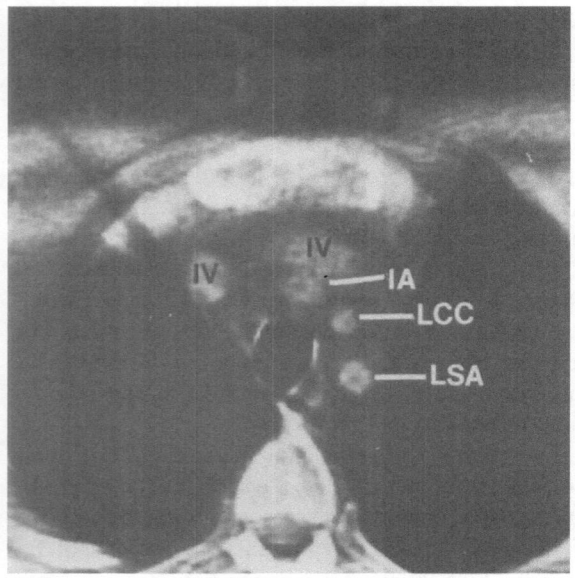

Figure 4.1(c)

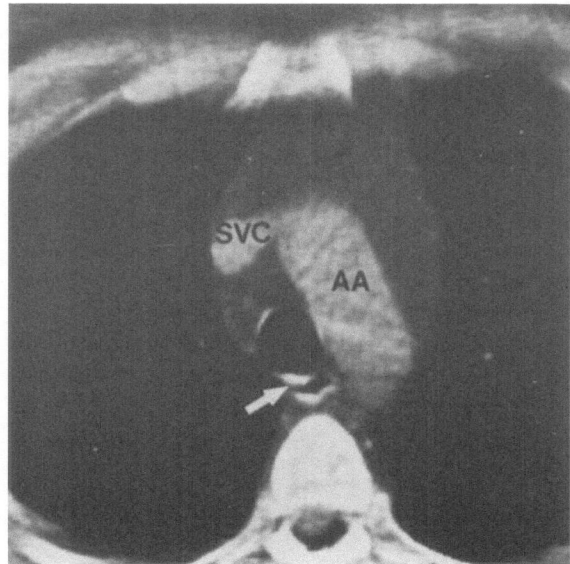

Figure 4.1(d)

Figure 4.1   Normal scans through the mediastinum at 1 cm intervals. Innominate veins (IV), innominate artery (IA), left common carotid artery (LCC), left subclavian artery (LSA), superior vena cava (SVC), aortic arch (AA); air-containing oesophagus is arrowed in (d)

structure, usually lying in front of the left innominate vein or arch of the aorta (figure 4.3a). When seen as a defined structure, it conforms to the normal contours of the space, unlike a tumour, which usually has rounded margins and tends to distort the mediastinal outline.

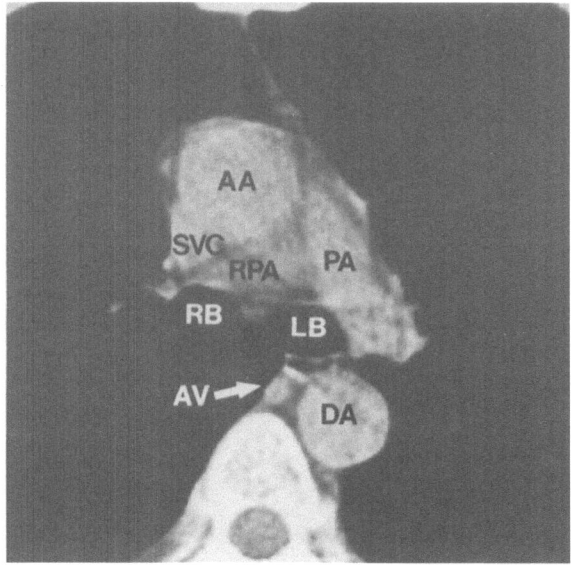

Figure 4.2(a)

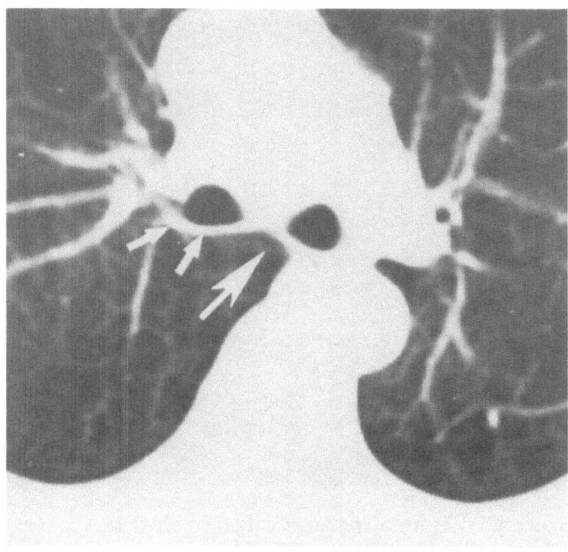

Figure 4.2(b)

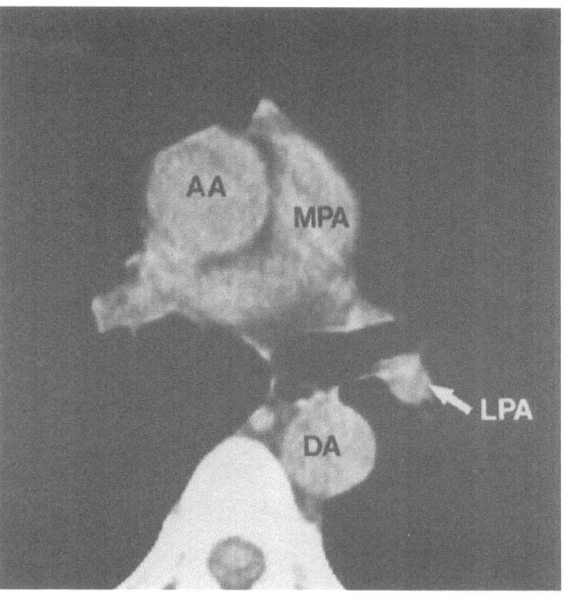

Figure 4.2(c)

Figure 4.2 (a) Normal scan through the mediastinum showing the junction of the main pulmonary artery and left pulmonary artery (PA). Right pulmonary artery (RPA), superior vena cava (SVC), right bronchus (RB), left bronchus (LB), ascending aorta (AA), descending aorta (DA), azygos vein (AV). (b) At a low window level the posterior wall of the right main bronchus is seen (small arrows). It forms the anterior border of the azygo-oesophageal recess (large arrow). (c) At a slightly lower level, the descending branch of the left pulmonary artery (LPA) lies behind the left main bronchus. Main pulmonary artery (MPA), ascending aorta (AA), descending aorta (DA)

The anatomy of the hila is not shown particularly well in axial section, but the main vessels and their branches can usually be identified.

Extensions of lung tissue between the major vascular structures give the mediastinum its characteristic appearance. For example, a tongue of lung parenchyma separates the left pulmonary artery from the descending aorta (the aortic pulmonary window) (figure 4.4). Normal lung also extends into the azygo-oesophageal recess behind the intermediate and right main bronchus, the wall of which is normally only a few millimetres thick (figure 4.4). Obliteration of these air-filled spaces

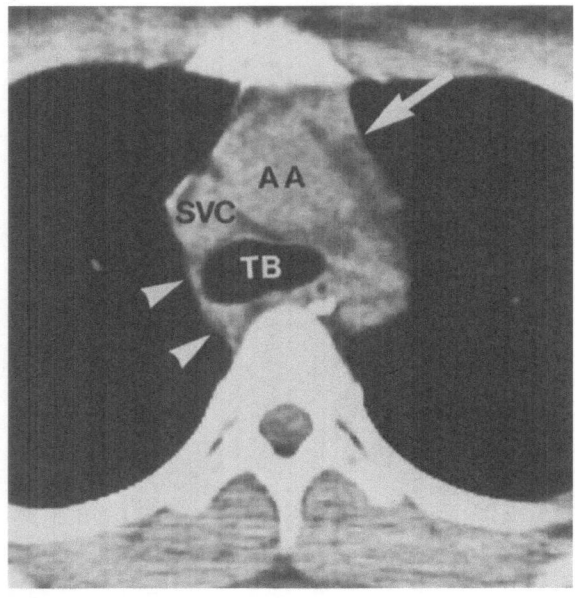

Figure 4.3(a)

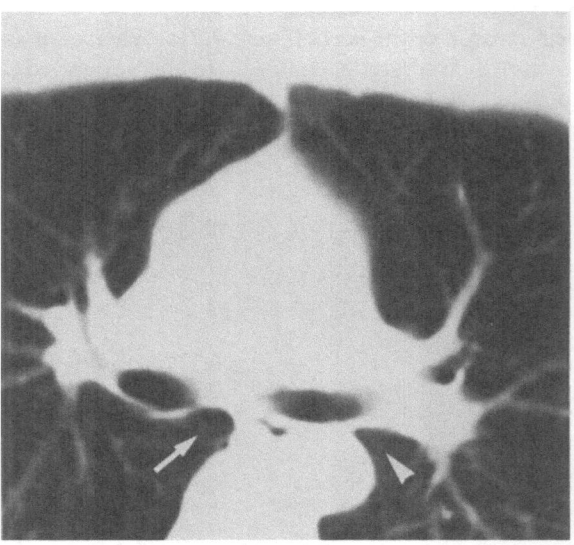

Figure 4.4   Aortic pulmonary window (arrowhead), and azygo-oesophageal recess (arrowed). Note posterior wall of right main bronchus

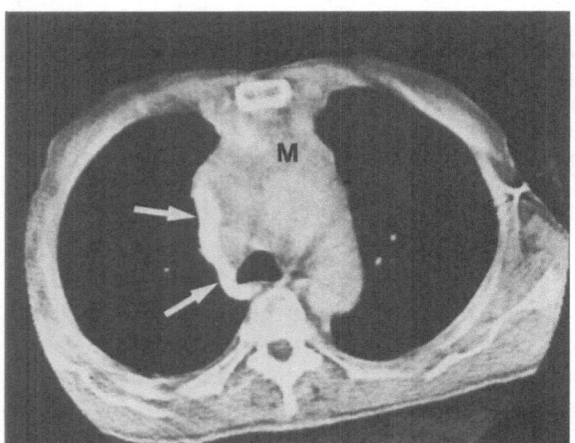

Figure 4.3(b)

Figure 4.3   (a) Normal azygos vein (arrowheads) seen as it enters the superior vena cava (SVC). Residual thymic tissue (large arrow), aortic arch (AA), tracheal bifurcation (TB). Note residual contrast medium from lymphography. (b) Superior vena cava obstruction showing retrograde flow of intravenous contrast medium into the azygos vein (arrowed) from the superior vena cava. The patient has a large mediastinal mass (M)

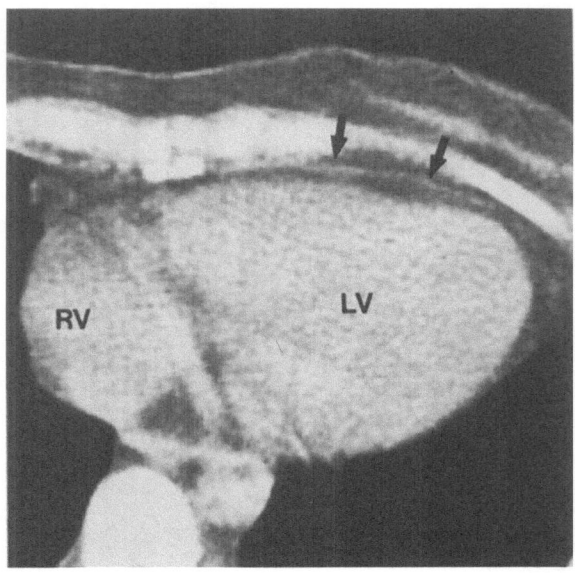

Figure 4.5   Normal pericardium (arrowed) in a patient with abundant pericardial fat. Left ventricle (LV), right ventricle (RV)

suggests lymph node enlargement (Goldwin *et al.*, 1977).

Above the level of the azygos vein, the soft tissue between the trachea and the right lung should not be more than a few millimetres thick and, if wider, is likely to be abnormal.

CT sections through the heart provide little, if any, useful information that cannot be gleaned from the conventional chest radiograph. This is largely because it is not possible to define the anatomy of individual cardiac chambers, although their general shape can be recognised. The normal pericardium is seen as a structure a few millimetres thick, separated from the heart by a layer of fat (figure 4.5). It appears most prominent anteriorly, usually on the right (Houang *et al.*, 1979). The inferior vena cava produces a characteristic convex bulge on the posterior aspect of the right heart border where it enters the right atrium at the level of the ninth thoracic vertebra (figure 4.6).

The diaphragmatic crura are seen as they arch over the descending aorta as it passes through the diaphragm. The azygos vein, thoracic duct, lymph vessels and nerves pass with the aorta through this hiatus (figure 4.7).

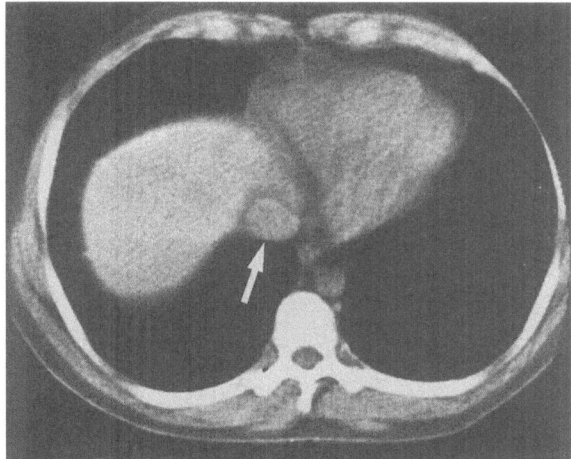

Figure 4.6 Inferior vena cava produces a bulge on the posterior aspect of the right heart border at the level of the ninth thoracic vertebra (arrowed)

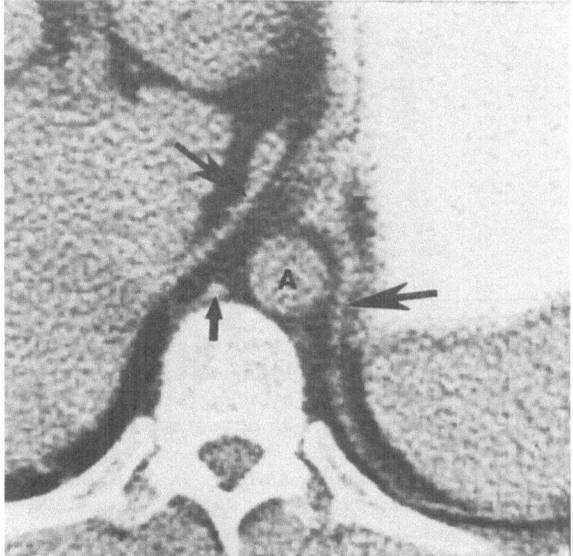

Figure 4.7 Normal diaphragmatic crura (large arrows). Note normal structures within the retrocrural space. Aorta (A), azygos vein (small arrow)

MEDIASTINAL MASSES

Provided there is a reasonable amount of fat, masses can usually be identified, even if they do not distort the mediastinal outline (figure 4.8). An intravenous contrast medium may have to be injected to distinguish a mass from a major vessel (figure 4.9). This is especially so in the thoracic inlet where the left innominate vein can itself look very much like a tumour (figure 4.10). The commonest masses in the upper mediastinum are thymic tumours, dermoid cysts and enlarged lymph nodes. Thymic tumours and dermoids sometimes calcify. The latter may contain fat. Malignancy may be indicated by lack of definition of the outline of the mass and by obliteration of the fat planes, making the vessels difficult to identify without enhancement (figure 4.11).

Enlarged lymph nodes are most easily detected when they alter the contours of the normal mediastinum because they are then silhouetted against the lung (figure 4.12).

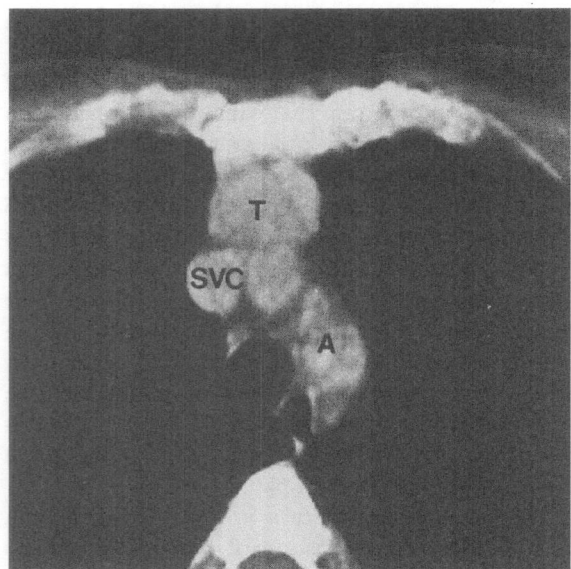

Figure 4.8(a)

Centrally placed lymph nodes are more difficult to identify, especially in the subcarinal region and at the thoracic inlet. Diagnosis of lymphadenopathy in these areas is easier in patients with abundant mediastinal fat and is facilitated by the use of intravenous contrast medium to enhance the normal vessels (figure 4.13).

The ability of CT to determine the nature of the lesion by examining tissue density is of particular value in the diagnosis of mediastinal masses, especially in the region around the heart. Lesions

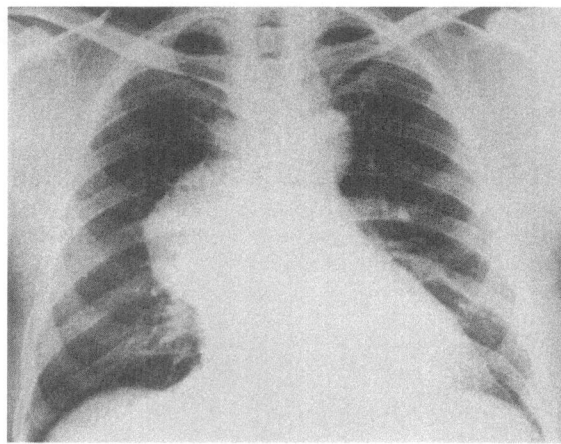

Figure 4.9(a)

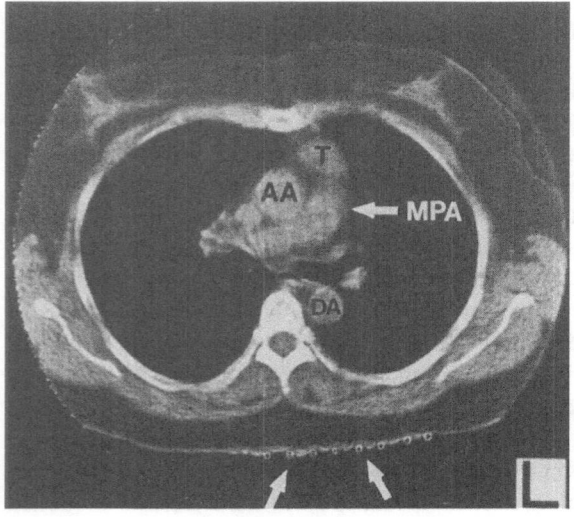

Figure 4.8(b)

Figure 4.8   (a) Thymoma (T) in a patient who presented with myasthenia gravis. This tumour was not detected on standard chest films. (b) Thymoma (T) in a patient with ectopic ACTH secretion. This tumour was also not visible on standard radiographs. Superior vena cava (SVC), aortic arch (A), ascending aorta (AA), descending aorta (DA), main pulmonary artery (MPA). Note catheters placed on patient's back (arrowed). Each catheter is 1 cm shorter than the next so that the number of catheters on the CT section can be correlated with the anatomical vertebral level on a plain chest film also taken with the catheters in position

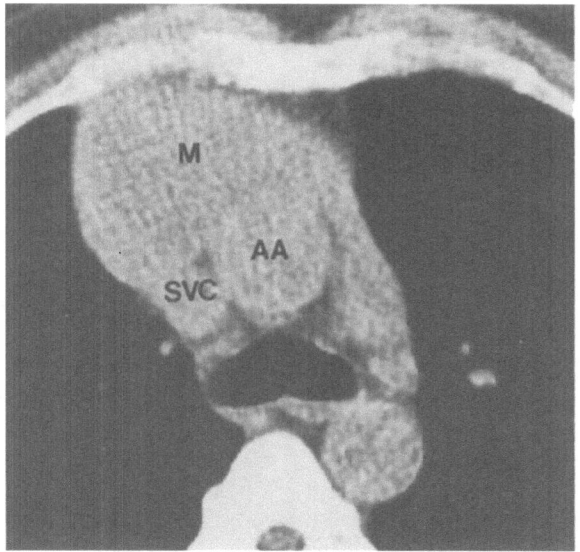

Figure 4.9(b)

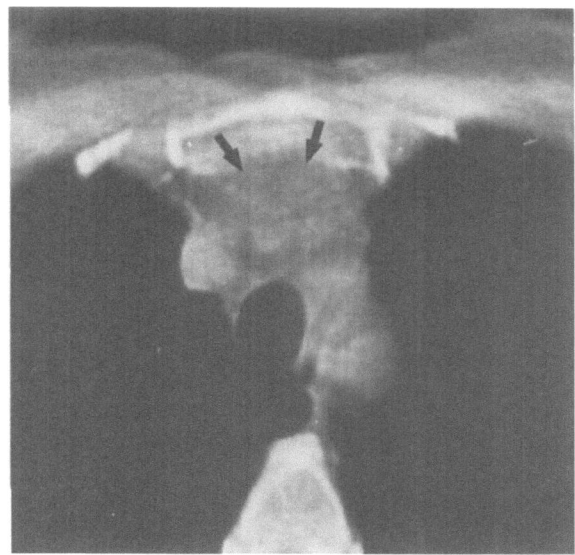

Figure 4.10(a)

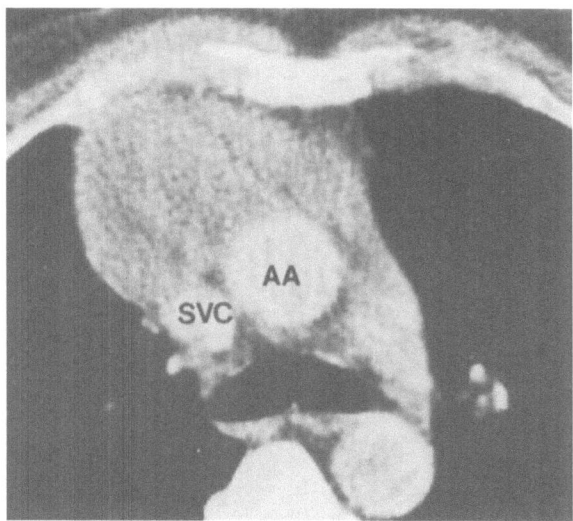

Figure 4.9(c)

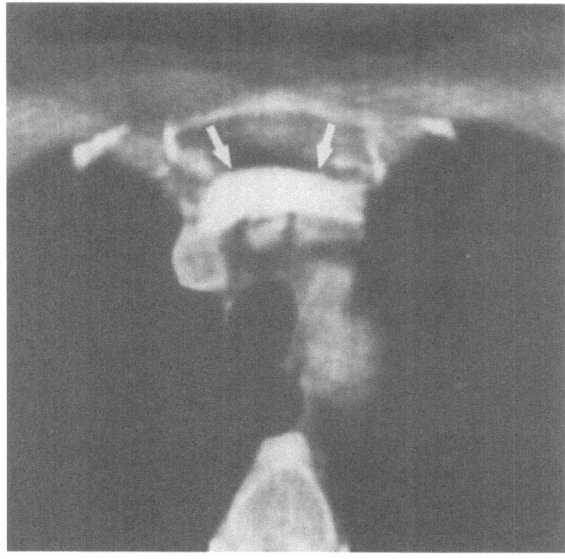

Figure 4.10(b)

Figure 4.9 Right anterior mediastinal mass on chest radiograph. Possibility of aneurysm considered. (a) Plain chest radiograph. (b) The unenhanced CT scan shows an anterior mediastinal mass (M) which appears to be separate from the ascending aorta (AA) and superior vena cava (SVC). (c) After injection of intravenous contrast medium, the major vessels have enhanced and the mass is clearly separate from the aorta. (Reproduced by kind permission of Pitman Press)

Figure 4.10 Normal mediastinum. The pre-contrast scan suggests an anterior mediastinal mass (arrowed). (b) Post-contrast scan shows that the apparent mass represents the left innominate vein (arrowed)

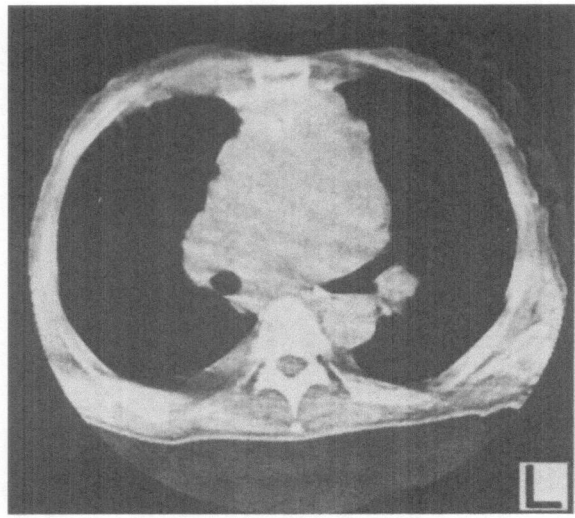

Figure 4.11(a)

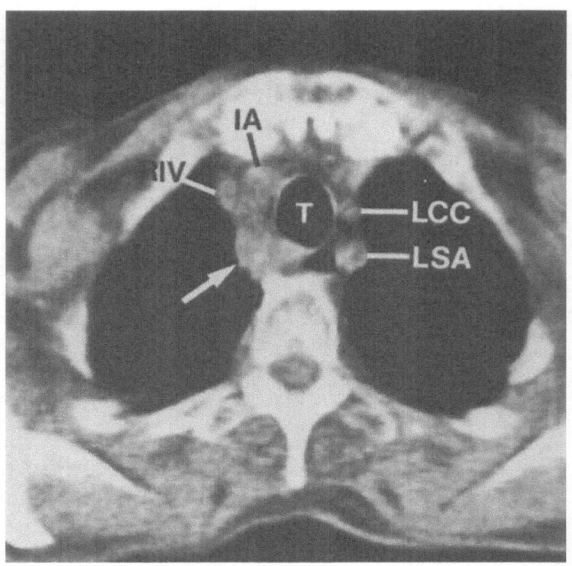

Figure 4.12(a)

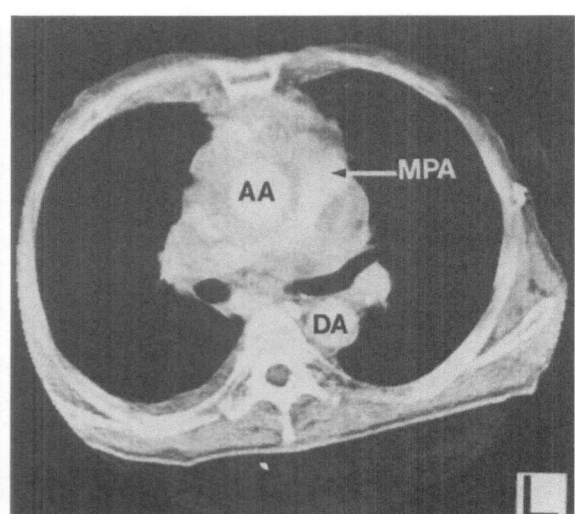

Figure 4.11(b)

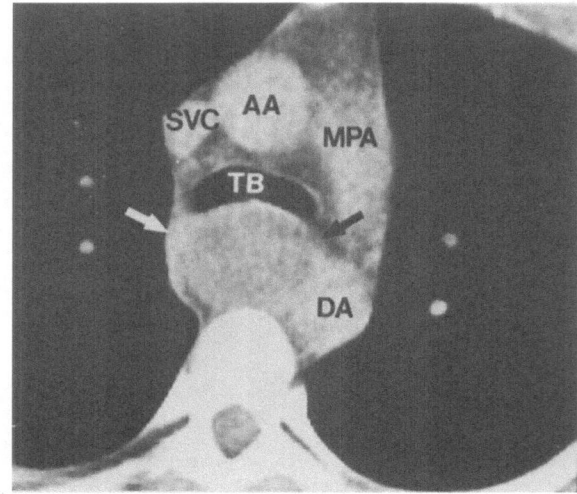

Figure 4.12(c)

Figure 4.11 Extensive mediastinal tumour: (a) pre-contrast; (b) post-contrast. There is obliteration of the mediastinal fat planes which makes it impossible to identify the vessels without contrast medium. Ascending aorta (AA), descending aorta (DA), main pulmonary artery (MPA)

Figure 4.12 Enlarged mediastinal nodes. (a) Widening of right paratracheal soft tissue due to lymph node enlargement in patient with bronchogenic carcinoma. Trachea (T), right innominate vein (RIV), innominate artery (IA), left common carotid (LCC), left subclavian artery (LSA). (b) Enlarged anterior mediastinal node (arrowed) in a patient with lymphoma. Superior vena cava (SVC), ascending aorta (AA), main pulmonary

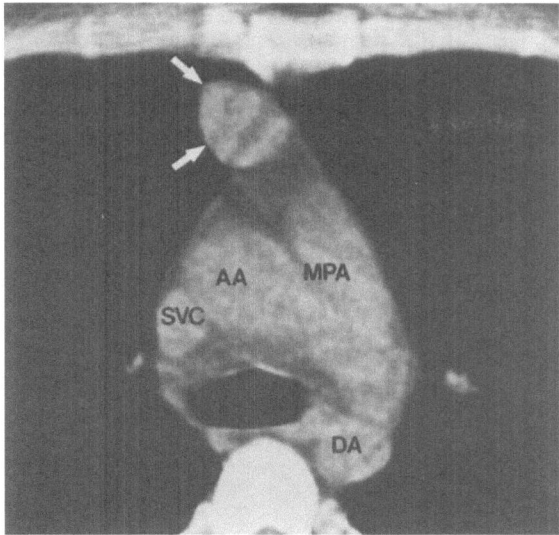

Figure 4.12(b)

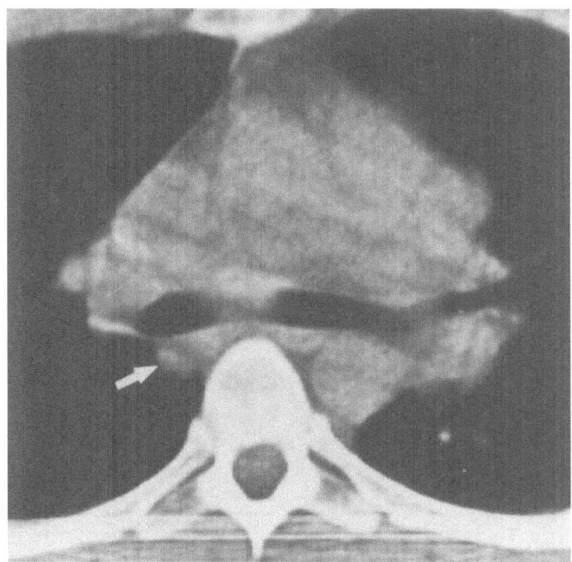

Figure 4.12(d)

consisting mainly of fat or fluid can be distinguished from solid tumours; for example, a prominent fat pad (figure 4.14) or a cystic lesion such as a parapericardial or pericardial cyst (figure 4.15) can be distinguished from a solid tumour (figure 4.16). It may thus be possible to confirm that a lesion is

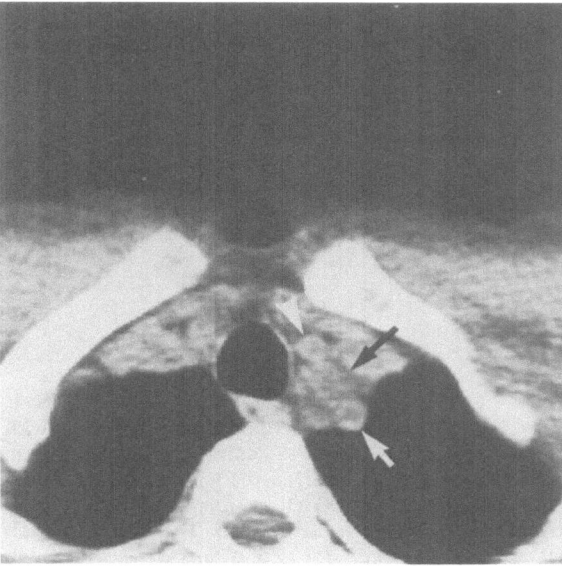

Figure 4.13(a)

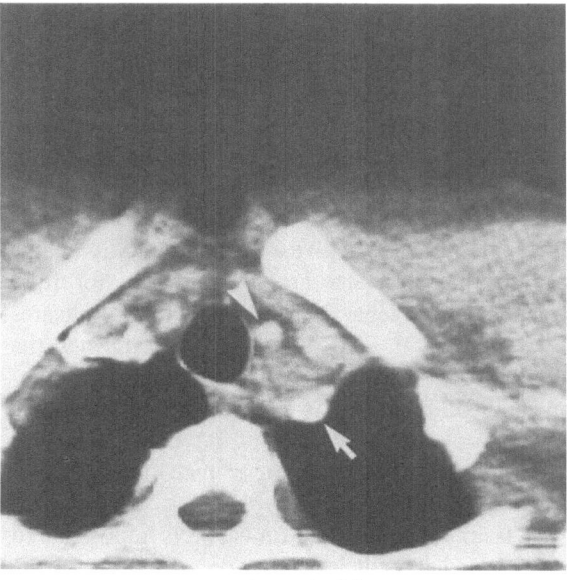

Figure 4.13(b)

artery (MPA), descending aorta (DA). (c) Enlarged posterior mediastinal node (arrowed) in a patient with testicular teratoma. Tracheal bifurcation (TB), descending aorta (DA), superior vena cava (SVC), ascending aorta (AA), main pulmonary artery (MPA). (d) Enlarged node occupying the azygo-oesophageal recess (arrowed). Transbronchial biopsy of this node showed sarcoidosis

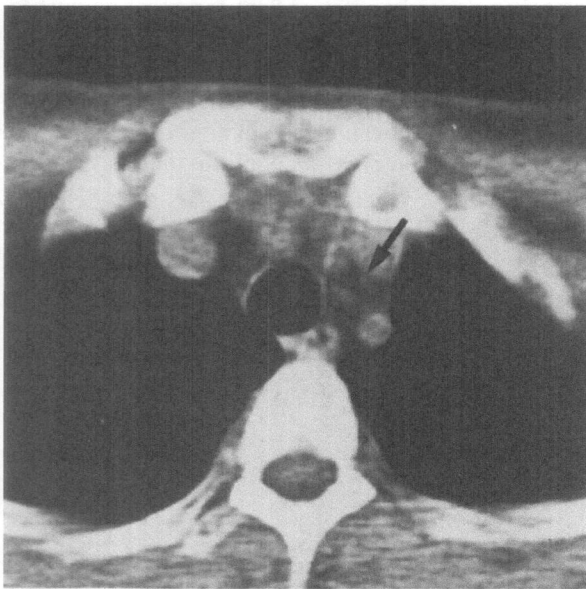

Figure 4.13(c)

Figure 4.13 Enlarged mediastinal node in a patient with testicular teratoma. (a) Pre-contrast scan shows an opacity (black arrow) between the left subclavian artery (small arrow) and the left common carotid artery (arrowhead). (b) Post-contrast scan. The normal vessels have been opacified. (c) Following six courses of chemotherapy, the lymph node has reduced in size leaving a fat-containing space

general rule, well circumscribed masses tend to be benign but those which infiltrate the fat planes are likely to be malignant, although Crowe *et al.* (1978) report that mediastinal bleeding, extensive sarcoidosis and other diseases can give similar appearances. The problem of distinguishing benign

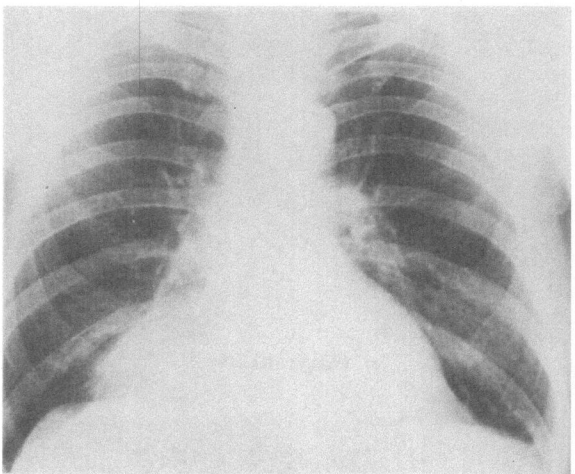

Figure 4.14(a)

benign. It is, however, important to recognise that CT examination close to the heart is not always satisfactory because of the artefacts due to cardiac pulsation. Not only may this degrade the image but it may also invalidate density measurements. Sometimes, a mixture of fat and soft tissue, as for instance in some dermoids, can give a mean attenuation value close to that of water and be mistaken for fluid (figure 4.17). In general, if the CT number indicates fat (−30 to −50 EMI units), this establishes the diagnosis of a fatty mass without further investigation. If the CT number is close to that of water, the lesion is probably a cyst but it may be necessary to prove this, depending on the clinical features and radiographic appearance.

If a lesion appears solid on CT, it is impossible to determine whether it is benign or malignant on the basis of the CT scan appearances alone. As a

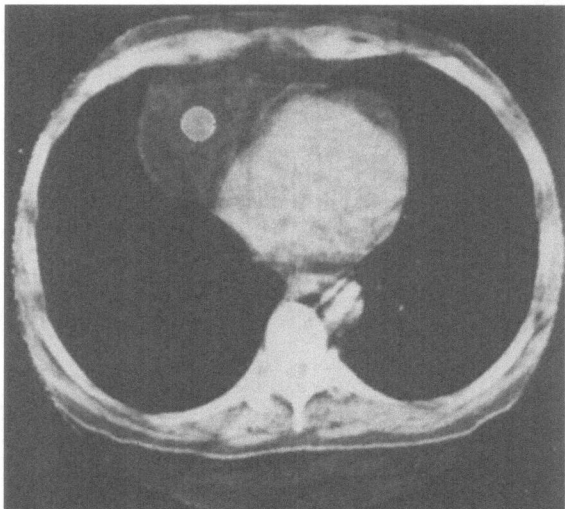

Figure 4.14(b)

Figure 4.14 Right paracardiac mass. (a) Routine chest radiograph. (b) The scan demonstrates that the mass represents a large pericardial fat pad (EMI number −40.5, standard deviation ±7.97). (Scan (b) reproduced by kind permission of Pitman Press)

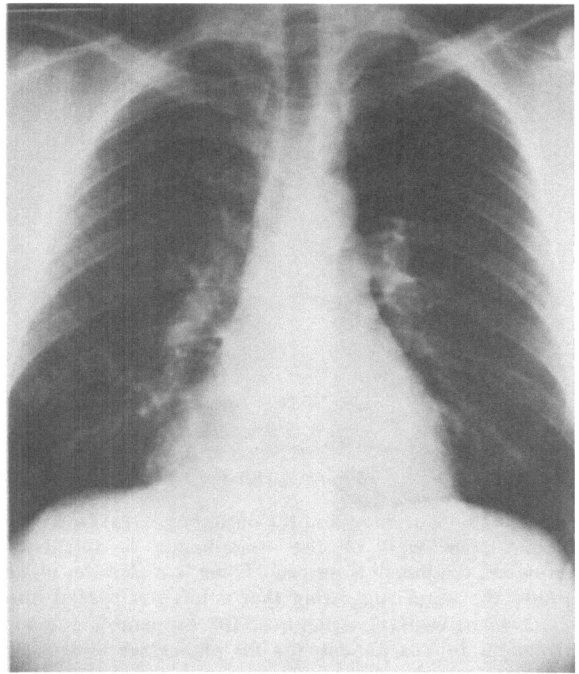

Figure 4.15(a)

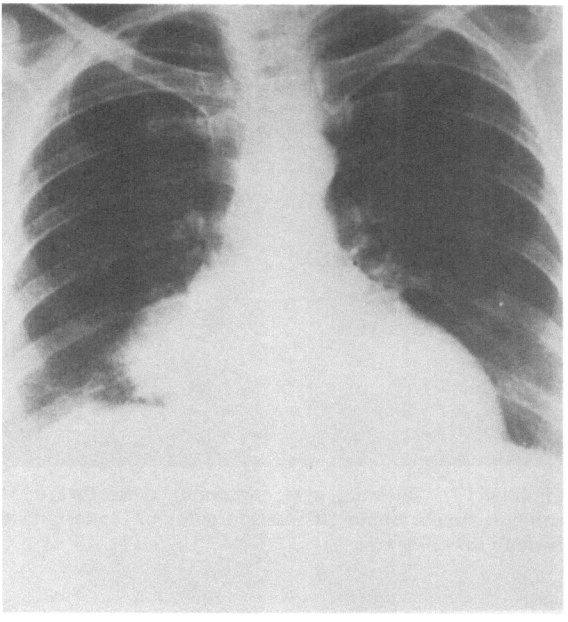

Figure 4.16(a)

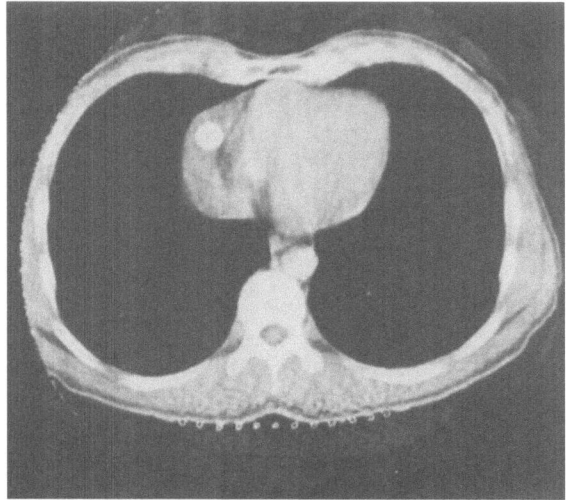

Figure 4.15(b)

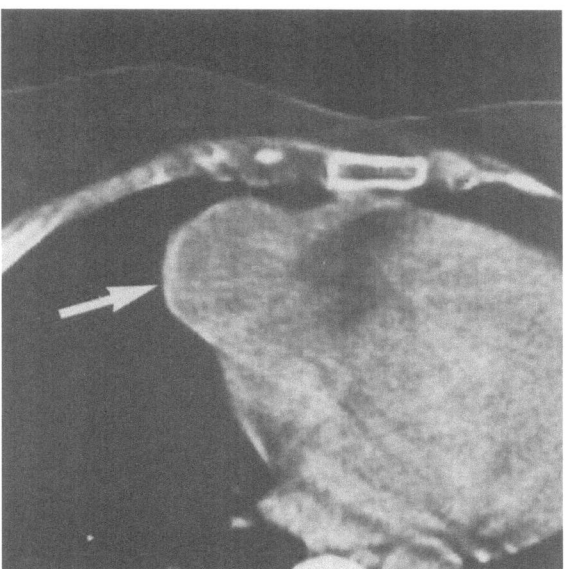

Figure 4.16(b)

Figure 4.15 Pericardial cyst. (a) The chest radiograph shows a right paracardiac mass. (b) The scan indicated that the mass contained fluid (EMI number +1.5, standard deviation ±7.72). A pericardial cyst was subsequently removed

Figure 4.16 Thymoma. (a) The chest radiograph shows a right paracardiac mass. (b) The mass (arrowed) has a density similar to soft tissue indicating a solid tumour. This was subsequently removed and shown to be a thymoma

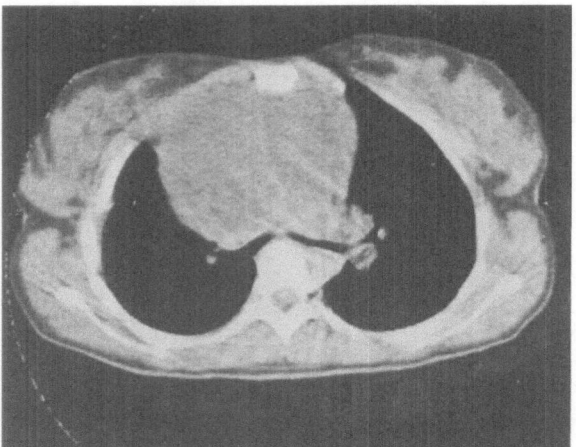

Figure 4.17   Dermoid cyst containing a mixture of fat and soft tissue. Mean attenuation value of the lesion was close to that of water

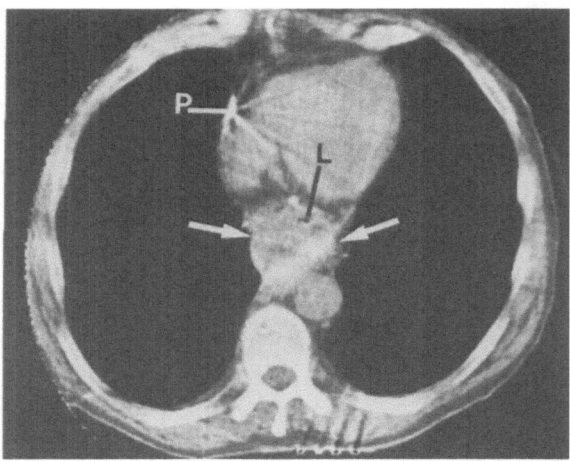

Figure 4.18(b)

from malignant lesions is one of the major limitations of CT, not only in the chest. If serious errors are to be avoided, interpretation of the scan should always be made in the light of clinical information.

In *carcinoma of the oesophagus* the narrow lumen and thickened oesophageal wall are seen (figure 4.18a). If the lesion spreads into the surrounding tissues, fat planes will become ill-defined and the tissue outlines will be lost (figure 4.18b).

Figure 4.18   Carcinoma of the oesophagus. (a) Operable tumour. The wall of the oesophagus is thickened (arrowed), the lumen is narrow. There is a clear fat plane around the mass suggesting that it has not spread into adjacent mediastinal structures. (b) Inoperable tumour (arrowed). In this patient, the fat planes are ill-defined, particularly posteriorly. The oesophageal lumen is displaced anteriorly (L). Note calcification in the pericardium (P)

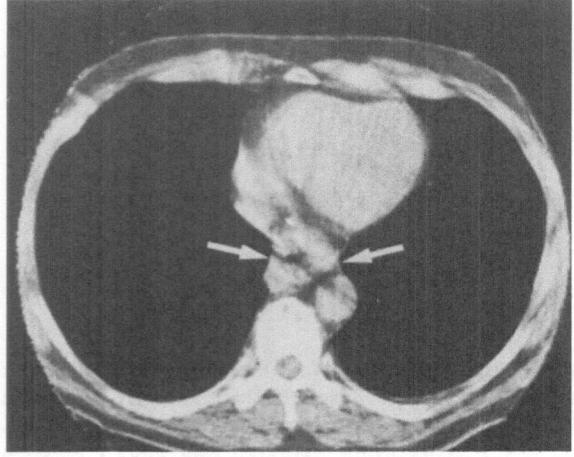

Figure 4.18(a)

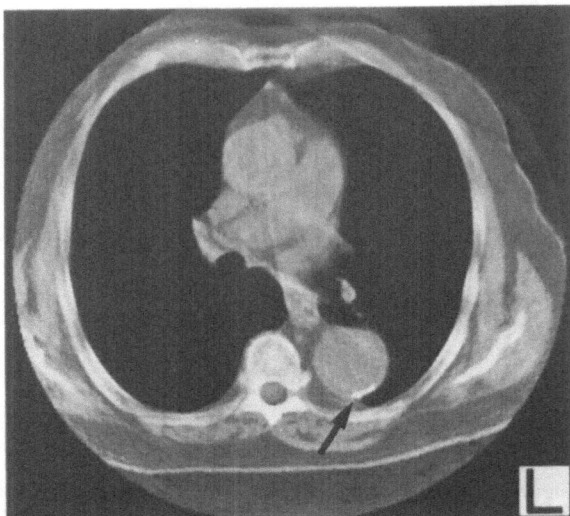

Figure 4.19   Diffuse aneurysmal dilatation of the aorta. Note calcification of the posterior wall of the descending aorta (arrowed)

Aneurysmal dilatation of the *major vessels* is easily seen (figures 4.19 and 4.20), together with calcification of the wall. If there is intraluminal thrombus, the injection of intravenous contrast medium shows the lumen separate from the thrombus. CT will also show the degree of displacement of neighbouring structures. The relation of intimal calcification of the wall of the aneurysm is easy to see. When calcification is displaced inwards, a

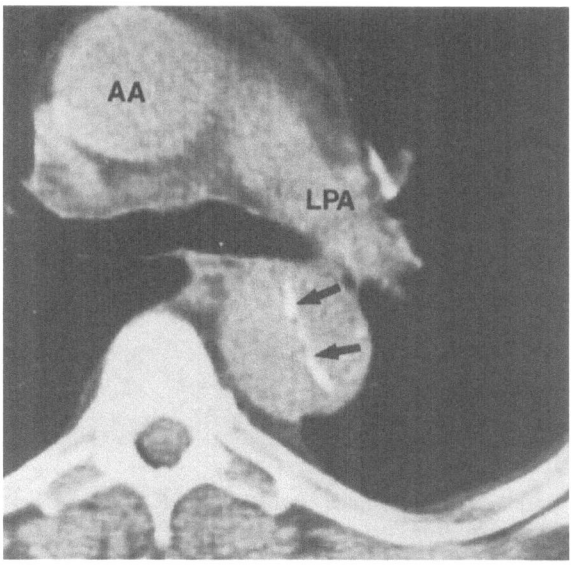

Figure 4.21 Dissecting thoracic aneurysm. Note medial displacement of the calcified aortic wall (arrowed). Ascending aorta (AA), left pulmonary artery (LPA)

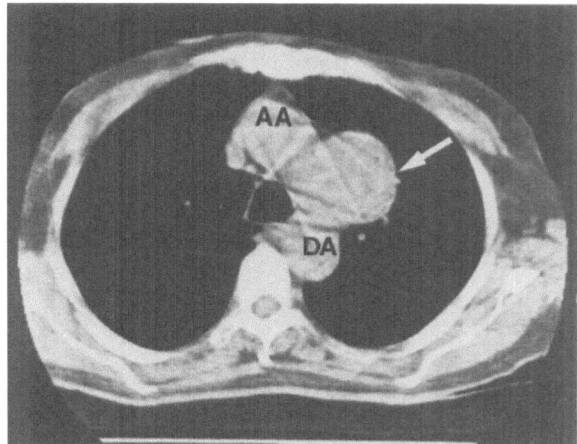

Figure 4.20(a)

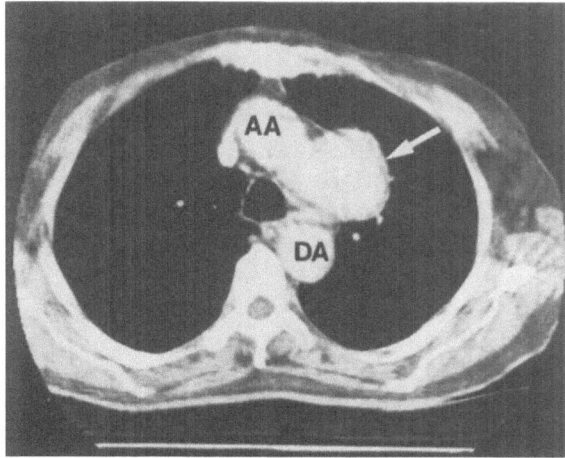

Figure 4.20(b)

Figure 4.20 Saccular aortic aneurysm: (a) pre-contrast; (b) post-contrast. After injection of intravenous contrast medium, the aneurysm (arrowed) has opacified to the same degree as the ascending aorta (AA) and descending aorta (DA)

diagnosis of dissection can be strongly suspected, even on the unenhanced scan (Gross *et al.*, 1980) (figure 4.21). The dissection may be seen after the injection of intravenous contrast medium as an opacified crescent (Gross *et al.*, 1980). In a proportion of patients with dissection, both the true and false lumen opacify and the intimal flap can be

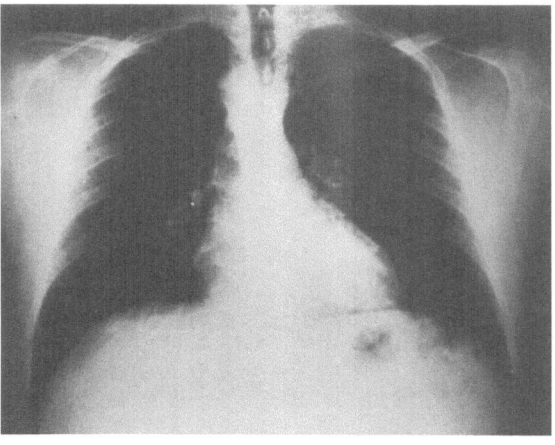

Figure 4.22(a)

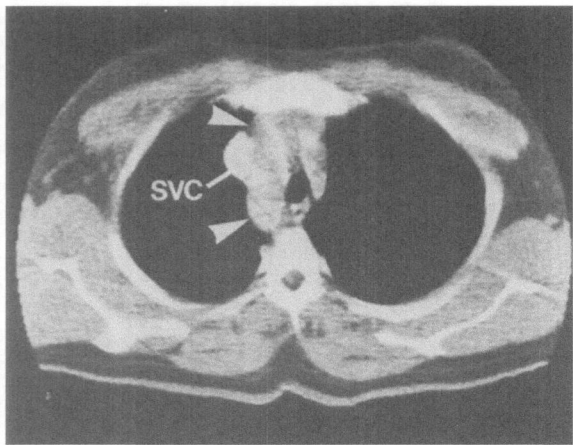

Figure 4.22(b)

**Figure 4.22   Right-sided   aortic   arch.   (a)   Chest
radiograph. (b) The anomaly is clearly shown (arrow
heads). Superior vena cava (SVC)**

identified; successful demonstration of this flap is
more likely when it is possible to obtain rapid
sequential scans (Godwin *et al.*, 1980). Congenital
abnormalities of the major vessels sometimes
produce abnormalities on the chest radiograph, the
nature of which can be resolved by CT (figure 4.22).

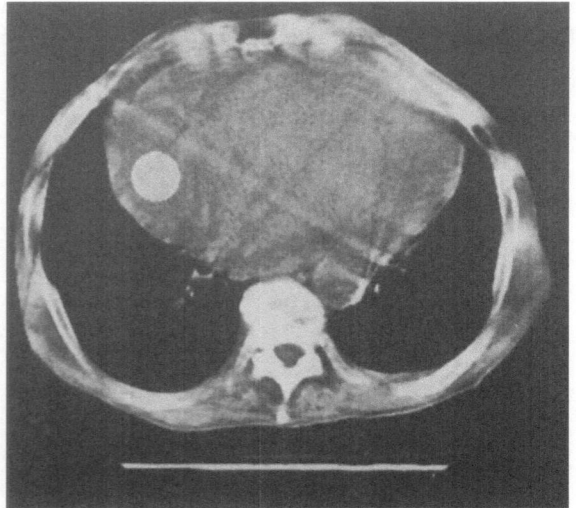

**Figure 4.23   Massive pericardial effusion (mean attenua-
ation value + 7 EMI units)**

HEART

There is so far very little experience of the CT
appearances in heart disease. In patients with
pericardial effusions, the effusion may be seen
(figure 4.23) and there may be some pericardial
thickening (Houang *et al.*, 1979). In animal studies,
CT shows ischaemically damaged myocardium as
an area of relatively low density compared with the
surrounding normal myocardium (Higgins *et al.*,
1979). It is reported that, after the insertion of
coronary artery bypass grafts, the patency of the
grafts can be indicated by opacification after the
injection of intravenous contrast medium (Guthaner
et al., 1980).

USE AND ACCURACY OF COMPUTED
TOMOGRAPHY

The Evaluation of a Known Mediastinal Mass

The reader is referred to Goldwin *et al.* (1977),
Livesay *et al.* (1978) and Pugatch *et al.* (1980). CT
will show the anatomical site of the mass and sometimes indicate its nature. In the upper mediastinum,
its main value lies in its ability to separate soft-tissue
masses from abnormalities of the great vessels (*see*
figures 4.9a and b and 4.13a and b). In many cases,
angiography   can   be   avoided.   In   the   lower
mediastinum, the site of the lesion is usually evident
from the chest radiograph. CT is useful because
many lesions close to the diaphragm are benign
incidental findings and CT may be able to show that
a mass is fatty or cystic.

Occult Mediastinal Disease

CT is particularly helpful in identifying primary
tumours in the retrosternal space when conventional
techniques have shown no abnormality or when the
results are equivocal. CT is, therefore, valuable in
the investigation of patients with myasthenia gravis
(Mink *et al.*, 1978). Sometimes quite large lesions
may be difficult to demonstrate on conventional
examinations. For instance, the thymoma shown in

figure 4.8a measured 5 cm × 3 cm in cross section. The tumour in figure 4.8b was of similar size. Neither could be seen with any confidence on the standard radiographs or tomograms. These tumours lay, respectively, at the upper and lower ends of the anterior mediastinum. It seems likely that these are sites where masses are liable to be missed because the anterior mediastinal space is at its smallest, the major vessels being close to the anterior chest wall.

CT is also valuable in patients suspected of harbouring occult nodal metastases (Crowe *et al.*, 1978). For instance, in a study of 62 patients with malignant teratoma, mediastinal lymphadenopathy was demonstrated in seven patients with CT but in only four of these by conventional tomography (Husband *et al.*, 1979).

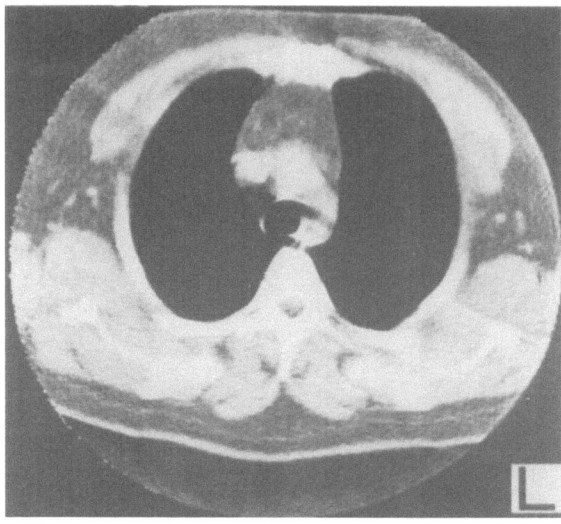

Figure 4.24(b)

Figure 4.24 Questionably   abnormal   upper   mediastinum. **(a)** Chest radiograph. **(b)** CT scan excludes a mass by demonstrating that the widened mediastinum is due to an excessive amount of mediastinal fat

The Questionably Abnormal Mediastinum

CT provides a simple method for resolving the problem of the chest radiograph in which the upper mediastinum looks a little wide but in which there is no definite evidence of disease. A few scans are sufficient to show whether there is a mass or whether the appearances are produced by an excessive amount of fat or by vessels that are more prominent than usual (figures 4.24 and 4.25).

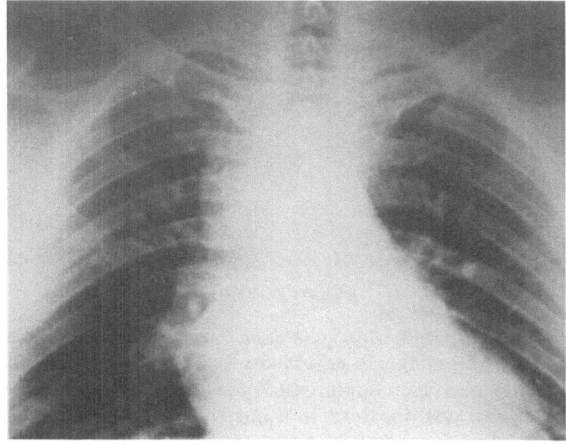

Figure 4.24(a)

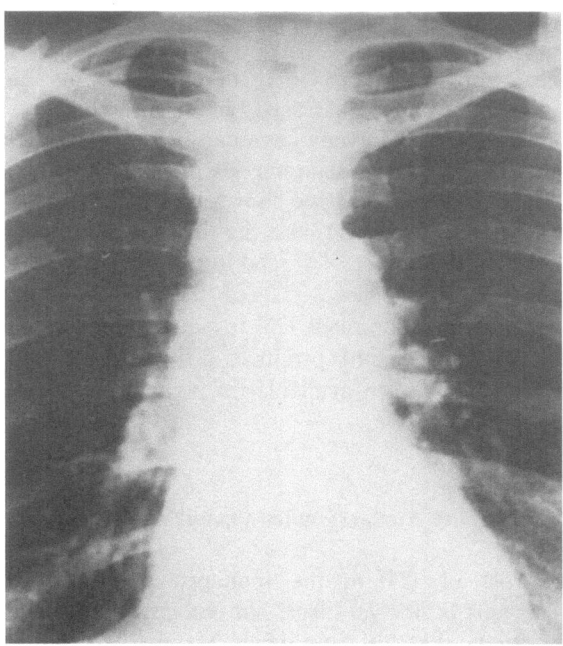

Figure 4.25(a)

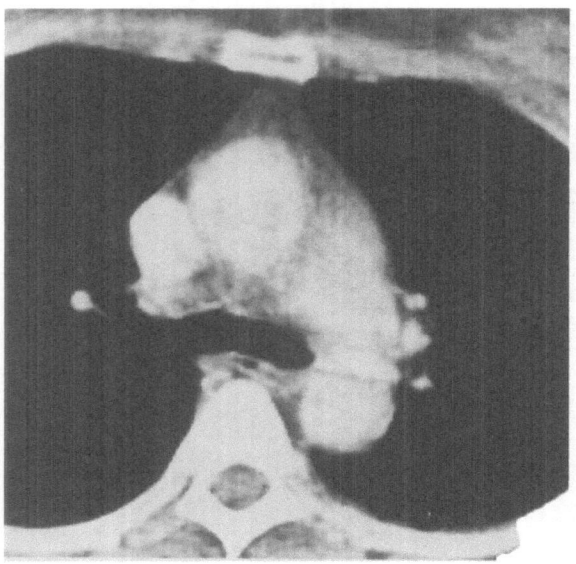

Figure 4.25(b)

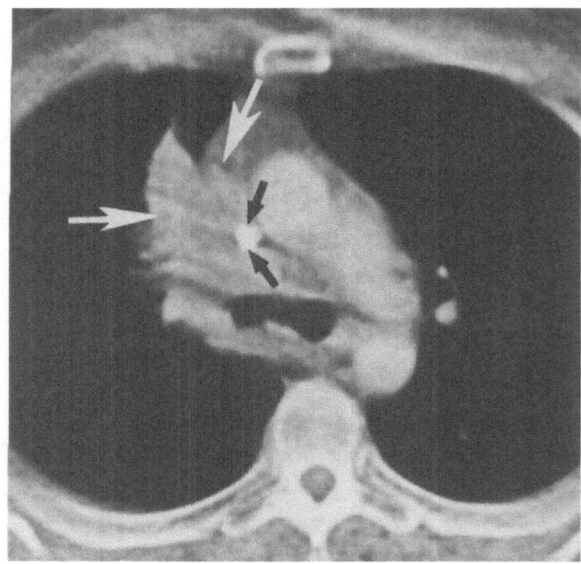

Figure 4.26(a)

Figure 4.25 Wide upper mediastinum. (a) Chest radiograph. (b) Enhanced CT scan demonstrates prominent vessels but there is no evidence of a mediastinal mass

The Extent of Malignant Disease

Direct spread of bronchial carcinoma into the mediastinum can be assessed by CT and compression of the superior vena cava can be demonstrated (figure 4.26). In carcinoma of the oesophagus, Daffner *et al.* (1979) have shown that there is good correlation between CT and the findings at surgery relating to the degree of spread into the surrounding tissues. In their view, CT of the mediastinum, together with abdominal CT to show lymph node and liver involvement, produces a firmer base than has previously been available for planning management.

Lesions of the Aorta, Greater Vessels and Heart

The role of CT in the management of aortic aneurysms is not yet clear, but recent reports have suggested that it is likely to replace some aortograms, especially when rapid serial scans can

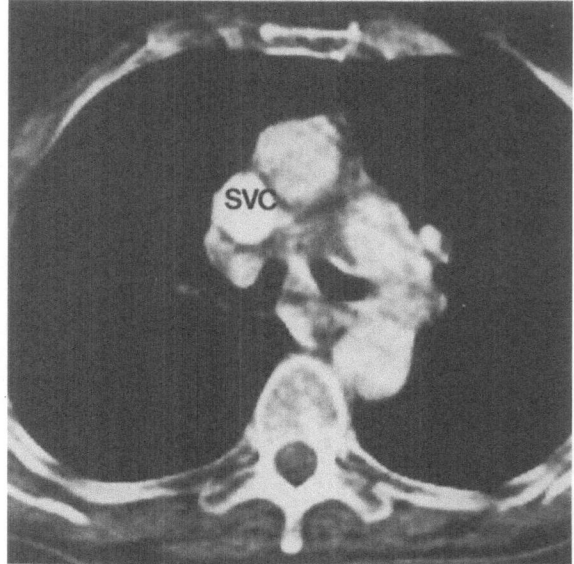

Figure 4.26(b)

Figure 4.26 Superior vena cava compression. (a) Extension of bronchogenic carcinoma (white arrows) into the mediastinum has compressed the superior vena cava (black arrows). (b) Scan in a normal patient through the same level for comparison showing opacified superior vena cava (SVC)

be obtained (Egan *et al.*, 1980; Godwin *et al.*, 1980). Similarly, the fact that coronary artery bypass grafts can be shown to opacify after intravenous contrast medium has led to reports that CT may avoid the need for angiography in the follow-up of a proportion of patients (Brundage *et al.*, 1980; Guthaner *et al.*, 1980). So far, CT imaging of the heart itself has no place in cardiac diagnosis. With the rapidly advancing technology, this seems unlikely to remain true for long.

REFERENCES

Brundage, B. H., Martin, M. J., Herfkens, R. J., Berninger, L. H., Redington, R. W., Chatterjee, K. and Carlsson, E. (1980). Detection of patent coronary bypass grafts by computed tomography. *Circulation*, **61** (4), 826–831

Crowe, J. K., Brown, L. R. and Muhm, J. R. (1978). Computed tomography of the mediastinum. *Radiology*, **128**, 75–89

Daffner, R. H., Halber, M. D., Postlethwaite, R. W., Korobkin, M. and Thompson, W. M. (1979). CT of the esophagus. II. Carcinoma. *American Journal of Roentgenology*, **133**, 1051–1055

Egan, T. J., Neiman, H. L., Herman, R. J., Malave, S. R. and Sanders, J. H. (1980). Computed tomography in the diagnosis of aortic aneurysm dissection of traumatic injury. *Radiology*, **136**, 141–146

Godwin, J. D., Herfkens, R. L., Skioldebrand, C. G., Federle, M. P. and Lipton, M. J. (1980). Evaluation of dissections and aneurysms of the thoracic aorta by conventional and dynamic CT scanning. *Radiology*, **136**, 125–133

Goldwin, R. L., Heitzman, E. R. and Proto, A. V. (1977). Computed tomography of the mediastinum. Normal anatomy and indications for CT. *Radiology*, **124**, 235–241

Gross, S. C., Barr, I., Eyler, W. R., Khaja, F. and Goldstein, S. (1980). Computed tomography in dissection of the thoracic aorta. *Radiology*, **136**, 135–139

Guthaner, D. F., Brody, W. R., Rice, M., Oyer, P. E. and Wexler, L. (1980). The use of computed tomography in the diagnosis of coronary artery bypass graft patency. *Cardiovascular and Interventional Radiology*, **3**, 3–8

Higgins, C. B., Siemers, P. T., Schmidt, W. and Newell, J. D. (1979). Evaluation of myocardial ischaemic damage of various ages by computerized transmission tomography. *Circulation*, **60** (2), 284–291

Houang, M. T. W., Arozena, X. and Shaw, D. G. (1979). Demonstration of the pericardium and pericardial effusion by computed tomography. *Journal of Computer Assisted Tomography*, **3** (5), 601–603

Husband, J. E., Peckham, M. J., Macdonald, J. S. and Hendry, W. F. (1979). The role of computed tomography in the management of testicular teratoma. *Clinical Radiology*, **30**, 243–252

Livesay, J. J., Mink, J. H., Fee, H. J., Bein, M. E., Sample, W. F. and Mulder, D. G. (1978). The use of computed tomography to evaluate suspected mediastinal tumours. *Annals of Thoracic Surgery*, **27**, 305–311

Mink, J. H., Bein, M. E., Sukov, R., Hermann, C., Winter, J., Sample, W. F. and Mulder, D. G. (1978). Computed tomography of the anterior mediastinum in patients with myasthenia gravis and suspected thymoma. *American Journal of Roentgenology*, **130**, 239–246

Pugatch, R. D., Faling, L. J., Robbins, A. H. and Spira, R. (1980). CT diagnosis of benign mediastinal abnormalities. *American Journal of Roentgenology*, **134**, 685–694

5

The Thorax – Lungs, Pleura and Chest Wall

The standard chest radiograph shows the lungs so well that CT has so far found few applications in patients with lung disease in spite of the striking way in which the lung fields are displayed. The capacity of CT to detect finer variations in density than conventional radiography does, however, mean that CT can detect small lesions such as metastases or minimal parenchymal changes when these are not visible or only suspected on the standard radiograph. CT may also occasionally help to clarify the nature of abnormal lung shadowing.

Lesions of the chest wall and pleura are shown in profile so that their extent is readily defined and minor abnormalities may be detected when not otherwise visible.

TECHNIQUE OF EXAMINATION

The number of scans and the intervals between scans will depend on the problem being examined. A relatively small number of scans may be sufficient to solve a localised problem. Multiple contiguous scans throughout the lung are needed if small lesions such as metastases are not to be missed. The number of scans required is less if the breath is held in mid-inspiration, but the lung fields, like the mediastinum, are more clearly displayed on full inspiration. Most lung scans are, therefore, best carried out on full inspiration, especially as the mediastinum is usually being scanned at the same time. The patient nor-

mally lies supine. Repeat scans with the patient lying prone or lying on one side are frequently helpful, especially when trying to distinguish fluid from pleural thickening or from underlying parenchymal disease.

Air-filled lungs have a very low attenuation value which accentuates the problem of partial volume averaging of pulmonary parenchymal structures, a small quantity of normal lung within the scan leading to a marked reduction of attenuation value. For these reasons, density measurements of small soft-tissue structures in the lung are unreliable and contrast enhancement is likely to be unhelpful (Kollins, 1977).

Interpretation of a thoracic scan can be very time-consuming because it entails viewing each scan with the full range of window levels to ensure that the bones, lungs and soft tissues have all been properly evaluated.

CT ANATOMY

The cross-sectional CT image permits examination of the lungs without superposition of overlying structures such as the ribs and sternum. At an appropriately low window setting, the pulmonary vasculature can be seen as a network of relatively high-density structures passing from the hilum through the lung parenchyma (figure 5.1a). At the

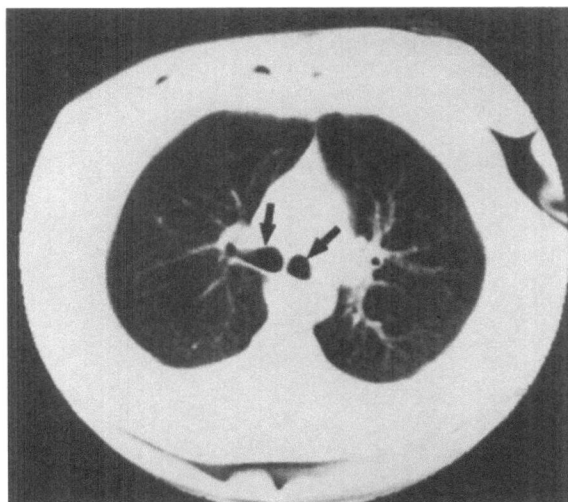

Figure 5.1(a)

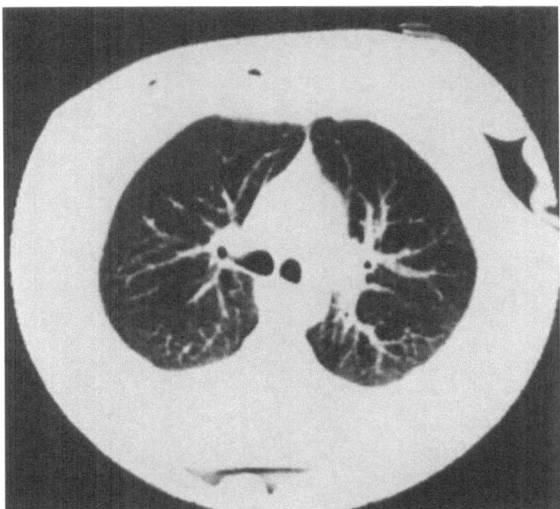

Figure 5.1(b)

Figure 5.1 Normal lungs. (a) The section is at the level of the carina, the origins of the air-filled right and left main bronchi appear black (arrowed). The mediastinum and the soft tissues and bones of the chest wall are white. The pulmonary vessels can be seen out to the periphery contrasted against the lung parenchyma. Wide window width. (b) The same scan. Narrower window width, showing a relatively greater density and greater vascularity of the dependent parts of the lungs

periphery of the lung, vessels as small as 2–3 mm in diameter can be seen close to the pleural surface. The bronchi are only recognised in the central parts of the lung.

Perfusion is greater in the more dependent parts of the lung so that, with the patient supine, the posterior part of the lung appears denser and the posteriorly lying vessels are fuller and appear to be more numerous. This is more clearly seen with a narrower window width (figure 5.1b). When the patient turns to the prone position, the reverse

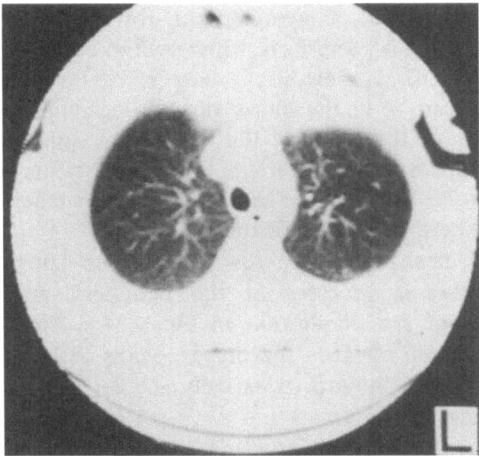

Figure 5.2(a)

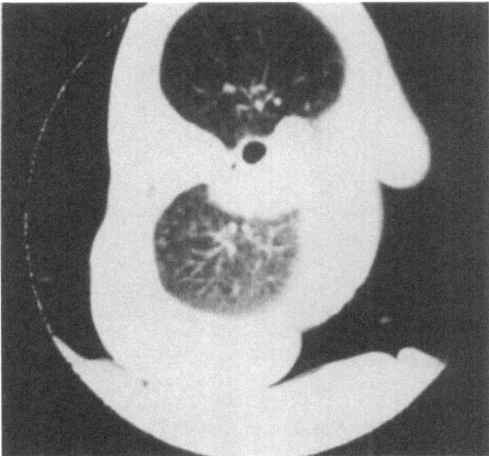

Figure 5.2(b)

Figure 5.2 Normal lungs. Gravity perfusion effect: (a) supine, and (b) lying on the side

occurs. This effect is less marked on scans done on full inspiration than on 'neutral' inspiration (Kreel, 1979). When the patient is lying on one side, the difference in density and in vascular pattern between the two lungs can be very obvious (figure 5.2). When the gravity perfusion changes are prominent, they are often associated with some fluffy increase in density in the most dependent part of the lung, even in patients without evidence of parenchymal disease or circulatory insufficiency (figure 5.3).

Vessels running upwards in the apical segments of the lower lobes produce the characteristic appearance of a symmetrical row of apparent nodules lying posteriorly when seen in cross section (figure 5.4). Vessels at the base of the lung sometimes seem to be the source of spiky densities on the surface of the dome of the diaphragm (figure 5.5). The appearance is an artefact, presumably the result of cardiac pulsation. When small, these artefacts can look like spots of calcification.

CT scans through the lung bases show the costophrenic recesses at the periphery and the domes of the diaphragm in the centre. Since the lungs taper towards the apices, scans through the upper chest show progressively smaller portions of the lung.

Several normal structures indent the pleural surface of the lungs. The internal mammary vessels

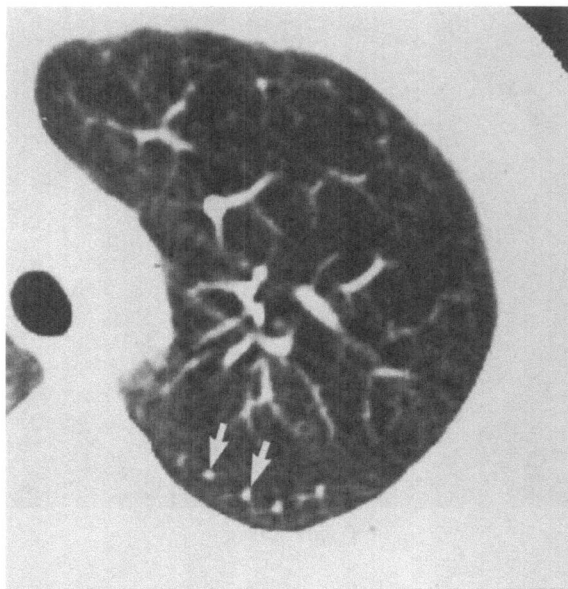

Figure 5.4   Normal vessels running up an apical segment of lower lobe (arrowed)

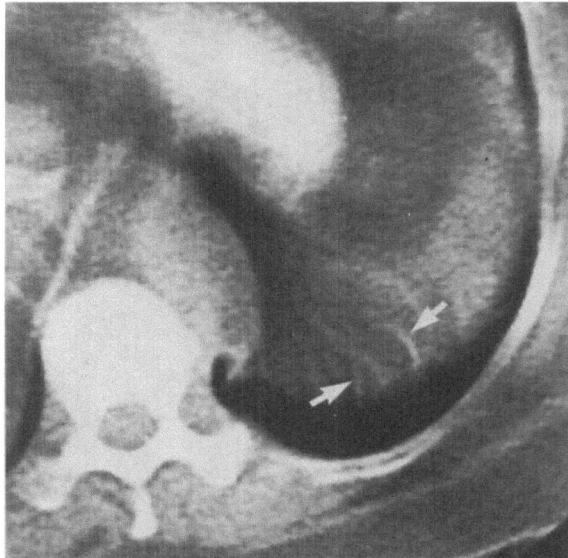

Figure 5.5   Spiky densities on the surface of the diaphragm due to overlying vessels (arrowed)

are seen as symmetrical, soft-tissue indentations lying anteriorly just lateral to the sternum (figure 5.6). In normal subjects, the oblique fissure is sometimes seen as a small triangular soft-tissue structure

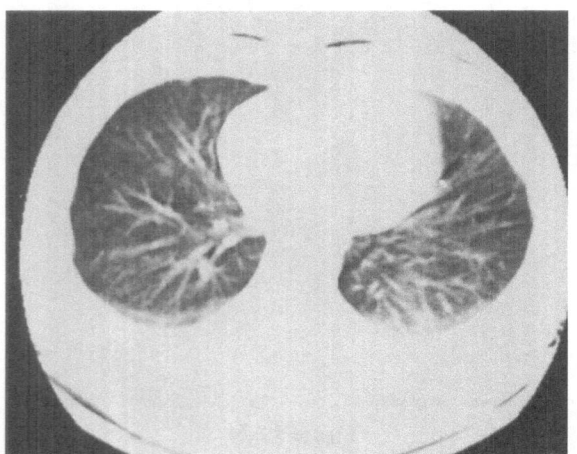

Figure 5.3   Prominent vascularity in dependent part of lungs with symmetrical fluffy increase in density

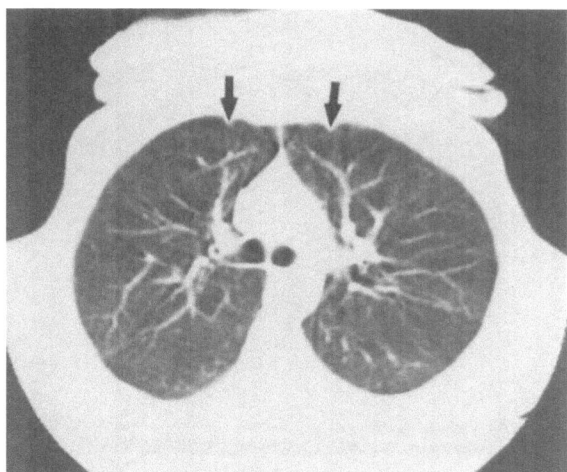

Figure 5.6   Internal mammary arteries (arrowed)

at the point where it intercepts the costal margin. If it is thickened or contains fluid, it can be seen extending far into the central portions of the lung. The lesser fissure separating the middle lobe from the right upper lobe is not usually seen unless displaced by disease, because it passes horizontally towards the hilum in the same plane as the CT section. Anomalous fissures may be shown, the azygos fissure is elegantly demonstrated (figure 5.7).

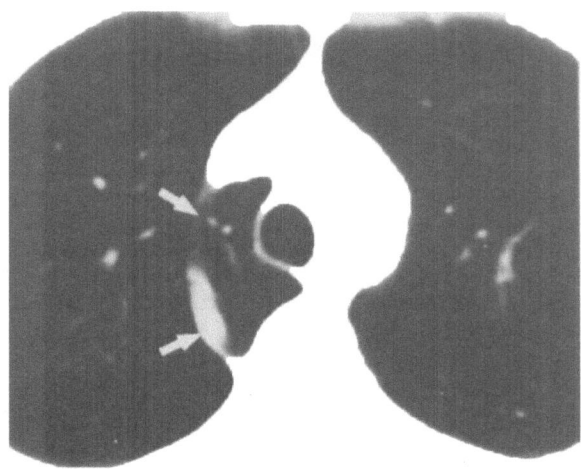

Figure 5.7   Azygos lobe (arrowed)

Partial volume averaging of the anterior parts of the upper ribs, especially the first rib, can provide an appearance suggesting symmetrical, apparently sub-pleural densities lying anteriorly (figure 5.8). When symmetrical, the appearance creates no diagnostic

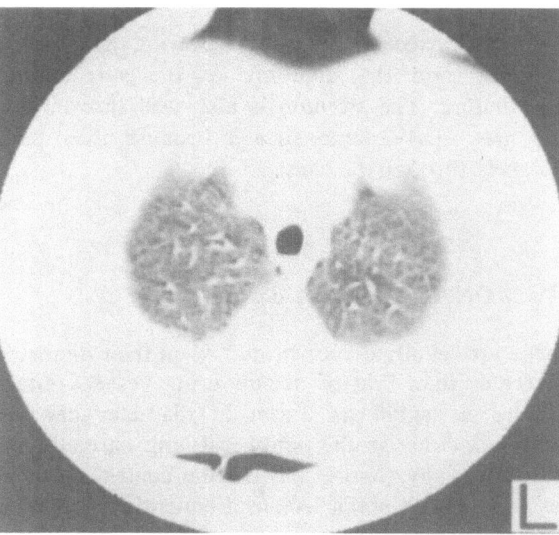

Figure 5.8(a)

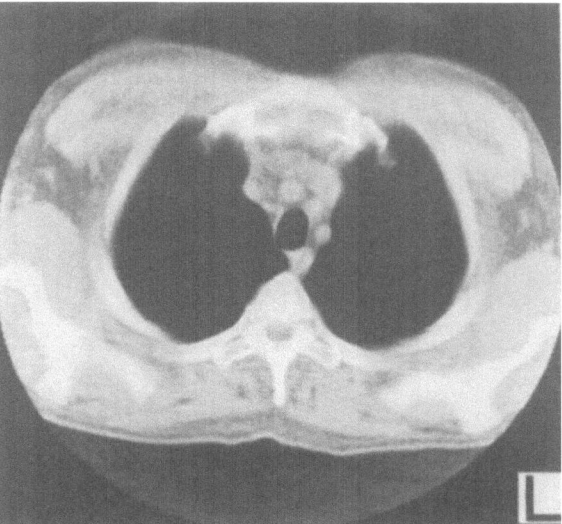

Figure 5.8(b)

Figure 5.8   Anterior ends of first ribs producing apparent soft-tissue shadows: (a) at low window level; and (b) the same section at a higher window level showing the ends of the ribs articulating with the sternum

difficulty, but, if the patient is not quite straight, the density may only be seen on one side and may be misinterpreted as a subpleural nodule. A similar density can be produced by the anterior end of the clavicle. Awareness of the possibility of these appearances is usually sufficient to avoid diagnostic confusion.

CT is an excellent method of showing the thoracic vertebrae and the anatomy of the surrounding musculature. The sternum is also well shown. The ribs are poorly demonstrated because they pass obliquely through the chest.

PULMONARY NODULES

These are readily demonstrated when their diameter is greater than that of neighbouring vessels. Thus, nodules as small as 3 mm in diameter can be identified, either in the peripheral lung parenchyma or subpleurally (figure 5.9). In the central parts of the lungs, such small lesions frequently cannot be distinguished from pulmonary vessels. Fortunately, the majority of metastases lie peripherally in the lung or subpleurally. It may sometimes be difficult to distinguish a small metastasis from a vessel seen end-on, but the problem can usually be resolved by observ-

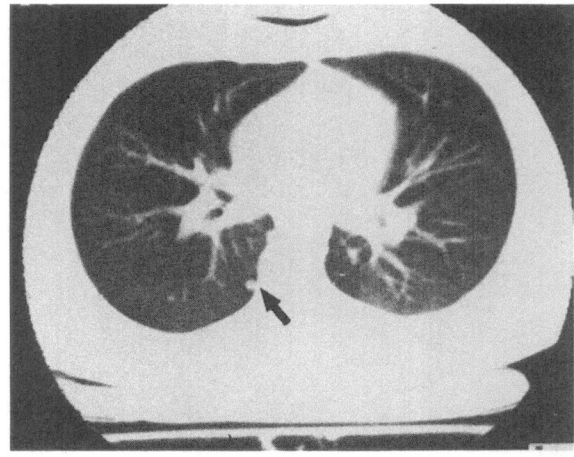

Figure 5.9(b)

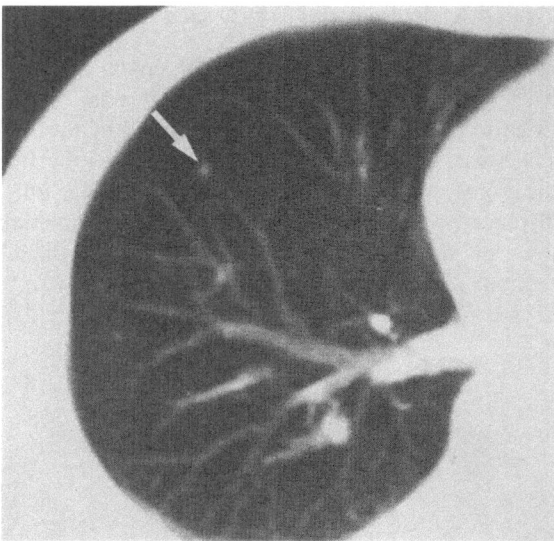

Figure 5.9(c)

Figure 5.9 Small metastases. (a) One peripherally in the right lung, another subpleurally anteriorly on the left. (b) Metastases in the right paraspinal region invisible on the chest radiographs. (c) Small metastasis detectable because it is just larger than the neighbouring vessels (arrowed)

ing contiguous scans. If caused by a vessel, the opacity will be continuous with a vessel on the neighbouring scan. If there is still doubt, a scan with the patient prone or lying on one side may resolve the problem because of the way in which the vessels change size with position (figure 5.10).

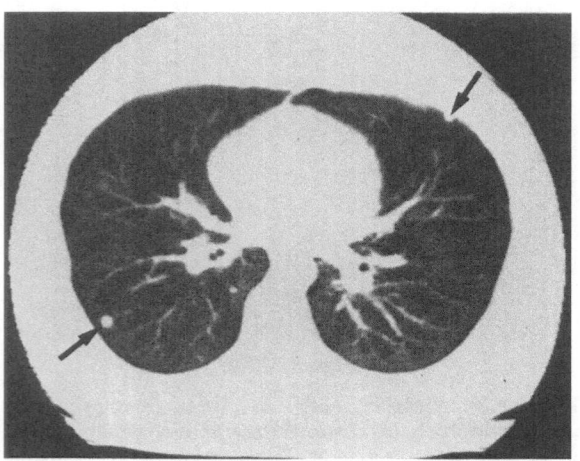

Figure 5.9(a)

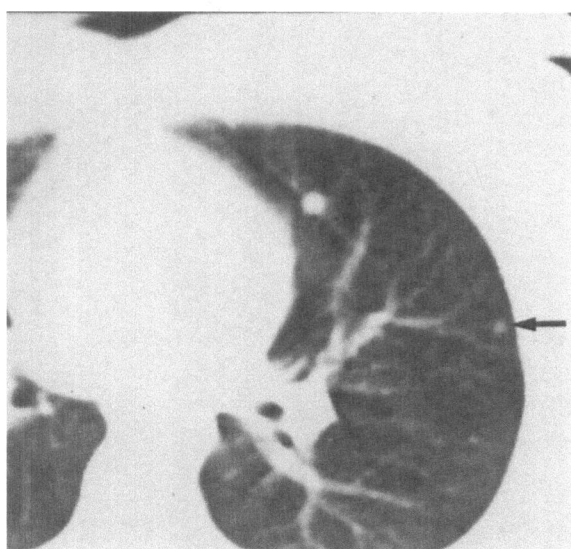

Figure 5.10(a)

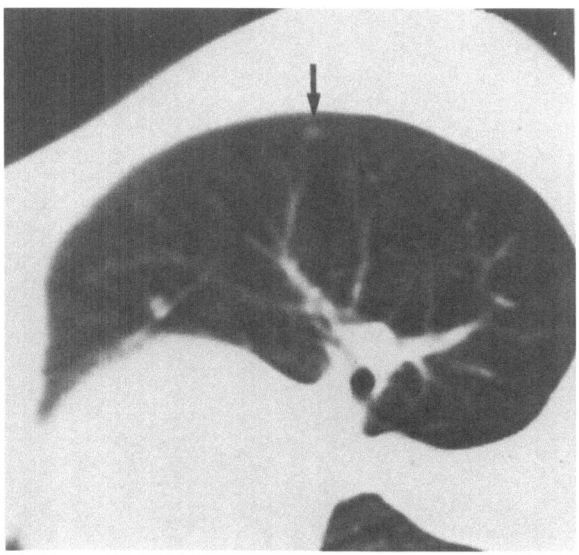

Figure 5.10(b)

Figure 5.10 Metastasis. Use of position to prove nodule separate from vessel. (a) The peripheral opacity is only questionably larger than the neighbouring vessels. (b) Patient lying on the right side. The vessels are smaller and the opacity is more clearly not a vessel (arrowed)

Sometimes relatively large nodules greater than 1 cm in diameter are revealed by CT when not shown by standard radiography, especially in the area behind the heart (figure 5.11), and in the posterior costophrenic recesses. The latter are a

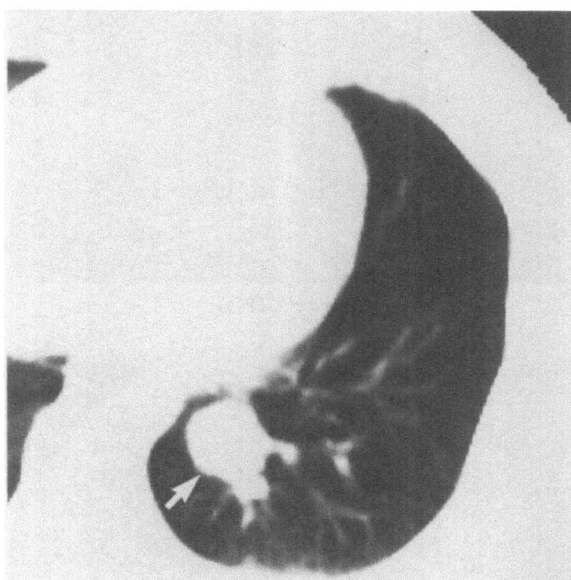

Figure 5.11 A 3 cm metastasis behind the heart, difficult to detect on the chest radiograph (arrowed)

particularly common site for metastases and should always be viewed carefully on the upper sections of an abdominal scan (figure 5.12).

Sometimes small parenchymal scars may be confused with metastases, but metastases are almost always seen as smoothly rounded lesions whilst scars are frequently angular. Nevertheless, one of the disadvantages of CT scanning is that it is not tissue-specific and so cannot differentiate a benign from a malignant nodule. Thus, subpleural lymph nodes and benign granulomata cannot be distinguished from small metastases (Schaner *et al.*, 1978).

When the scans are viewed on window settings appropriate to the lung fields, a small calcified nodule has the same appearance as a metastasis. Even when the window settings are manipulated, the density of the nodule may be misleadingly low because of partial volume averaging. A glance at the

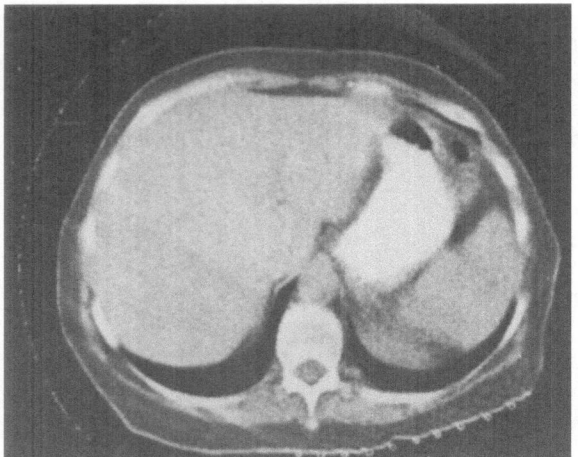

Figure 5.12(a)

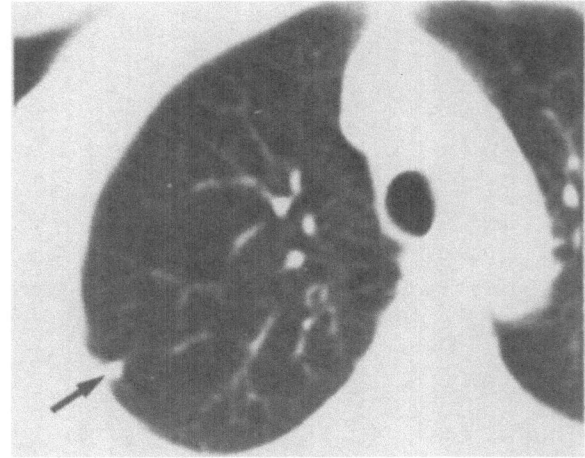

Figure 5.13(a)

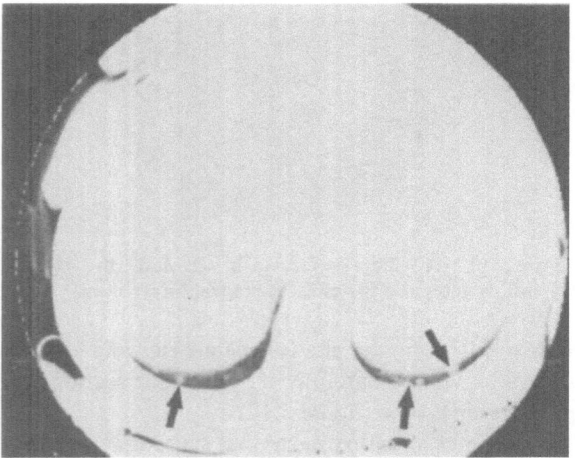

Figure 5.12(b)

Figure 5.12   Numerous small metastases deep in the costophrenic recesses. The highest scan from an examination of the abdomen in a patient scanned to elucidate the nature of a mass which proved to be a renal cell carcinoma. (a) Window level appropriate to soft tissues. (b) Window level appropriate to lung fields. The metastases are arrowed

Figure 5.13   Pulmonary nodule. (a) With CT the nodule has a similar appearance to a metastasis. (b) Chest radiograph clearly demonstrates calcification within the lesion (arrowed)

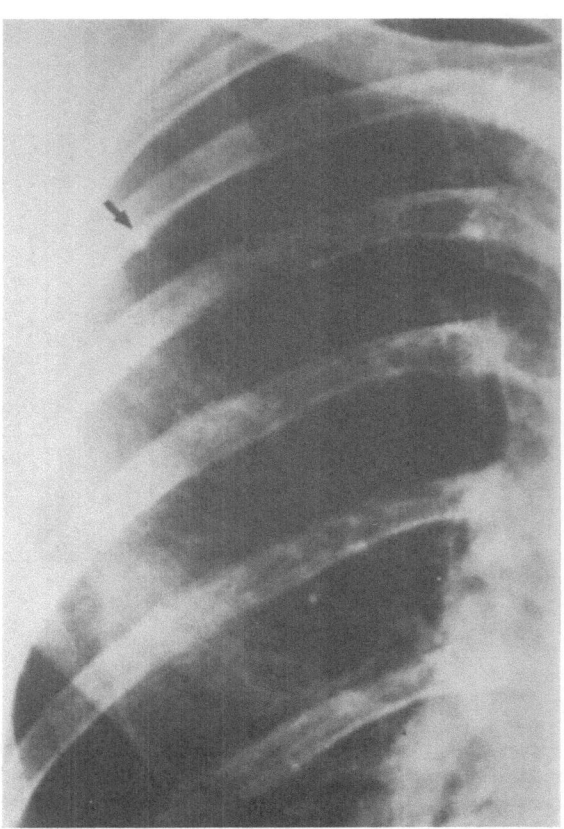

Figure 5.13(b)

chest radiograph resolves the problem (figure 5.13) provided there is sufficient calcification.

When the chest radiograph shows a solitary lung nodule and there is reason to suspect that it might be metastatic, CT can be helpful in showing other lesions confirming metastatic disease. The value of CT is less clear in the differential diagnosis of a solitary nodule in a patient in whom there is no reason to suspect a metastasis. Calcium can be detected when not visible on standard tomograms (Ratopoulos *et al.*, 1978; Jost *et al.*, 1978). Siegelman *et al.* (1980), using thin slices, have suggested that even when no calcification is visible on the chest film, high CT numbers indicate a benign lesion – presumably due to minor degrees of calcification. However, it seems unlikely that with present techniques CT will determine the nature of a solitary lesion with sufficient confidence to avoid the need for biopsy.

GENERAL LUNG DISEASE

Airless lung has a similar density to that of other soft tissues and contrasts sharply with the surrounding normal lung parenchyma (figure 5.14). Its density distinguishes it from fluid in the pleural space. When consolidation is present with a patent bronchus, the air bronchogram is strikingly shown (figure 5.15). Fibrosis, shrinkage cavities and emphysematous bullae are likewise well seen (figures 5.16, 5.17 and 5.18). Such gross abnormalities are usually clearly delineated on standard chest radiography and tomography, but there are occasions when CT is helpful in clarifying the underlying pathology (figure 5.19).

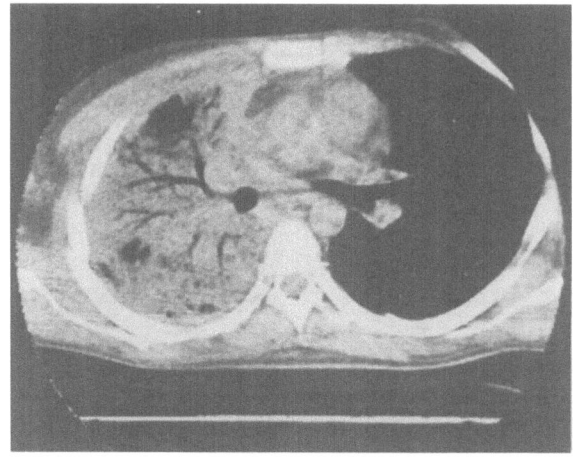

Figure 5.15 Consolidation with air bronchogram. Patient with mesothelioma

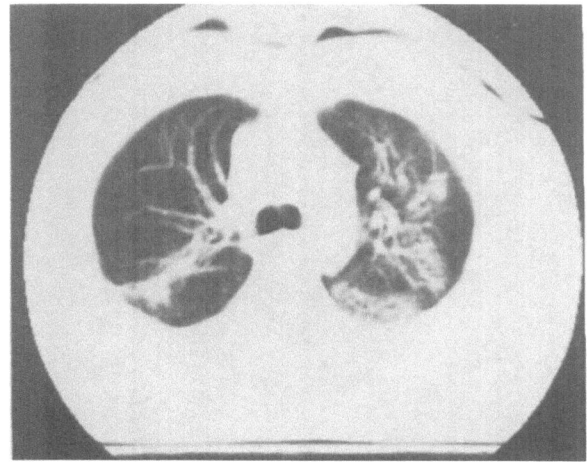

Figure 5.14 Patchy consolidation

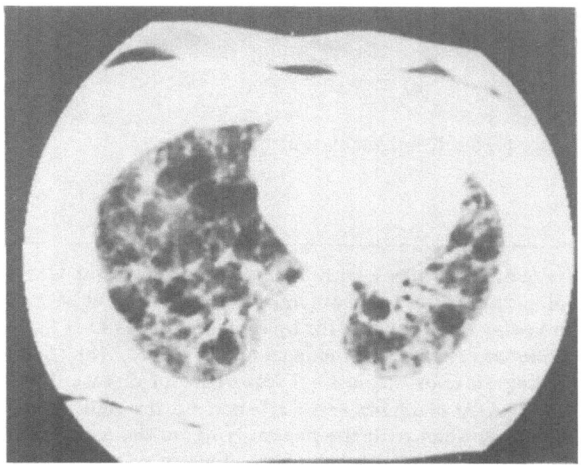

Figure 5.16 Interstitial pulmonary fibrosis

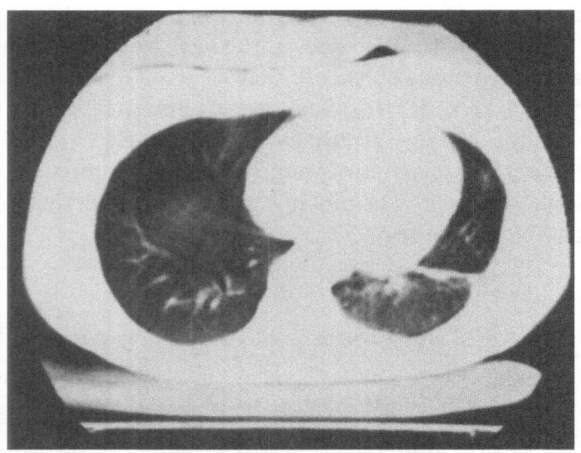

Figure 5.17   Shrunken left lower lobe. Fissure thickened. Relative increase in density of less well aerated lobe

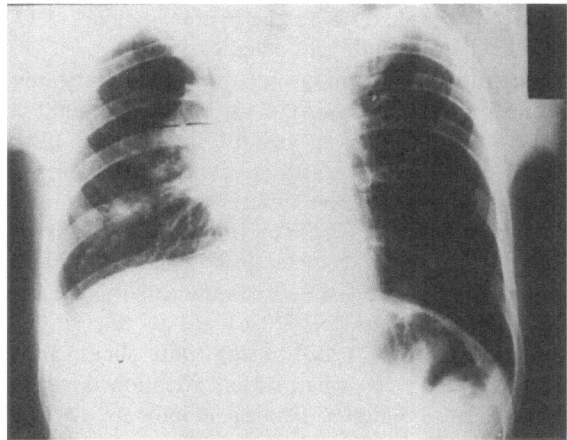

Figure 5.19(a)

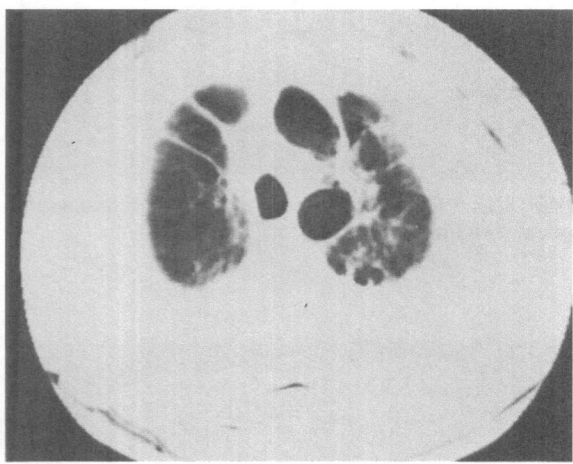

Figure 5.18   Emphysematous bullae

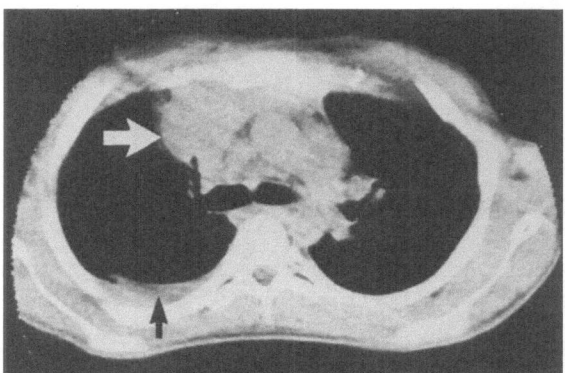

Figure 5.19(b)

Figure 5.19   Patient with Hodgkin's disease. (a) Chest radiograph after radiotherapy. Can the abnormal shadowing be accounted for by radiation fibrosis? Is there additional recurrent mediastinal disease? (b) Scan showing anterior mediastinal recurrence of disease (large arrow). Also probable small effusion on the right (small arrow). (c) Scan with the patient lying on the side. Fluid has moved to dependent part, therefore not pleural thickening or deposit

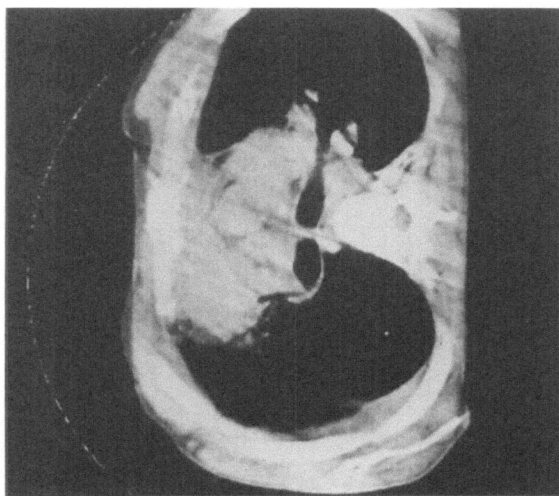

Figure 5.19(c)

PLEURAL DISEASE

Effusions appear as smooth, elliptical shadows of water density situated posteriorly if the patient is supine (figure 5.20 and 5.21). Small effusions can be demonstrated with CT when they are not evident on

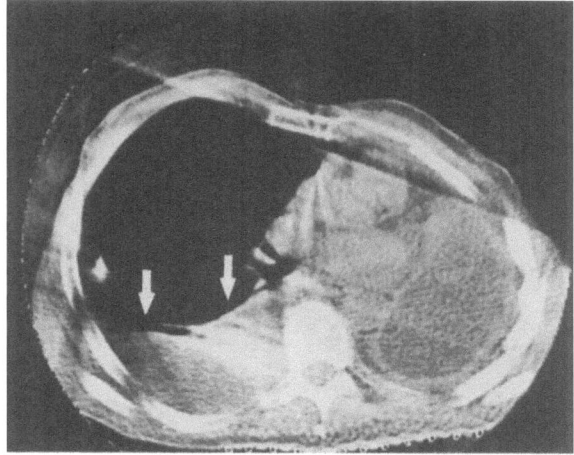

Figure 5.20(c)

Figure 5.20   Moderate-sized right subpulmonary effusion in patient with left pneumonectomy. Scan to exclude recurrent mediastinal disease. (a) Postero-anterior (PA) radiograph; (b) decubitus view. (c) Scan showing the effusion (arrowed). The pneumonectomy cavity has a thick capsule and is filled with fluid

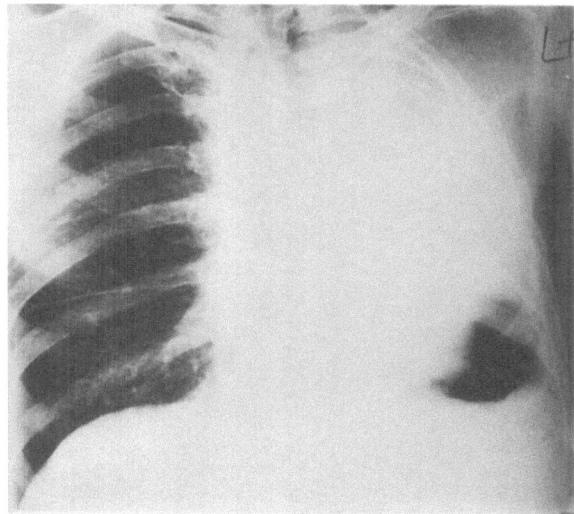

Figure 5.20(a)

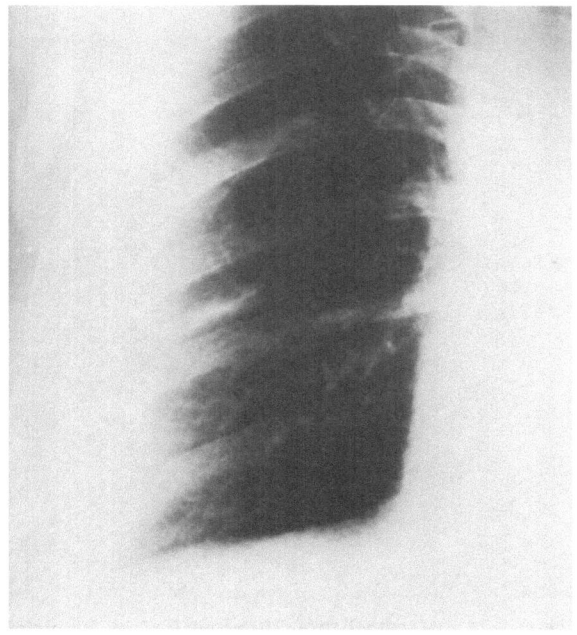

Figure 5.20(b)

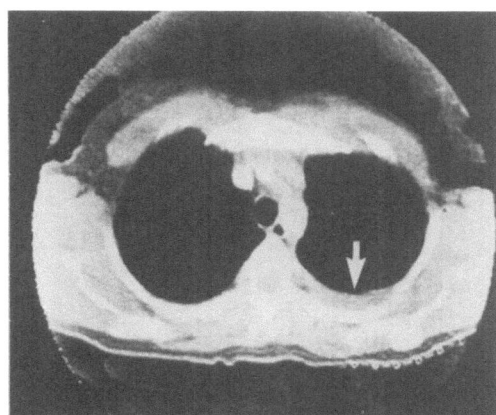

Figure 5.21   Small right effusion (arrowed)

plain chest radiographs. Sometimes it is difficult to distinguish between an effusion and pleural thickening, especially when the effusion is small. The problem can be resolved by moving the patient into the prone or lateral decubitus position, allowing fluid to move to the most dependent part (*see* figure 5.19c).

Pleural thickening and tumours are well displayed

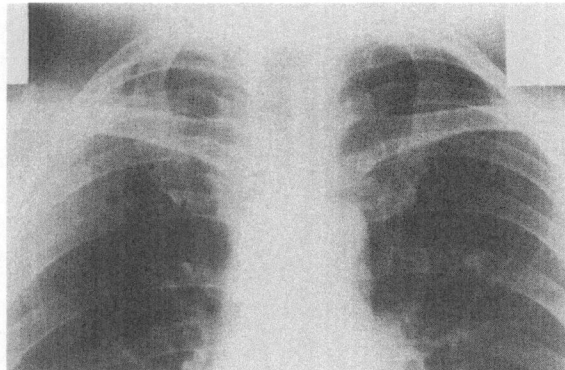

Figure 5.22(a)

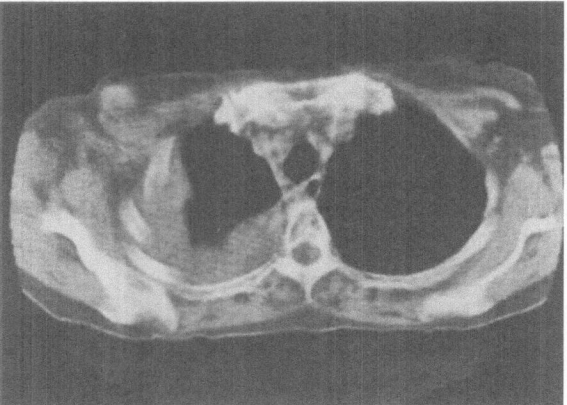

Figure 5.22(b)

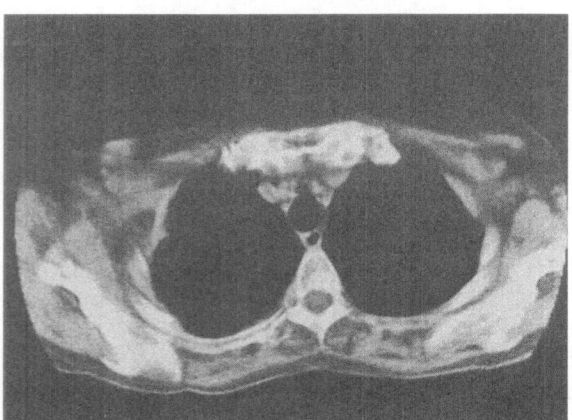

Figure 5.22(c)

Figure 5.22 Carcinoma of the breast. (a) Chest radiograph. Only hazy shadowing at the right apex. (b) Scan showing plaque of tumour encasing upper part of right lung. (c) Scan at same level five months later, showing response to treatment

because they are shown in profile and are sharply defined against the low-density lung (figure 5.22). Katz and Kreel (1979), when investigating patients exposed to asbestos, found that pleural plaques and

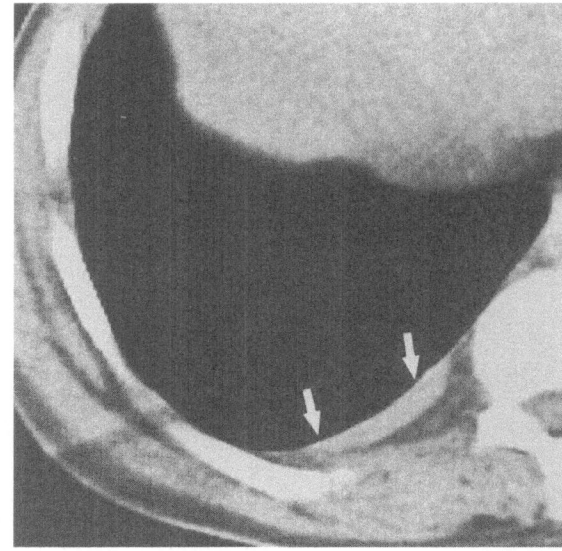

Figure 5.23   Pleural plaque with calcification in patient with exposure to asbestos (arrowed)

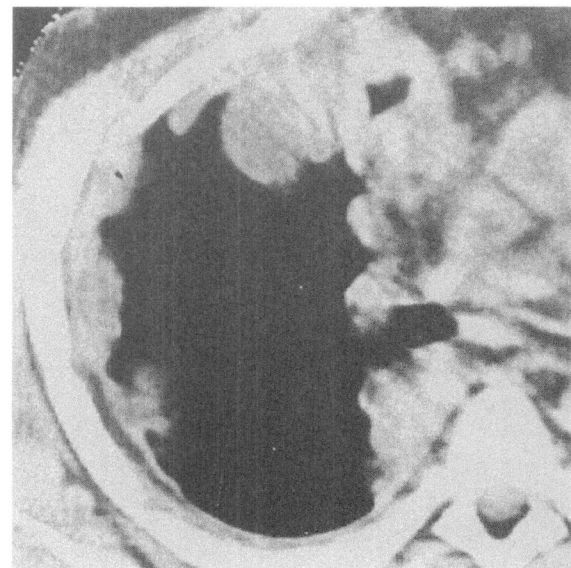

Figure 5.24   Mesothelioma showing typical lobulated outline

calcification, as well as the interstitial changes, were more common and appeared more extensively on CT than on conventional radiography (figure 5.23). Mesothelioma has a characteristic lobulated outline (figure 5.24).

CHEST WALL

The chest wall may be the site of tumours which can spread into the pleural cavity or retrosternal space, and the extent of the tumour is readily shown on CT (figures 5.25 and 5.26). The demonstration of internal mammary node enlargement in patients with inner-quadrant breast tumours is possible with CT since the internal mammary chain is silhouetted against the air-filled lungs (figure 5.27). CT could, therefore, provide a means of staging in those breast cancers which spread to the internal mammary nodes.

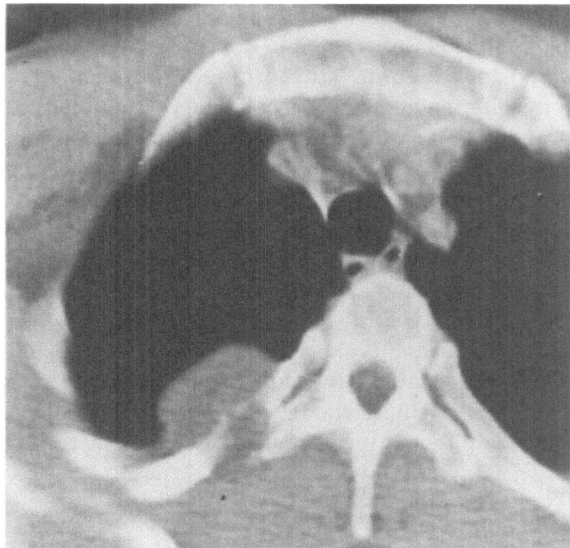

Figure 5.25   Chondrosarcoma arising from neck of ribs. Note bone destruction and extrapleural soft tissue mass

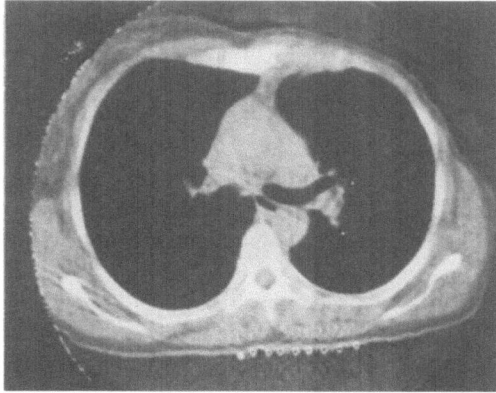

Figure 5.27(a)

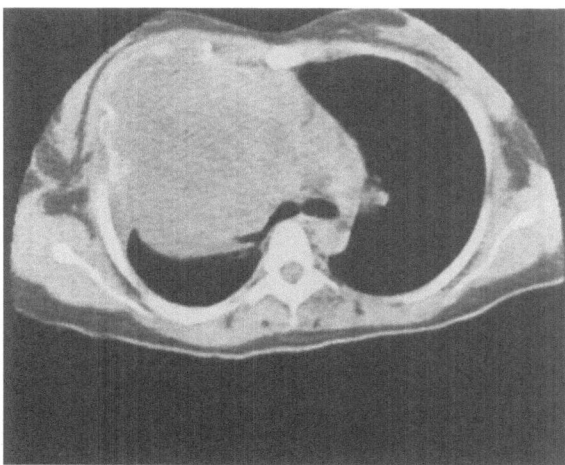

Figure 5.26   Large tumour arising from rib filling much of the right hemithorax. Note the lack of any tissue plane between the mass and the mediastinum indicating extension into the mediastinum

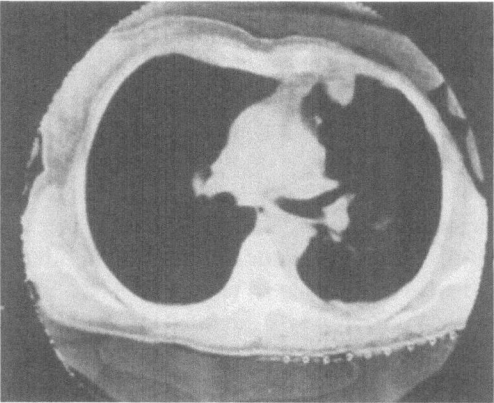

Figure 5.27(b)

Figure 5.27   Carcinoma of the breast. (a) Enlarged internal mammary nodes with erosion of the left side of the sternum. (b) Scan at the same level four months later, showing response to treatment

USE AND ACCURACY OF COMPUTED TOMOGRAPHY

The commonest indication for CT examination of the lung is for the detection of metastases when the chest radiograph is normal. When used for this purpose, computed tomography is more sensitive than conventional whole-lung tomography (Jost *et al.*, 1978). At the Royal Marsden Hospital, the results of CT scanning of the lungs were compared with whole-lung tomography in 62 patients with malignant testicular teratoma (Husband *et al.*, 1979). In 22 patients with known pulmonary metastases, 15 were shown to have a greater number of pulmonary nodules on CT than on whole-lung tomograms. In addition, multiple pulmonary nodules were demonstrated on CT in five patients in whom whole-lung tomography showed no abnormality. Similarly, Muhm *et al.* (1978) reported that more nodules were detected by CT than by whole-lung tomography in 32 out of 91 patients with malignant disease. In five of these patients, nodules were seen on CT although whole-lung tomography was negative.

The lack of tissue specificity has limited the role of CT in detecting pulmonary metastases in the United States of America where benign granulomata are commoner than in this country. In our own experience, round nodules are rarely seen as incidental findings in the lung fields in patients without evidence of malignant disease. When multiple rounded nodules are seen in a patient with known malignant disease, the overwhelming likelihood is that they are metastases. It is, however, wise to be cautious if there are only one or two nodules, especially if they are not round or do not lie at the periphery. Under these circumstances, it is worth repeating the examination after an interval to see whether there is any change in size. Even so, from the point of view of management, even one or two round nodules in a patient with malignant disease liable to metastasise to the lung should be regarded as metastatic until proven otherwise. It is perhaps worth emphasising that a negative CT scan does not exclude the smallest metastases. Creagan *et al.* (1978) reported that some metastases up to 5 mm in diameter were found at surgery which had not

been detected on CT; a few patients had numerous very small metastases.

Very occasionally, CT will reveal a small primary tumour in the lung, suspected on clinical, biochemical or cytological grounds, which is not visible on the standard radiographs (figure 5.28). CT examination should, however, be limited to those patients in whom the grounds for suspicion are strong. It is not warranted as a screening test.

CT does not at present seem to be of much value in the differential diagnosis of solitary lung lesions. It may, however, have a place in the staging of bronchogenic carcinoma once the diagnosis is established (Shevland *et al.*, 1978; Harper *et al.*, 1979; Mintz *et al.*, 1979). Metastases can be detected below the diaphragm as well as in the pleura, lung and mediastinum (Dunnick *et al.*, 1979). The size of the neoplasm itself may be difficult to define because it may not be distinguishable from contiguous collapse or consolidation (figure 5.29). Underwood *et al.* (1979) found CT less accurate than mediastinoscopy for detecting mediastinal node involvement.

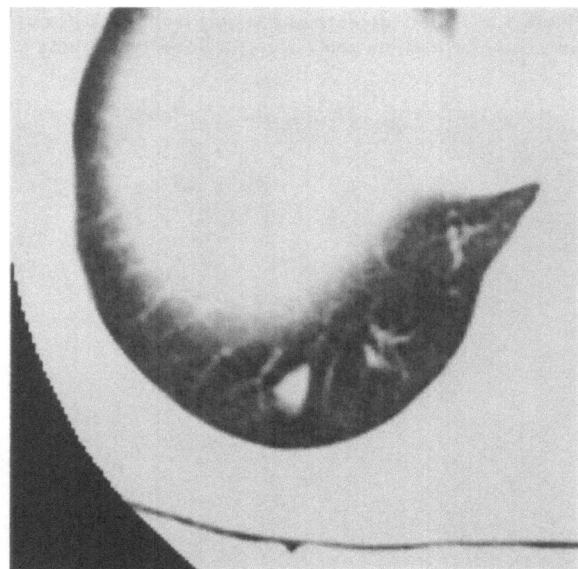

Figure 5.28 An 0.5 cm mass in right costophrenic recess in a patient with ectopic ACTH secretion. Chest x-ray and tomography were normal. At operation the mass was found to be a small carcinoid tumour

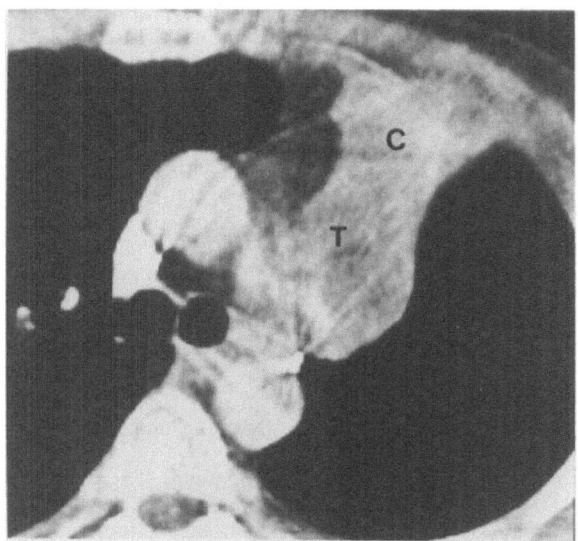

Figure 5.29   Carcinoma of the bronchus (T). Rounded mass close to the hilum corresponding to the tumour merging with the soft-tissue density of distal collapse/consolidation (C)

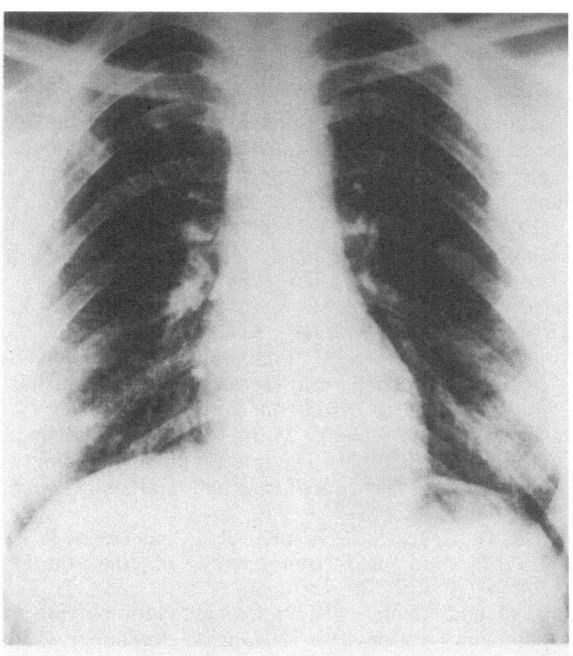

Figure 5.30(a)

Not only is CT more sensitive than the chest radiograph for detecting pulmonary nodules, but there is also evidence to suggest that it is more sensitive for detecting early parenchymal disease (figure 5.30). Thus, Katz and Kreel (1979) reported that in patients with asbestosis the changes of interstitial fibrosis were more easily visible and appeared to be grosser on CT. Twelve out of 34 patients showed parenchymal changes on CT, of whom only six showed changes on the chest radiograph. Likewise, parenchymal involvement can be seen in patients with sarcoidosis when not visible on the chest radiograph (Putman *et al.*, 1977; Solomon *et al.*, 1979). CT is also a sensitive method of detecting emphysematous bullae (Kreel, 1979). Although CT is a sensitive indicator of the presence of parenchymal disease, there is no evidence that it is any more helpful than the chest radiograph in distinguishing one type of parenchymal disease from another.

The ability of CT to detect small differences in lung density raises the possibility that CT might have a place in demonstrating variations in perfusion and ventilation of the lung (Rosenblum *et al.*, 1978; Robinson and Kreel., 1979).

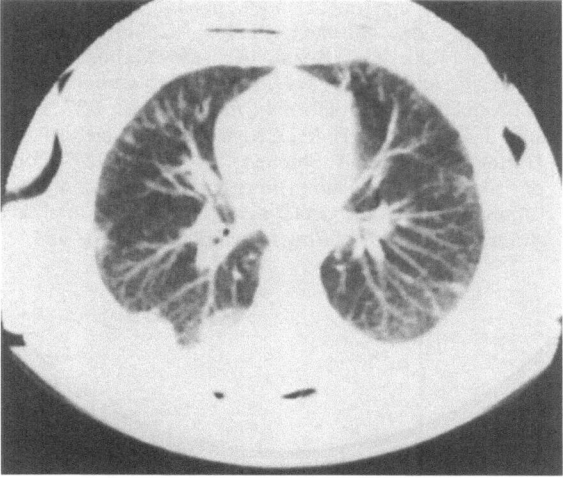

Figure 5.30(b)

Figure 5.30   Bleomycin   toxicity.   The   peripheral pulmonary changes are difficult to see on the PA chest film (a) but are clearly shown with CT (b)

REFERENCES

Creagan, E. T., Frytak, S., Pairolero, P., Hahn, R. G. and Muhm, J. R. (1978). Surgically proven pulmonary metastases not demonstrated by computed tomography. *Cancer Treatment Reports*, **62**, 1404–1405

Dunnick, N. R., Ihde, D. C. and Johnston-Early, A. (1979). Abdominal CT in the evaluation of small cell carcinoma of the lung. *American Journal of Roentgenology*, **133**, 1085–1088

Harper, R. G., Houang, M., Spiro, S. G., Souhami, R. L., Geddes, D. N., Morgan, P. G. and Smyth, J. F. (1979). Computerised tomography in the initial staging of oat (small cell) carcinoma of the bronchus. *British Journal of Diseases of the Chest*, **73**, 416

Husband, J. E., Peckham, M. J., Macdonald, J. S. and Hendry, W. F. (1979). The role of computed tomography in the management of testicular teratoma. *Clinical Radiology*, **30**, 243–252

Jost, R. G., Sagel, S. S., Stanley, R. J. and Levitt, R. G. (1978). Computed tomography of the thorax. *Radiology*, **126**, 125–136

Katz, D. and Kreel, L. (1979). Computed tomography in pulmonary asbestosis. *Clinical Radiology*, **30**, 207–213

Kollins, S. A. (1977). Computed tomography of the pulmonary parenchyma and chest wall. *Radiologic Clinics of North America*, **15** (3), 297–308

Kreel, L. (1979). Computed tomography of the abdomen and thorax. In *Recent Advances in Radiology and Medical Imaging*, eds. T. Lodge and R. E. Steiner, Churchill Livingstone, London, p. 61

Mintz, U., de Meester, T. R., Golomb, H. M., Cimochowski, G., Rezai, K., MacMahon, M. B., Sovik, C. and Bitran, J. D. (1979). Sequential staging in bronchogenic carcinoma. *Chest*, **76**, 653–657

Muhm, J. R., Brown, L. R., Crowe, J. K., Sheedy, P. F., Hattery, R. R. and Stephens, D. H. (1978). Comparison of whole lung tomography and computed tomography for detecting pulmonary nodules. *American Journal of Roentgenology*, **131**, 981–984

Putman, C. E., Rothman, S. L., Littner, M. R., Allen, W. E., Schachter, E. N., McLoud, T. C., Bein, M. E. and Gee, J. B. (1977). Computerised tomography in pulmonary sarcoidosis. *Computerised Tomography*, **1**, 197–209

Raptopoulos, V., Schellinger, D. and Katz, S. (1978). Computed tomography of solitary pulmonary nodules: experience with scanning times longer than breath-holding. *Journal of Computer Assisted Tomography*, **2** (1), 55–60

Robinson, P. J. and Kreel, L. (1979). Pulmonary tissue attenuation with computed tomography: comparison of inspiration and expiration scans. *Journal of Computer Assisted Tomography*, **3** (6), 740–748

Rosenblum, L. J., Mauceri, R. A., Wellenstein, D. E., Bassano, D. A., Cohen, W. N. and Heitzman, R. E. (1978). Computed tomography of the lung. *Radiology*, **129**, 521–524

Schaner, E. G., Chang, A. E., Doppman, J. L., Conkle, D. M., Flye, M. W. and Rosenberg, S. A. (1978). Comparison of computed and whole lung tomography in detecting pulmonary nodules: a prospective radiologic–pathologic study. *American Journal of Roentgenology*, **131**, 51–54

Shevland, J. E., Chiu, L. C., Schapiro, R. L., Young, J. A. and Rossi, N. O. (1978). The role of conventional tomography and computed tomography in assessing the resectability of primary lung cancer: a preliminary report. *Journal of Computed Tomography*, **2**, 1–19

Siegelman, S. S., Zerhouni, E. A., Leo, F. P., Khouri, N. F. and Stitik, S. P. (1980). CT of the solitary pulmonary nodule. *American Journal of Roentgenology*, **135**, 1–13

Solomon, A., Kreel, L., McNicol, M. and Johnson, N. (1979). Computed tomography in pulmonary sarcoidosis. *Journal of Computer Assisted Tomography*, **3** (6), 754–758

Underwood, G. H., Hooper, R. G., Alexander, S. P. and Goodwin, D. W. (1979). Computed tomography scanning of the thorax in the staging of bronchogenic carcinoma. *New England Journal of Medicine*, **300**, 777–778

6

The Abdomen – Kidney

Intravenous urography and ultrasound are very effective methods of imaging the kidneys. CT is not, therefore, usually needed for the initial diagnosis of renal disease. It is, however, an excellent way of demonstrating the renal and perirenal areas and is a valuable tool for elucidating problems which have not been resolved by simpler methods.

TECHNIQUE OF EXAMINATION

The general technique is that already described for abdominal scans. Intravenous contrast medium is frequently used either for its nephrographic effect or to display the pelvicalyceal system. We use a bolus injection of 50 ml sodium iothalamate (Conray 325).

CT ANATOMY

The kidneys are exceptionally well displayed with CT because they are surrounded by perinephric fat, and even in thin patients this fat plane is usually preserved. They appear as smooth structures of uniform density with attenuation values in the range 15 to 25 EMI units. The hilum of the kidney is seen as a central area of low density caused partly by urine in the renal pelvis and major calyces but mainly by fat in the renal sinus (figure 6.1). The amount of sinus fat varies greatly from patient to

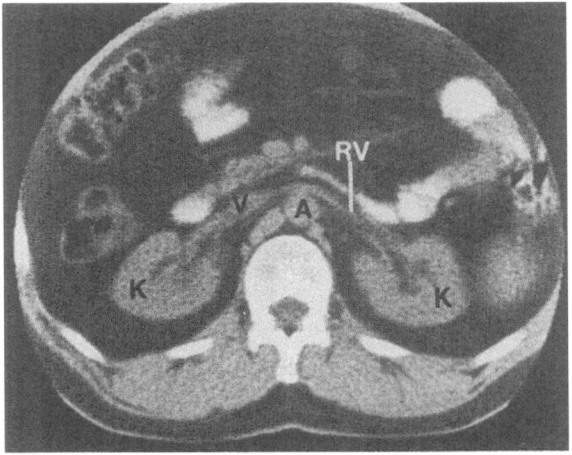

Figure 6.1 Normal kidneys (K), renal vein (RV), inferior vena cava (V), aorta (A)

patient. Sometimes it is sufficient to produce large symmetrical low-density filling defects at the hilum (figure 6.2). The calyces are not seen without the injection of contrast medium unless they are dilated. Contrast medium outlines the major parts of the pelvicalyceal system but little or no papillary/calyceal detail is shown (figure 6.3).

After the injection of intravenous contrast medium, the normal renal parenchyma enhances uniformly except when examined immediately after a rapid bolus injection when only the cortex is opacified (figure 6.4). Since the increase in attenuation value after the injection is a measure of the amount of contrast medium in the kidney, CT can be used to quantify the nephrogram. As a result of studies in dogs, Brennan *et al.* (1979a,b) have suggested that sequential studies of the nephrogram using CT might be used as an indicator of renal function, particularly as the density changes in the cortex can be separated from those in the medulla.

The vascular pedicles are almost invariably seen. The veins lie anteriorly and are more commonly seen as individual structures than are the arteries. The right renal vein enters the inferior vena cava

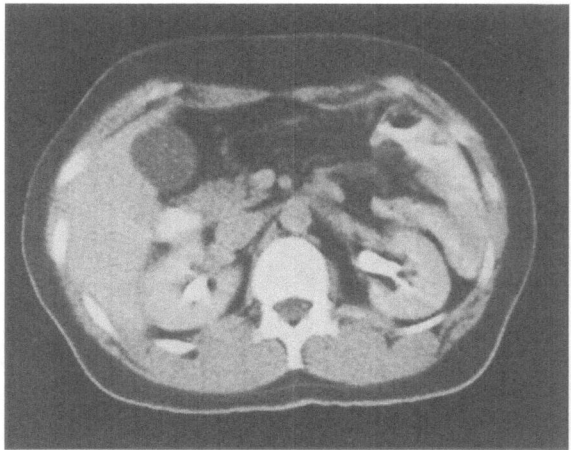

Figure 6.3(b)

Figure 6.3 Normal kidneys: (a) pre-contrast, and (b) post-contrast. After injection of intravenous contrast medium, the pelvicalyceal system is shown separate from the renal sinus fat

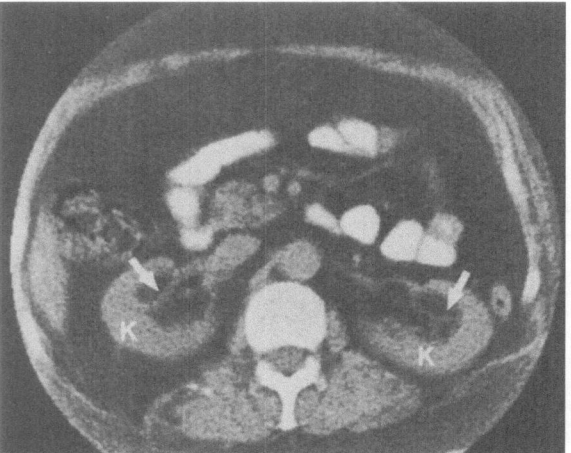

Figure 6.2 Normal kidneys (K) in a patient with abundant renal sinus fat (arrowed)

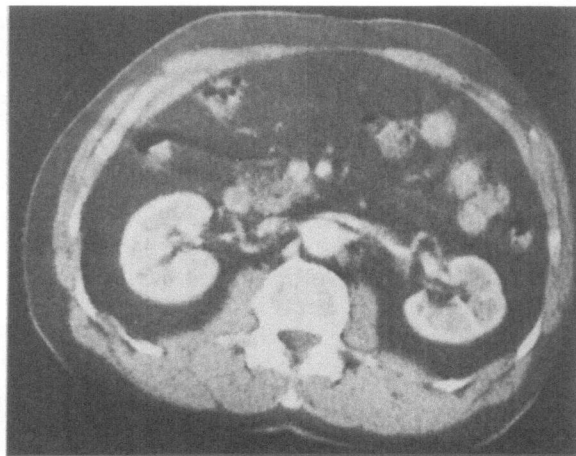

Figure 6.4 Cortical nephrogram. Scan immediately after rapid bolus injection of intravenous contrast medium using fast scanner. Note opacification of major vessels. (Reproduced by kind permission of Dr R. J. Stanley, Edward Mallinckrodt Institute of Radiology, St Louis)

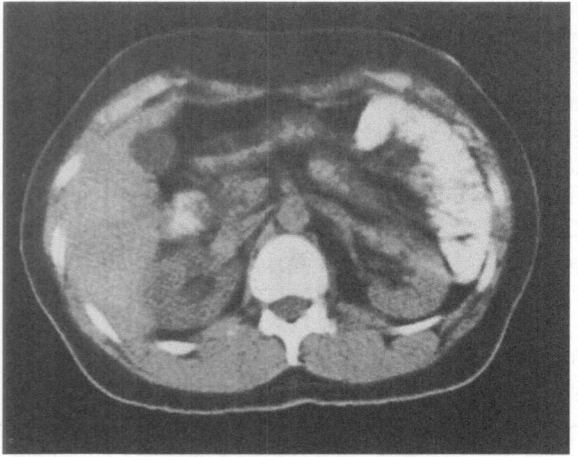

Figure 6.3(a)

directly. The left is a useful landmark, passing in front of the aorta and behind the superior mesenteric artery to join the inferior vena cava behind the head of the pancreas (figure 6.5, and *see* figure 6.1).

The upper pole of the right kidney is closely

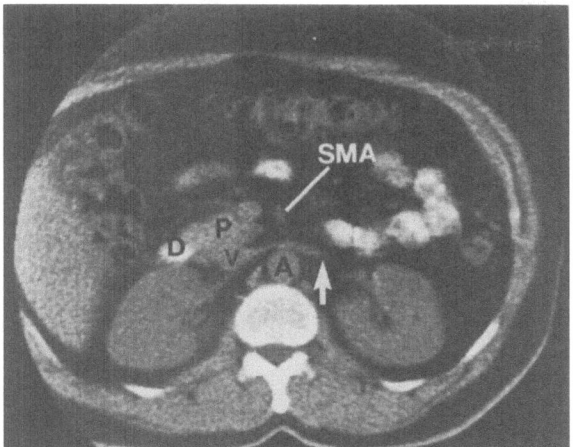

Figure 6.5 Normal kidneys. Left renal vein (arrowed). Aorta (A), inferior vena cava (V), superior mesenteric artery (SMA), head of pancreas (P), duodenum (D)

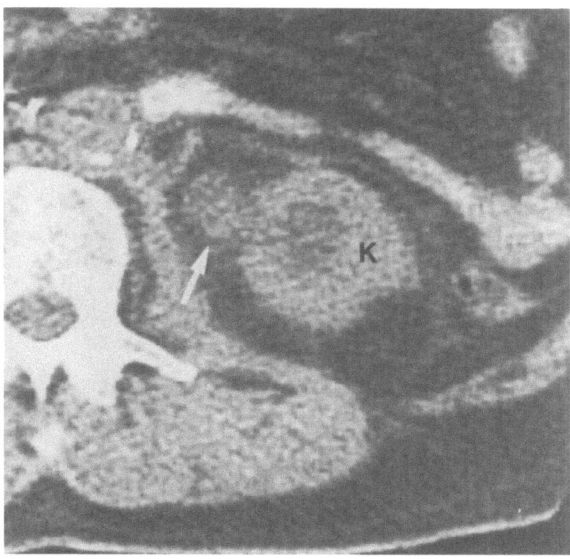

Figure 6.7(a)

related to the posterior aspect of the right lobe of the liver, but the fat plane between these organs can usually be demonstrated. This is helpful because the origin of lesions arising in this area is not always clear using other imaging techniques. Even the normal kidney can indent the right lobe and be mistaken for a lesion in the liver on isotope scans (figure 6.6).

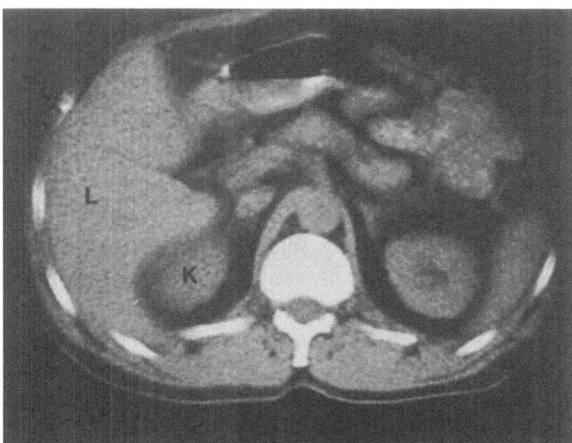

Figure 6.6 Normal scan showing the upper pole of the right kidney (K) indenting the right lobe of the liver (L). Note the clear fat plane between these two organs

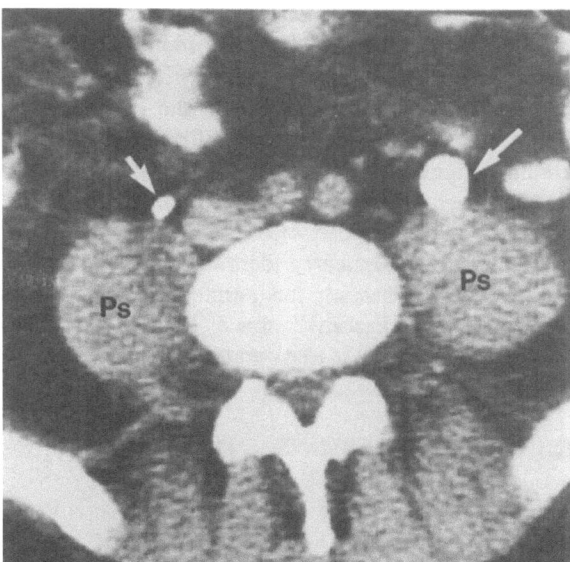

Figure 6.7(b)

Figure 6.7 Two patients with dilated left ureter. (a) Without intravenous contrast medium, the ureter is seen as a rounded shadow with a density close to that of water (arrowed). Note also the hydronephrotic left kidney (K). (b) Dilated left ureter after the injection of intravenous contrast medium (larger arrow). Ureter on the right is normal (small arrow). Psoas muscles (Ps)

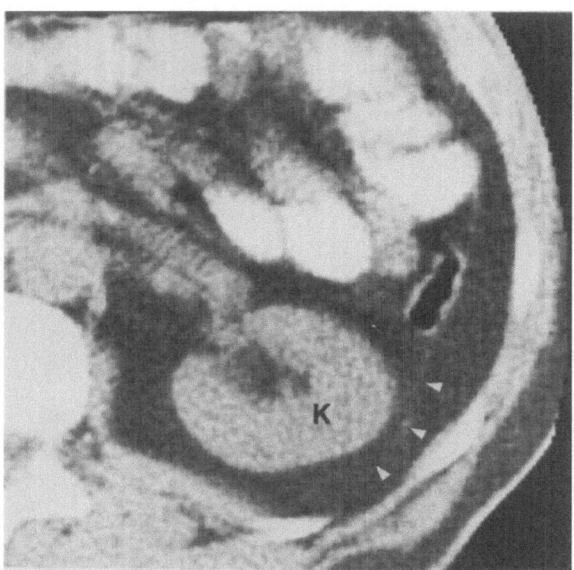

Figure 6.8   Posterior renal fascia (arrow heads). Left kidney (K)

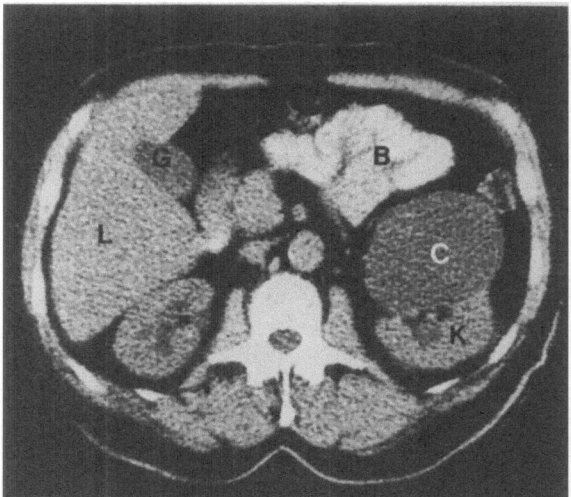

Figure 6.9   Renal cyst (C) arising from the anterior aspect of the left kidney (K). Liver (L), gall-bladder (G), bowel (B). (Reproduced by kind permission of Pitman Press)

The renal pelvis is not always identifiable but, if large, can be seen as a water-density mass at the hilum. The ureter runs down on the psoas muscle but is not seen unless dilated or filled with contrast medium (figure 6.7).

The fascia separating the compartments in the posterior abdomen can often be visualised on CT. The one most frequently identified is the posterior renal fascia separating the perinephric space from the posterior pararenal space (figure 6.8). The anterior renal fascia is less commonly seen.

RENAL MASS LESIONS

The commonest use of CT in renal disease is in the differential diagnosis and management of patients with renal mass lesions in whom there is doubt about the diagnosis or the extent of disease.

Simple Cysts

Simple cysts of the kidney have the same CT appearance as cysts elsewhere, being seen as sharply defined masses with attenuation values close to that of water (0 to 10 EMI units) (figure 6.9). Cysts smaller than 2 cm may be subject to partial volume averaging and may appear denser than expected. When lying wholly within the parenchyma, such small cysts may be difficult to detect without enhancement. After enhancement, even small intrarenal cysts can usually be detected (figure 6.10). Small cysts are readily detected when they present on the surface of the kidney and are outlined by perirenal fat.

Cyst contents do not enhance after the injection of intravenous contrast medium, but there may be some apparent enhancement of small cysts when a part of the enhanced surrounding parenchyma is included in the slice. The wall of a superficial cyst may be identified as a fine rim of slightly greater density than the cyst contents, but a thick wall must raise suspicion of a neoplasm, as it does on urography (figure 6.11). Hydatid cysts also have a thick wall (figure 6.12). Occasionally cysts arising from the upper or lower pole of the kidney may appear to have a thick wall if the section is taken through the beak of renal tissue surrounding its base as it arises from the kidney (figure 6.13) (Segal and Spitzer, 1979).

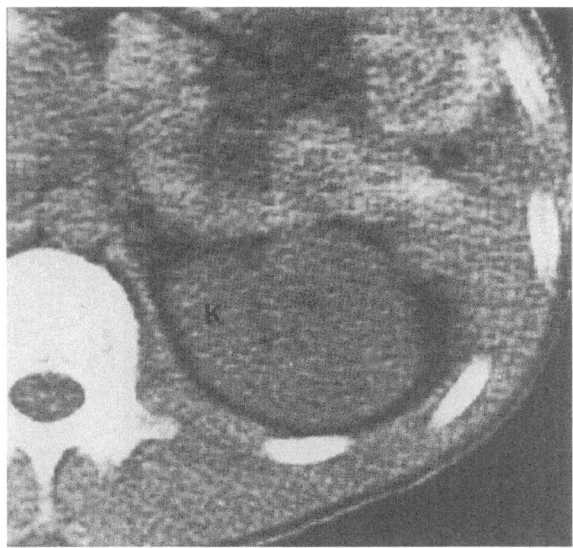

Figure 6.10(a)

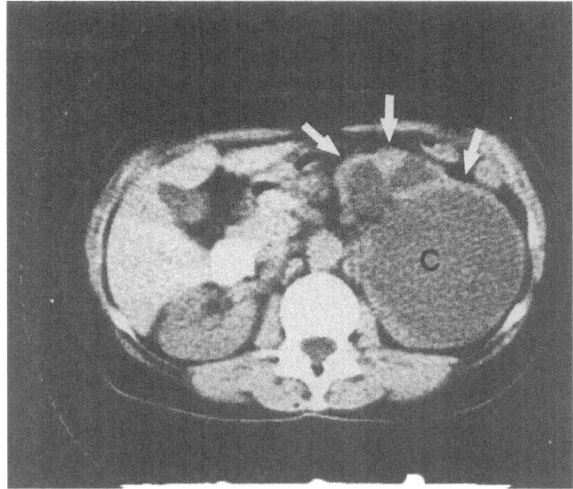

Figure 6.11   Left renal cell carcinoma (C). This lesion is multiloculated and has a thick wall (arrowed)

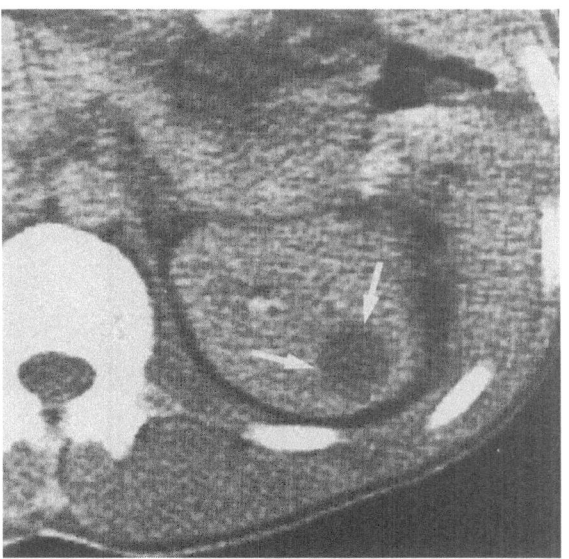

Figure 6.10(b)

Figure 6.10   (a) Pre-contrast scan. No abnormality can be identified in the left kidney (K). (b) After enhancement, well defined cyst (arrowed) is shown lying within the renal parenchyma

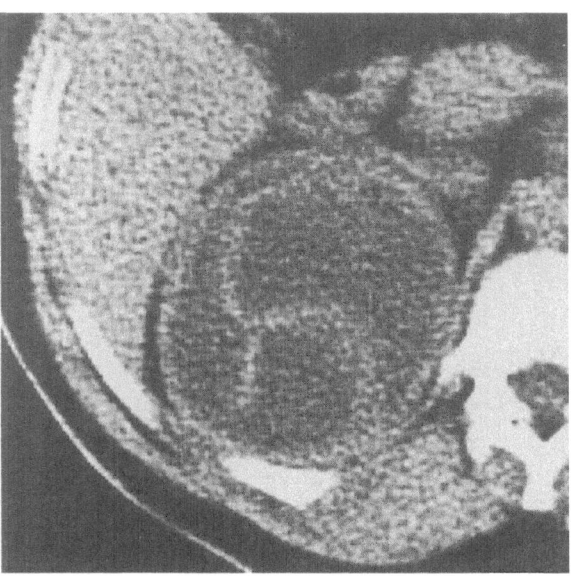

Figure 6.12   Hydatid cyst of the right kidney. Note the thick wall

A parapelvic cyst may be mistaken for hydro-nephrosis unless contrast medium is injected, and then the calyces will be seen to be splayed around the cyst (figure 6.14).

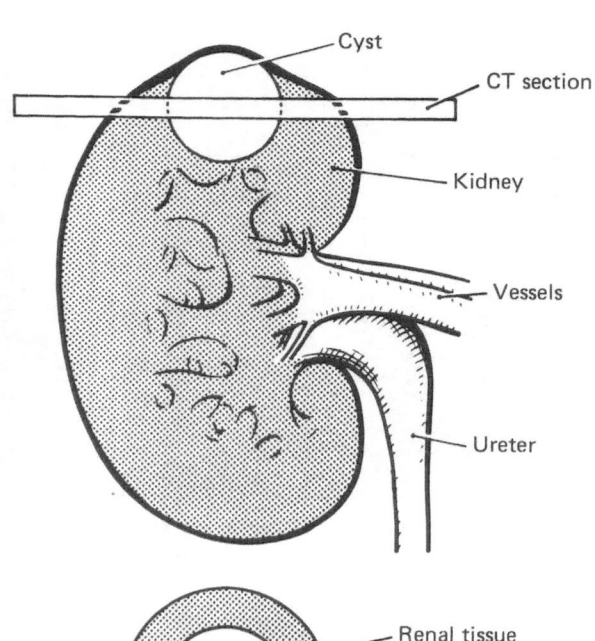

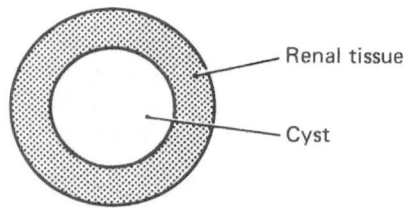

Figure 6.13(a)

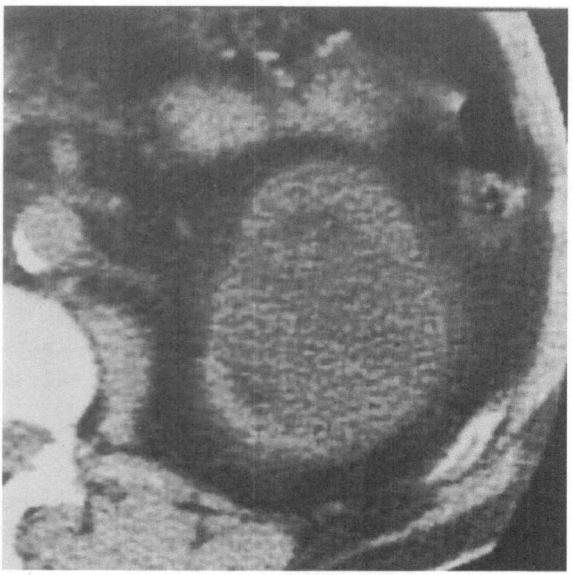

Figure 6.13(b)

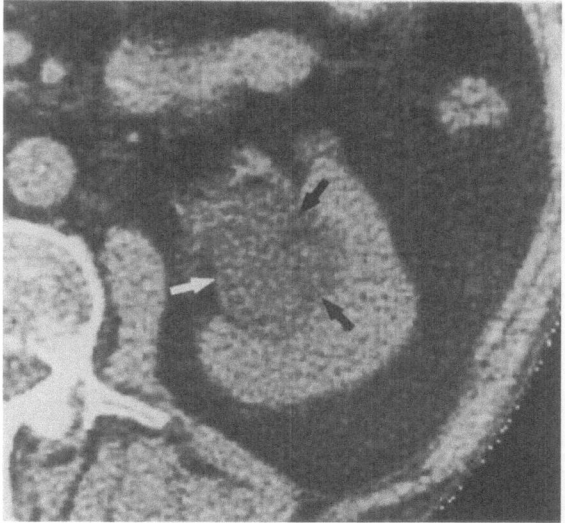

Figure 6.14(a)

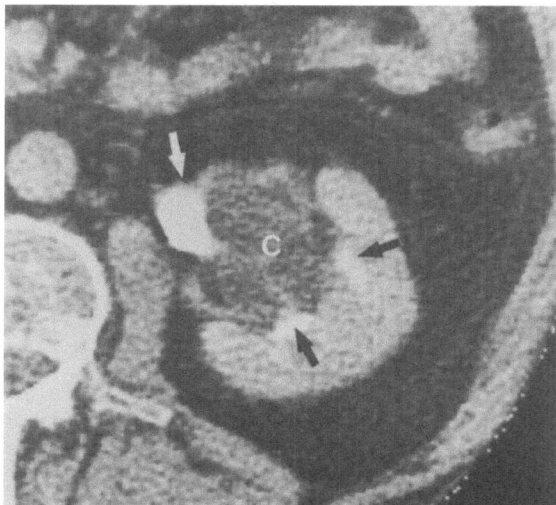

Figure 6.14(b)

Figure 6.14   Parapelvic cyst. (a) The pre-contrast scan shows a low-density mass at the left renal hilum (arrowed). (b) Post-contrast scan shows distortion of the opacified collecting system (arrowed) due to a large parapelvic cyst (C)

Figure 6.13   (a) Diagram to show CT section taken through the beak of renal tissue surrounding a renal cyst. (b) CT scan in a patient with a left renal cyst arising from the upper pole of the left kidney. Note the appearance of a thick wall representing a beak of normal renal tissue

Tumours

Tumours are usually similar in density to normal renal parenchyma (figure 6.15) but the density may not be uniform, especially in larger tumours which commonly contain low-density areas representing necrosis (figure 6.16). Some tumours show calcification and this may be visible on CT when not visible on plain abdominal radiographs. The margins of a tumour are less well defined than those of a cyst.

Tumours are readily detected if they distort the renal outline. Tumours too small to distort the outline may go undetected on unenhanced scans.

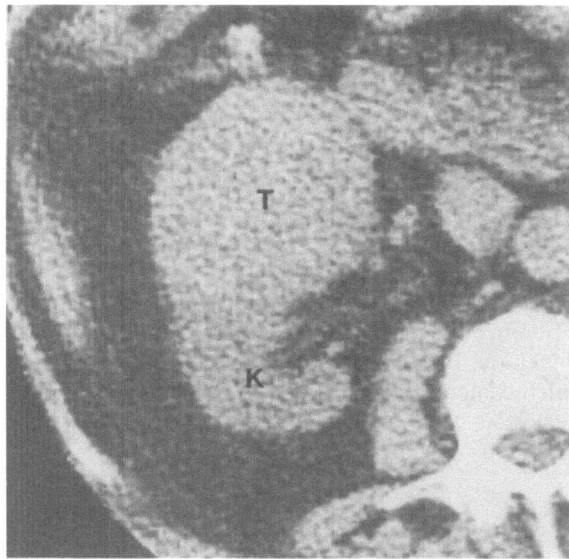

Figure 6.15   Carcinoma of the right kidney (T). This tumour has a similar density to normal renal parenchyma (K)

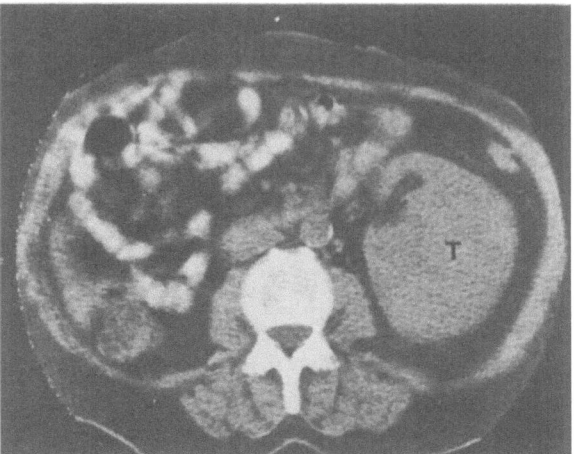

Figure 6.17(a)

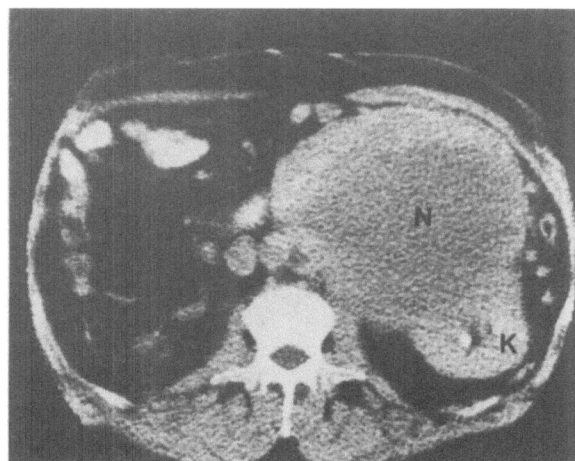

Figure 6.16   Large carcinoma of the left kidney. Scan taken after injection of intravenous contrast medium shows that the tumour contained a central area of low density (N). Normal part of left kidney (K)

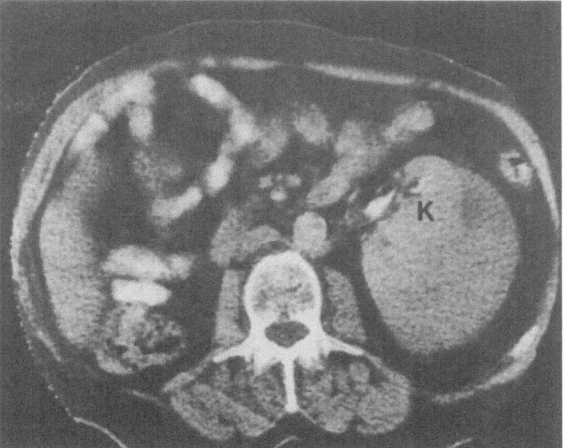

Figure 6.17(b)

Figure 6.17   Carcinoma of the left kidney. (a) Before enhancement, the tumour (T) has a similar density to normal renal tissue. (b) After enhancement, the tumour opacifies but to a lesser extent than normal renal tissue (K)

The majority of renal tumours take up contrast medium but to a lesser extent than the surrounding normal renal parenchyma (figure 6.17). Some tumours which are not readily detectable on an unenhanced scan may be seen clearly after the injection of contrast medium. Even so, with small

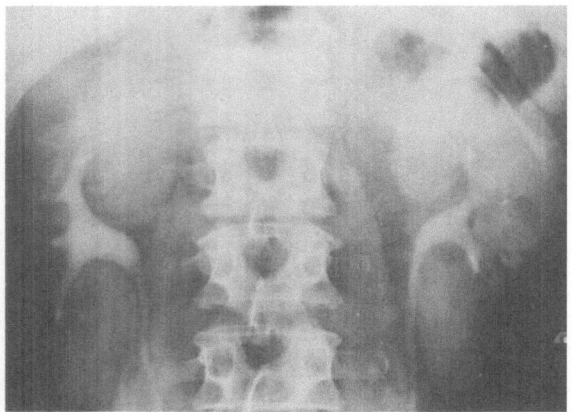

Figure 6.18(a)

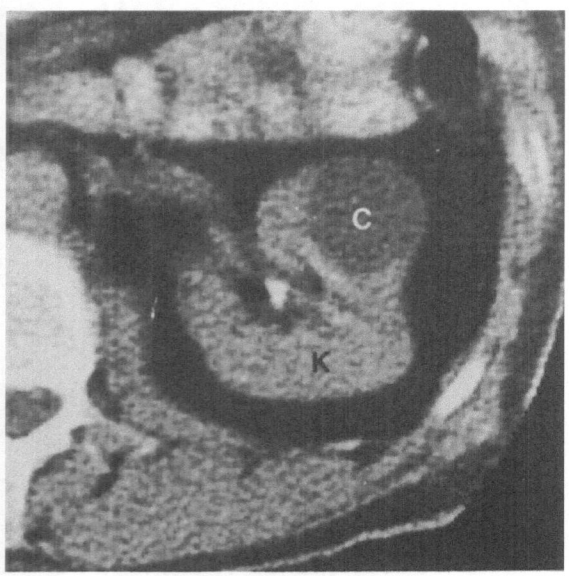

Figure 6.18(b)

Figure 6.18   Patient with left loin pain. (a) Intravenous urogram showing normal calyces and normal outline of the upper pole. (b) CT scan in the same patient showing a well defined cyst (C) arising from the anterior aspect of the left kidney (K)

tumours the partial volume effect of the enhanced normal tissue may influence the attenuation values so that small intrarenal tumours cannot be confidently excluded on CT evidence alone.

Masses may be shown on CT which have not been suspected on urography. Such masses usually originate from the anterolateral surface of the kidney growing outwards and causing very little calyceal deformity (figure 6.18).

Differential Diagnosis

The differential diagnosis between cysts and tumours 2 cm or more in diameter is usually simple, even on unenhanced scans, because of the differences in density, sharpness of margin and wall thickness. If in doubt, a scan can be obtained after enhancement. Even in tumours which are considered avascular at angiography, some enhancement can usually be detected by CT.

Evaluation of the Nature and Extent of a Mass

As in other organs, it is not always possible to determine whether a solid mass is benign or malignant on the basis of CT scan appearances alone, but some cases show unequivocal signs of malignancy. These include the presence of metastases in para-aortic lymph nodes or liver and extension of tumour beyond the renal capsule into the perinephric fat (figure 6.19). CT can demonstrate thrombus in the inferior vena cava (pp. 124–5). Renal vein involvement may be obvious, especially on the left, in which case tumour is seen spreading along the vascular pedicle. It is possible with the development of CT angiography that lesser degrees of involvement may be detected.

Not all non-cystic masses are renal cell carcinomas. Abscesses, haematomas, granulomatous pyelonephritis, hamartomas and other benign tumours may all have appearances which might be mistaken for carcinoma on CT. Inflammatory masses and arteriovenous malformations may enhance. Although an abscess might be expected to have a density between that of cyst and

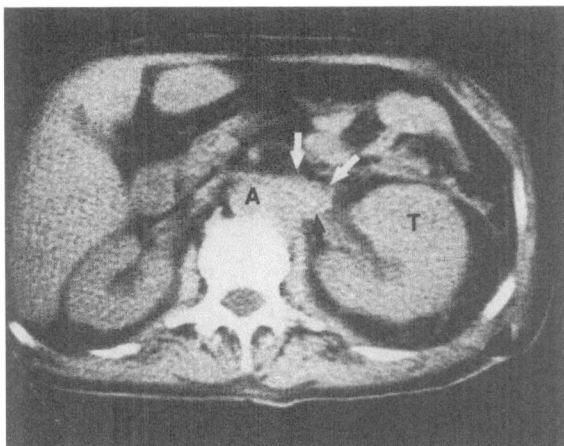

Figure 6.19(a)

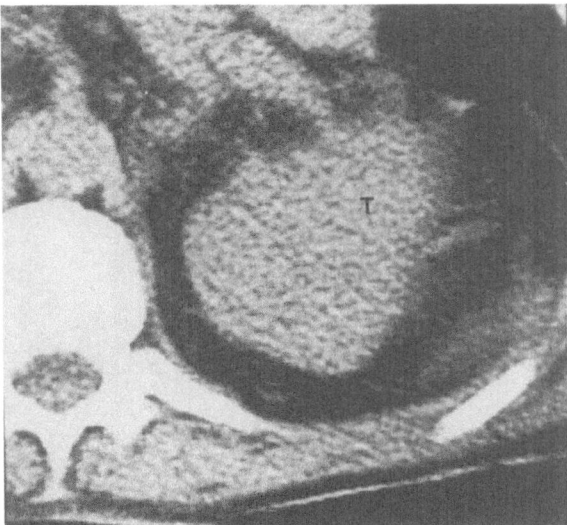

Figure 6.19(b)

Figure 6.19   Carcinoma of the left kidney. (a) Well
encapsulated tumour lying anteriorly (T). Note enlarged
para-aortic lymph nodes (arrowed) adjacent to the aorta
(A). (b) The scan taken 2 cm higher shows the tumour
(T) extending into the perinephric fat

solid tumour, in practice the density varies widely,
and on CT grounds alone there may be no clear
distinction between an abscess and a necrotic
tumour. Both may have a thick wall. Magilner and
Ostrum (1978) reported six patients with renal
masses which were avascular on angiography and in

which the attenuation values were unusually low for
a solid tumour. Four proved to be renal cell carcinomas and two were abscesses.

Xanthogranulomatous pyelonephritis is usually
associated with calculous disease and some degree
of hydronephrosis (figure 6.20a). The associated

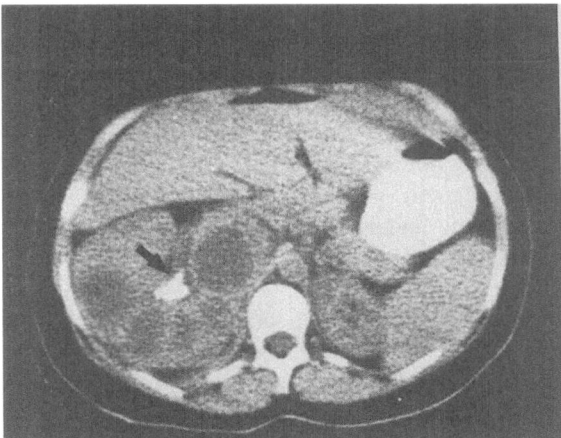

Figure 6.20(a)

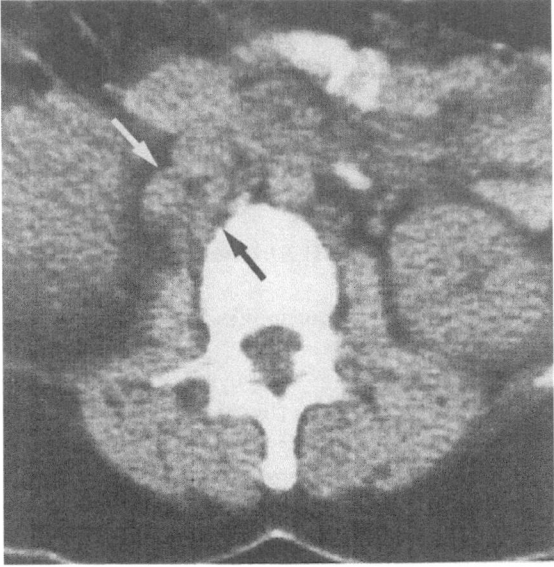

Figure 6.20(b)

Figure 6.20   Xanthogranulomatous pyelonephritis. (a)
The right kidney is large and there is hydronephrosis.
There is thickening of the renal substance. A calculus lies
centrally (arrowed). (b) Enlarged para-aortic lymph node
in the same patient (arrowed)

lymph node enlargement due to inflammatory changes could easily be misdiagnosed as evidence of metastatic spread (figure 6.20b). This topic is discussed in more detail in chapter 11.

The density of a haematoma may vary with its age, being initially denser than normal renal tissue and becoming less dense with time. Benign tumours are likely to be indistinguishable from carcinomas on CT evidence alone, except for fat-containing tumours, such as angiomyolipomas, which may have a characteristically low density (Sagel *et al.*, 1977). One might also expect CT to be helpful in establishing the diagnosis of renal sinus fibrolipomatosis which can sometimes lead to an appearance suggesting a renal mass lesion on urography.

Foetal lobulation and renal pseudotumours characteristically take up contrast medium to the same degree as normal renal tissue. Occasionally, however, a renal cell carcinoma is also isodense with normal tissue, even after injection of contrast medium, so that care should be taken when diagnosing a possible tumour as a normal variant.

Retroperitoneal tumours arising in sites other than the kidney cannot always be differentiated from a primary renal tumour, particularly when there is invasion of renal parenchyma. In cases of difficulty, it is worth investigating to see if a fat plane can be detected between the mass and the kidney.

OTHER RENAL AND PERIRENAL LESIONS

Major Congenital Abnormalities

Such abnormalities as polycystic kidneys (figure 6.21), horseshoe kidneys (figure 6.22) and presacral kidneys are demonstrated with CT but are usually adequately shown by simpler techniques. In polycystic disease, associated hepatic involvement is also demonstrated (*see* figure 6.21).

Scarred Kidneys

These are well shown, the scars being seen clearly because the whole of the kidney surface is seen in

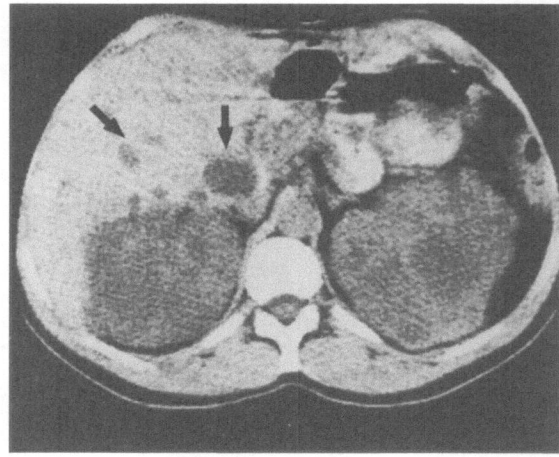

Figure 6.21 Polycystic kidneys. Both kidneys are grossly enlarged and contain multiple low-density lesions. The liver also contains multiple cysts (arrowed)

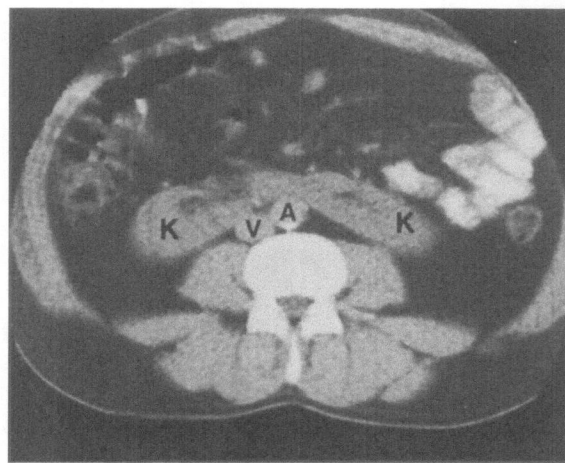

Figure 6.22 Horseshoe kidney. The kidneys (K) are joined anteriorly in front of the aorta (A) and inferior vena cava (V)

profile except at the poles (figure 6.23). Even very small kidneys are easy to see if there is a reasonable amount of perinephric fat (figure 6.24).

Hydronephrosis

Hydronephrosis is shown on CT even without contrast medium because the pelvis appears as a mass

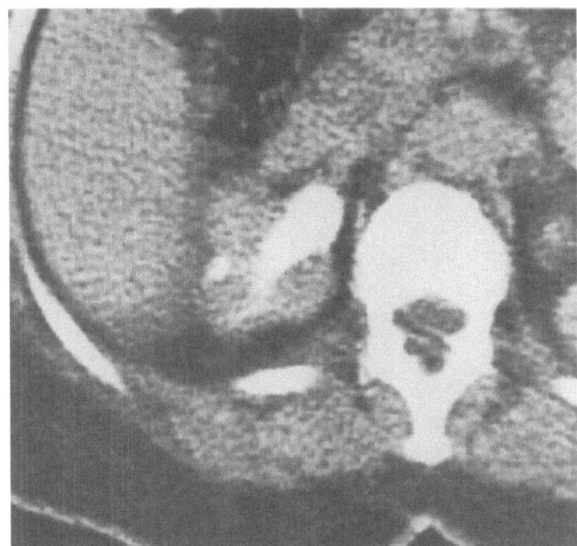

Figure 6.23 Post-contrast scan showing small scarred kidney due to chronic pyelonephritis

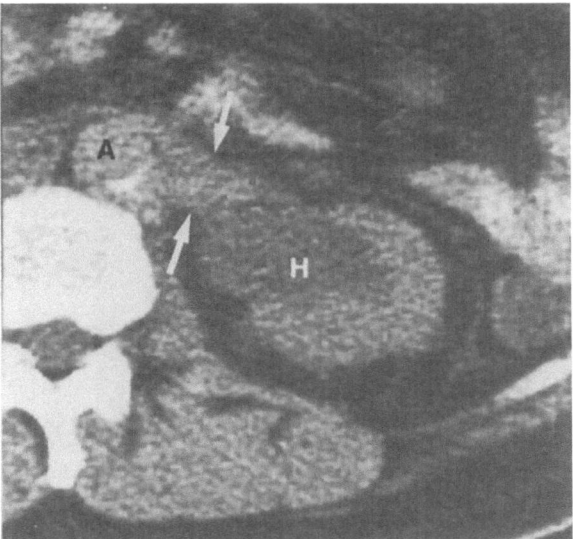

Figure 6.25(a)

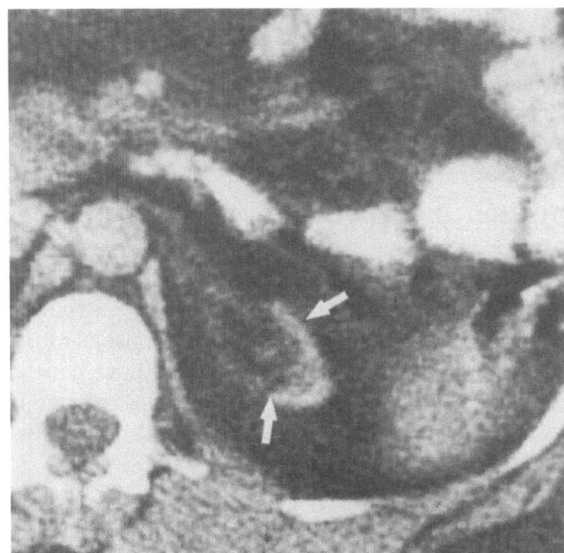

Figure 6.24 Post-contrast scan showing vestigial left kidney (arrowed). Note opacification of renal parenchyma

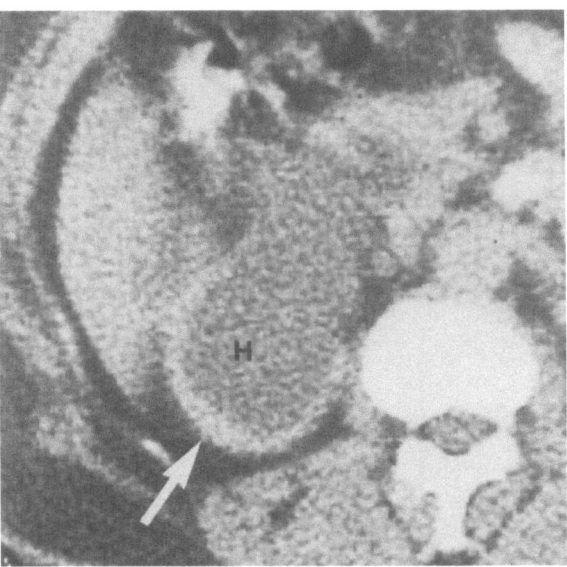

Figure 6.25(b)

Figure 6.25 Hydronephrosis. (a) Moderate hydro-nephrosis (H). Note enlarged para-aortic lymph nodes (arrowed) adjacent to the aorta (A). (b) Gross hydro-nephrosis (H). Note thin rim of renal parenchyma (arrowed)

of water density at the renal hilum and the dilated calyces are shown as a central area of low density within the normal renal substance (figure 6.25). Only fairly gross hydronephrosis can be diagnosed with confidence on CT. Even after the injection of con-trast medium, minor degrees of hydronephrosis can-not be excluded by CT alone.

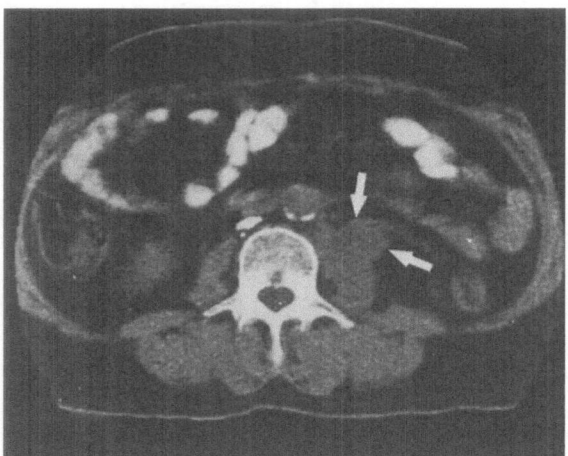

Figure 6.26   Left hydroureter (arrowed). The density measurement was close to that of water (4 EMI units)

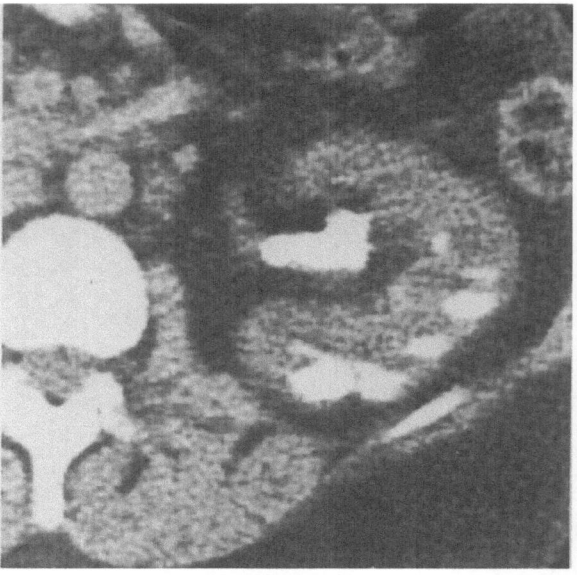

Figure 6.27(b)

Figure 6.27   Numerous renal calculi. (a) Intravenous urogram. (b) CT scan. The scan shows the posterior location of the majority of the calculi which lie in the renal substance. Demonstration in the axial plane simplifies the surgical approach

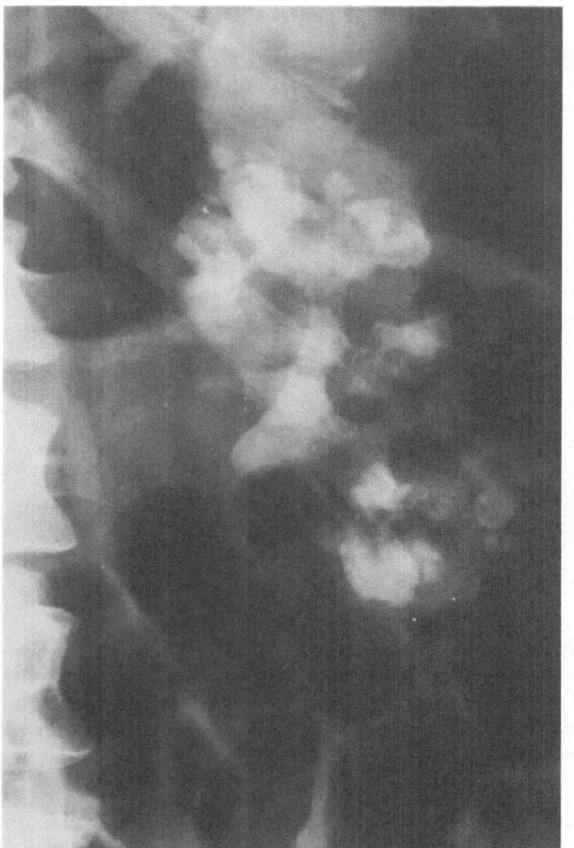

Figure 6.27(a)

Hydroureter

Hydroureter can often be seen even when unopacified, the dilated ureter appearing as a rounded structure of water density lying on the psoas muscle (figure 6.26, and *see* figure 6.7a). Without contrast medium even a dilated ureter is difficult to see once it crosses the pelvic brim and begins to run obliquely through the plane of the scans.

Calculi

These are obvious on CT even when 'non-opaque' on the plain radiograph. When taken together with the plain abdominal radiographs, demonstration of the position of calculi in the axial plane simplifies their localisation at surgery (figure 6.27) (Wickham *et al.*, 1980).

Renal Trauma or Suspected Renal Trauma

Such trauma may prove to be an important indication for CT. The extent of bleeding into the renal parenchyma and into the perinephric space can be clearly seen and the presence of a normal undamaged kidney on the opposite side may be confirmed. The extent of an intrarenal haematoma is best defined after injection of intravenous contrast medium.

Perinephric Lesions

Such lesions as abscess, haematoma and tumour spread are all visible with CT (figure 6.28). Figure 6.29 demonstrates a large mass arising in the perinephric space with attenuation values intermediate between cyst and tumour. A clinical diagnosis of an abscess was made. At operation, the lesion was found to be a necrotic secondary deposit.

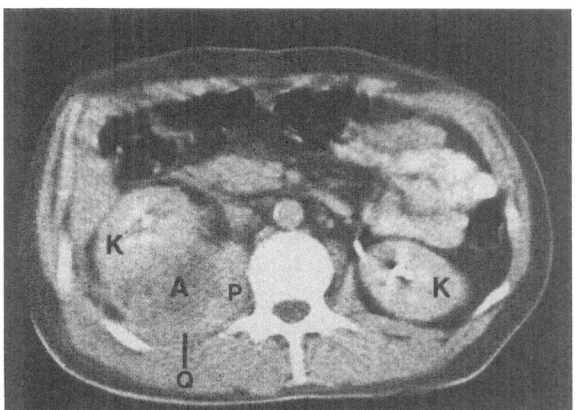

Figure 6.28(a)

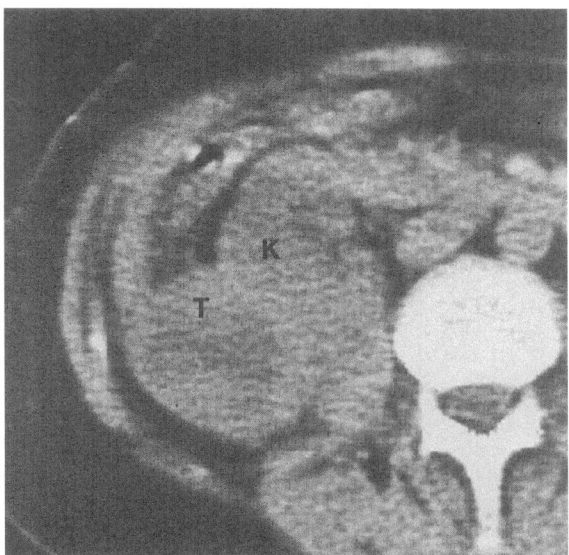

Figure 6.29 Necrotic secondary deposit (T) arising from the right kidney (K). The lesion has a similar appearance to a perinephric abscess

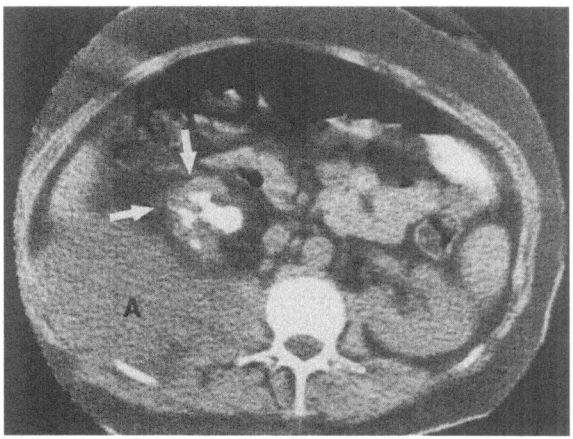

Figure 6.28(b)

Figure 6.28 Perinephric abscesses. (a) Post-contrast scan. Kidneys (K). The perinephric abscess (A) has a low-density centre and obliterates the margins of the psoas (P) and the quadratus lumborum (Q) muscles. (b) An abscess (A) associated with small scarred right kidney containing a stag-horn calculus (arrowed)

CT can be valuable in detecting fluid collections such as haematomas and abscess formation in relation to renal transplants (Kittredge *et al.*, 1978). The size of the transplanted kidney can be assessed better with CT than with conventional radiography because the location of the kidney frequently makes plain-film interpretation difficult. Figure 6.30 illustrates the scans in a patient with a transplant who was passing no urine. Ultrasound was inconclusive. CT shows contrast medium leaking from the transplanted kidney and tracking up the right paracolic gutter.

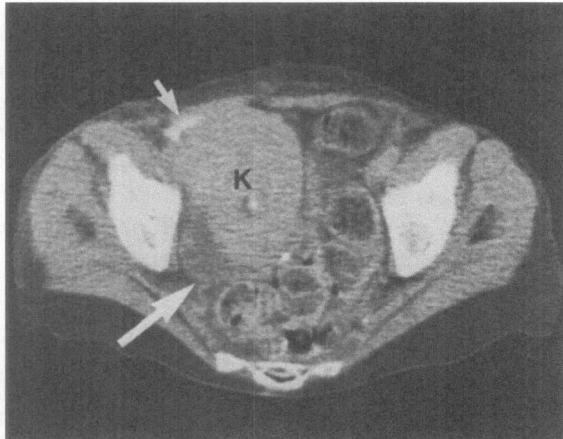

Figure 6.30(a)

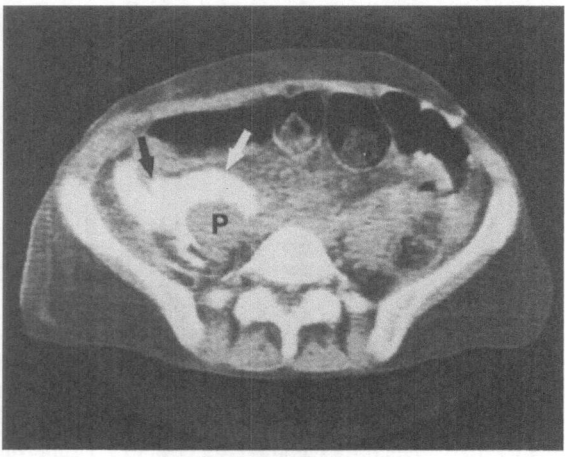

Figure 6.30(b)

Figure 6.30   Scans in a patient with a renal transplant who was not passing urine. The scans were taken after injection of intravenous contrast medium. (a) Transplanted kidney (K) is shown in the right iliac fossa. There is a low-density mass (large arrow) adjacent to the kidney. Note leaking contrast lying anterior to the kidney (small arrow). (b) The leaking contrast collected in the right paracolic gutter (arrowed). Right psoas muscle (P)

Abnormalities of the Ureter

CT may show the nature of abnormalities causing ureteric displacement or obstruction. CT also may be a great help for excluding disease in a patient in whom the ureter pursues an unusual course.

USE OF COMPUTED TOMOGRAPHY AND RELATIONSHIP TO OTHER TECHNIQUES

CT is an accurate method of distinguishing renal cysts from other masses. Thus, Magilner and Ostrum (1978) reported 145 consecutive renal masses with CT appearances characteristic of a cyst in which confirmation of the nature of the lesion was available. All proved to be cysts. This corresponds with our own experience. If CT shows unequivocal evidence that a mass is a cyst, we regard further investigations as unnecessary, especially when the lesion is an incidental finding. The great majority of lesions which appear to be non-cystic will prove to be renal cell carcinomas, but other possibilities must be borne in mind and the clinical presentation must always be taken into account.

Ultrasound is also an accurate method of distinguishing cysts from solid masses and is normally the first investigation to be carried out when a mass has been shown on the urogram. If ultrasound conclusively demonstrates the existence of a cyst, there is usually no need for CT, although in some circumstances CT may be considered preferable to percutaneous cyst puncture to confirm the diagnosis. If ultrasound is inconclusive or unsuccessful, CT is indicated.

If ultrasound shows an echogenic mass that suggests a renal cell carcinoma, CT can be used to confirm the diagnosis of a solid mass and to provide information about the extent and stage of a tumour. Lowe *et al.* (1979) have suggested that CT might provide sufficient information to replace renal arteriography as a preoperative investigation. This is a matter for debate and depends on the questions to which the surgeon needs answers. CT provides no information about the anatomy of the arterial supply to the kidney and cannot yet be used with confidence to exclude venous spread. Venacavography is still required if there is no obvious venous involvement. It is also important to remember that CT does not give as much information about the *nature* of a solid mass as can be obtained by arteriography.

Ultrasound examination is particularly liable to fail to display the upper poles of the kidneys, especially on the left. Figure 6.31a shows the urogram in such a patient with a mass lying medially

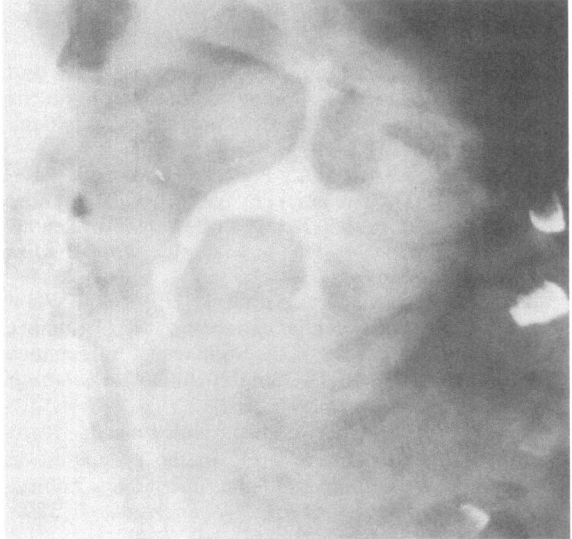

Figure 6.31(a)

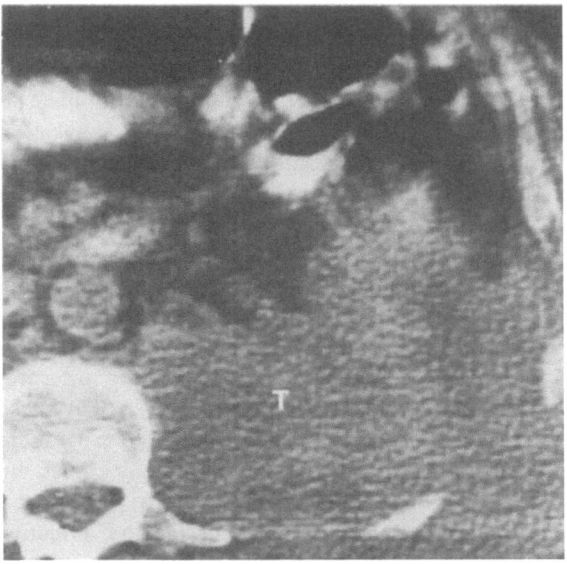

Figure 6.32(a)

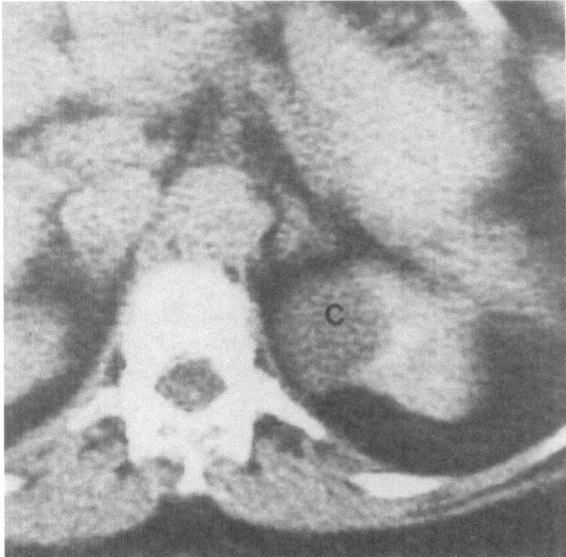

Figure 6.31(b)

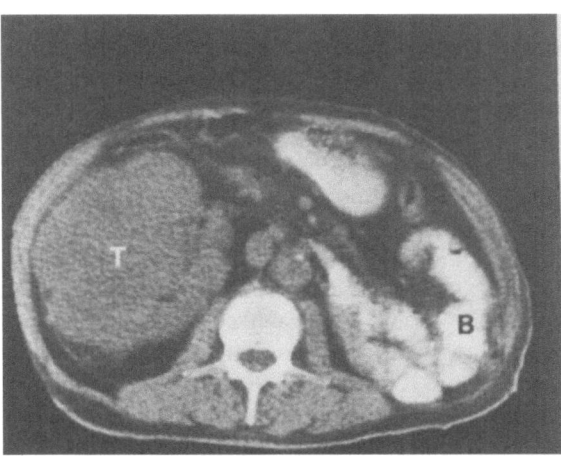

Figure 6.32(b)

Figure 6.32   (a) Recurrent tumour (T) in the left renal bed following nephrectomy for renal carcinoma. (b) Opacified bowel (B) occupying the left renal bed following nephrectomy for renal carcinoma. Note large tumour (T) arising from the right kidney

Figure 6.31   Renal cyst. (a) Intravenous urogram showing mass on medial aspect of left upper pole displacing the upper calyx. Ultrasound examination was unsuccessful. Residual barium is present in diverticula. (b) The CT scan showed a well defined cyst (C) arising from the upper pole of the left kidney

in the left upper pole, seen as an incidental finding during investigation for urinary tract infection. Ultrasound was unsuccessful. CT shows the typical appearance of a renal cyst (figure 6.31b).

Simple cysts are more commonly detected by CT

than by urography, and one or more cysts are commonly seen as incidental findings during examinations of the upper abdomen. Even quite large lesions can be missed on urography if they are situated on the anterolateral surface of the kidney. We have seen two renal cell carcinomas diagnosed by CT in patients having scans for the investigation of pyrexia of unknown origin when previous urography was reported as normal.

CT is the method of choice for demonstrating tumour recurrence after nephrectomy because conventional radiography is of little value and ultrasound can frequently be difficult to interpret (Bernardino *et al.*, 1979) (figure 6.32a). In these patients, it is important to ensure adequate opacification of the bowel as this now occupies the renal bed (figure 6.32b).

Ultrasound can be an accurate and effective technique in the diagnosis of perinephric lesions and in the postoperative investigation of renal transplants. CT may be useful in such patients where ultrasound shows no lesion or is inconclusive.

CT has been used for the investigation of kidneys which appear to be 'non-functioning' at urography (Forbes *et al.*, 1978). A retrograde examination can be used to solve this problem, but, if there is no other indication for cystoscopy, ultrasound is the next diagnostic step. This may show hydronephrosis or a shrunken kidney. If the diagnosis remains in doubt, CT may have a place, especially in showing that no kidney is present. CT can also be useful in some patients with severe renal failure in whom other methods are contra-indicated or have failed to demonstrate the shape and size of the kidneys and the presence or absence of obstruction.

REFERENCES

Bernardino, M. E., de Santos, L. A., Johnson, D. E. and Bracken, R. B. (1979). Computed tomography in the evaluation of the post-nephrectomy patient. *Radiology*, **130**, 183–187

Brennan, R. A., Curtis, J. A., Pollack, H. M. and Weinberg, I. (1979a). Sequential changes in the CT number of the normal canine kidney following intravenous contrast injection. I. The renal cortex. *Investigative Radiology*, **14**, 141–148

Brennan, R. A., Curtis, J. A., Pollack, H. M. and Weinberg, I. (1979b). Sequential changes in the CT number of the normal canine kidney following intravenous contrast injection. II. The renal medulla. *Investigative Radiology*, **14**, 239–245

Forbes, W. St C., Isherwood, I. and Fawcitt, R. A. (1978). Computed tomography in the evaluation of the solitary or unilateral non-functioning kidney. *Journal of Computer Assisted Tomography*, **2**, 389–394

Kittredge, R. D., Brensilver, J. and Pierce, J. C. (1978). Computed tomography in renal transplant problems. *Radiology*, **127**, 165–169

Lowe, L., Churchill, R., Reyne, S. C., Schuster, G. A., Moncada, R. and Kerkow, A. (1979). Computed tomography for the staging of renal cell carcinoma. *Urologic Radiology*, **1**, 3–10

Magilner, A. D. and Ostrum, B. J. (1978). Computed tomography in the diagnosis of renal masses. *Radiology*, **126**, 715–718

Sagel, S. S., Stanley, R. J., Levitt, R. G. and Geisse, G. (1977). Computed tomography of the kidney. *Radiology*, **124**, 359–370

Segal, A. J. and Spitzer, R. M. (1979). Pseudo thick walled renal cyst by CT. *American Journal of Roentgenology*, **132**, 827–828

Wickham, J. E. A., Fry, I. K. and Wallace, D. M. A. (1980). CT localisation of intrarenal calculi prior to nephrolithotomy. *British Journal of Urology*, **52** (6), 422–425

7

The Abdomen – Adrenals

Although small, the adrenal glands are surrounded by retroperitoneal fat and are usually easily seen. They are one of the structures for which CT appears at the present time to be the imaging technique of first choice in a high proportion of patients.

TECHNIQUE OF EXAMINATION

Scans should be obtained from a level just above the kidneys down to the level of the hilum of the left kidney using contiguous or even overlapping sections. When available, the use of a finely collimated beam giving thinner sections may allow the glands to be seen more clearly. The technique is otherwise the same as the general technique for abdominal scans. Intravenous contrast medium is not given routinely but may help to distinguish the kidney or neighbouring vascular structures, especially the inferior vena cava, from an adrenal mass. It should be remembered that glucagon is contra-indicated in patients with suspected phaeochromocytoma.

CT ANATOMY

Both glands can be visualised in the great majority of patients provided that there is sufficient retroperitoneal fat (Brownlie and Kreel, 1978; Karstaedt *et al.*, 1978; Montagne *et al.*, 1978). The glands are about 3 cm in length and are, therefore, seen on several scans. The right gland lies just above the right kidney and immediately behind the inferior vena cava, close to the point where this leaves the liver (figure 7.1). The gland is related medially to the right crus of the diaphragm and laterally to the bare area of the liver. It consists of a body and two limbs running posteriorly. The body is very short and often inconspicuous. It lies so close to the inferior

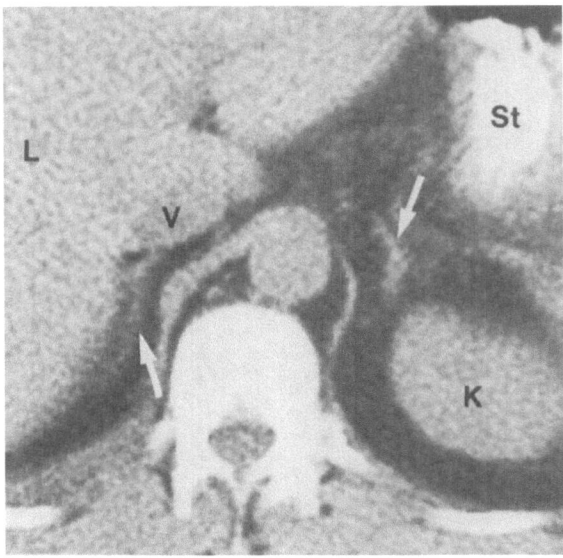

Figure 7.1 Normal adrenal glands (arrowed). Inferior vena cava (V), liver (L), left kidney (K), stomach (St)

vena cava that it usually appears to be in continuity with it. The medial limb is the part of the gland that is most commonly seen (*see* figure 7.1). It appears as a linear or curvilinear structure extending posteriorly for as much as 4 cm. The lateral limb of the gland is frequently indistinguishable from the liver. When both limbs are seen, the gland has the appearance of a wishbone seen from the side (figure 7.2).

The left gland lies anteromedially to the upper pole of the kidney (figure 7.3, and *see* figure 7.1). It may extend caudally nearly to the hilum of the kidney. It lies behind the tail of the pancreas and the splenic vessels and is related medially to the crus of the diaphragm and the aorta. The upper part of the gland lies close to the posterior aspect of the stomach. The appearance of the gland on the left is different to that on the right. Both limbs are usually visible, so that the gland may be seen as an inverted V- or Y-shaped structure (figure 7.4, and *see* figures 7.1 and 7.3). When the limbs are short or not seen, the gland may appear triangular (figure 7.5a). Whatever the shape, the margins of the gland are straight or concave. Convex margins must suggest a mass (Karstaedt *et al.*, 1978).

On both sides the medial limb lies at a more

cranial level than does the body, so that part of it may be seen as an isolated structure lying close to the crus on sections above the body (figure 7.5b). On the right, the gland is not likely to be confused with

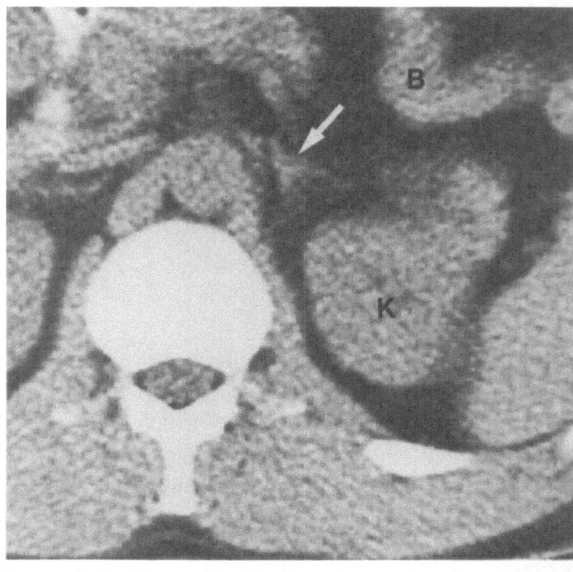

Figure 7.3 Normal left adrenal gland (arrowed). Left kidney (K), bowel (B)

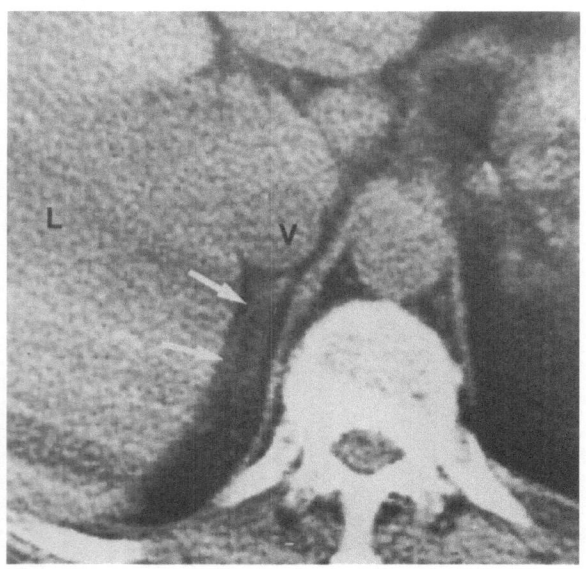

Figure 7.2 Normal right adrenal gland (arrowed) showing both limbs. Inferior vena cava (V), liver (L)

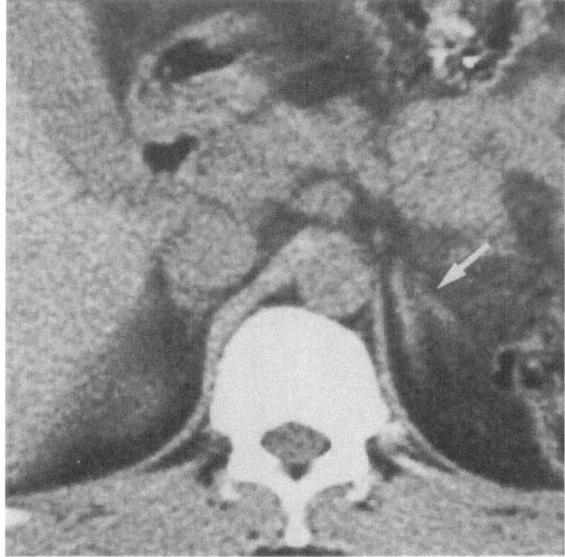

Figure 7.4 Normal V-shaped left adrenal gland (arrowed)

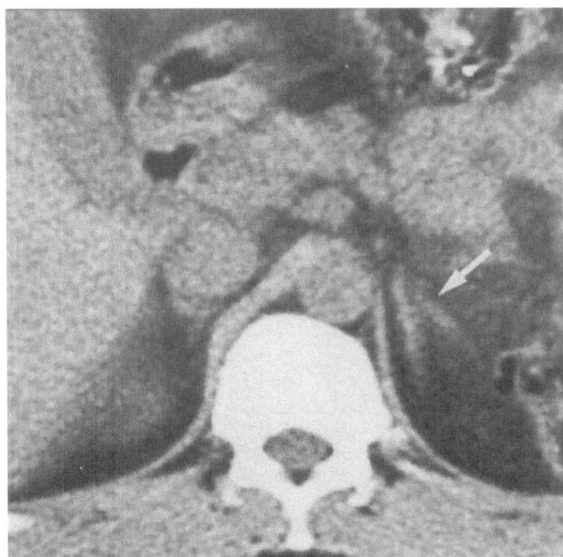

Figure 7.5(a)

other structures. On the left, the gland, particularly its lateral limb, may be confused with either splenic or renal vessels. Measurements of the thickness of normal V- or Y-shaped glands at the widest part have shown that the normal gland is rarely thicker than 1 cm and usually less, particularly on the right (Karstaedt *et al.*, 1978; Montagne *et al.*, 1978). Triangular-shaped glands appear thicker.

ADRENAL MASSES

The characteristic shape of the adrenal glands allows recognition of almost all tumours down to the size of 1.5 to 2 cm (figures 7.6, 7.7 and 7.8). Sometimes lesions as small as 0.5 cm can be detected in a patient with plenty of fat.

The density of most adrenal tumours is similar to that of other soft tissues. Some malignant tumours show central areas of low density caused by areas of necrosis (figure 7.9). A similar appearance can be seen in phaeochromocytomas due to haemorrhage (figure 7.10). Some cortical tumours are uniformly much less dense, probably owing to a high fat or

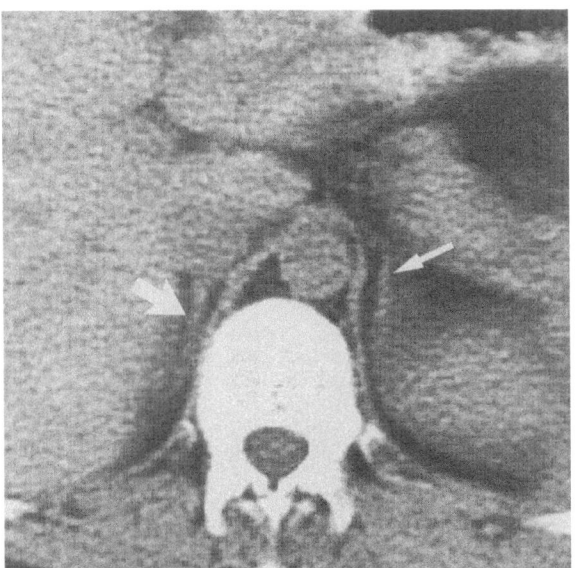

Figure 7.5(b)

Figure 7.5   Normal adrenal gland. (a) Body of left gland (arrowed) behind pancreas (P) and in front of left kidney (K). (b) Scan 2 cm above (a) showing medial limb only (arrowed) close to upper pole of kidney. The medial limb of the right adrenal gland is well shown (large arrow)

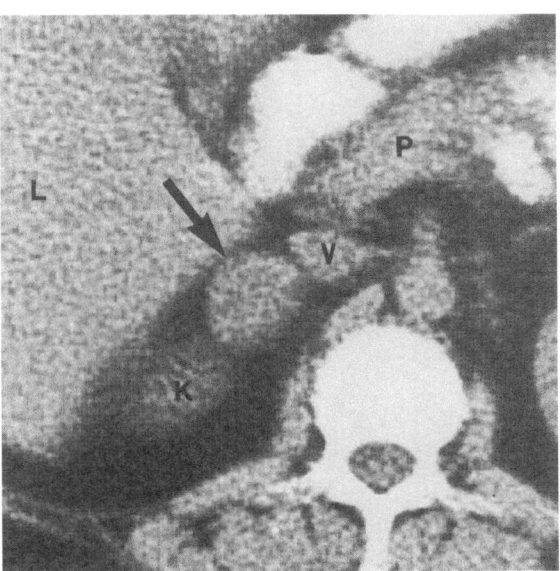

Figure 7.6   A 3.5 cm adrenal adenoma (arrowed) in patient with Cushing's syndrome. Liver (L), upper pole of right kidney (K), pancreas (P) and inferior vena cava (V)

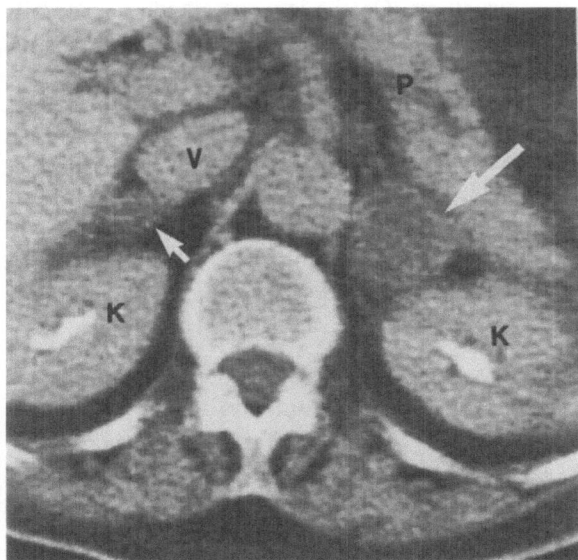

Figure 7.7 Bilateral adrenal masses (arrowed), 3.5 cm diameter on the left, 1.5 cm on the right. Pancreas (P), kidneys with contrast medium in the collecting system (K), inferior vena cava (V)

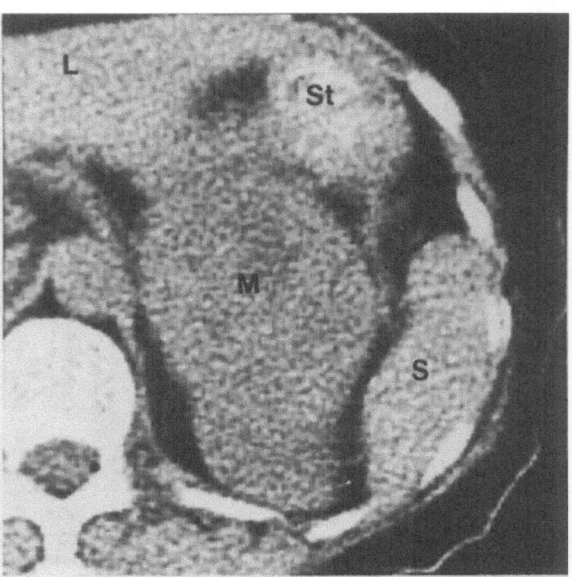

Figure 7.9 Left adrenal carcinoma with low-density areas representing necrosis (M). The tumour was invading the liver anteriorly. Spleen (S), liver (L), stomach (St)

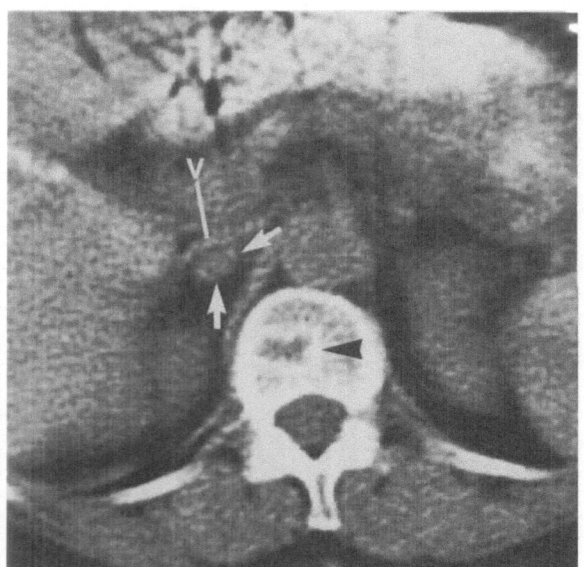

Figure 7.8 A 1.5 cm Conn's tumour in right adrenal (white arrows). Fine linear inferior vena cava (V). Note also possible Schmorl's node (arrowhead)

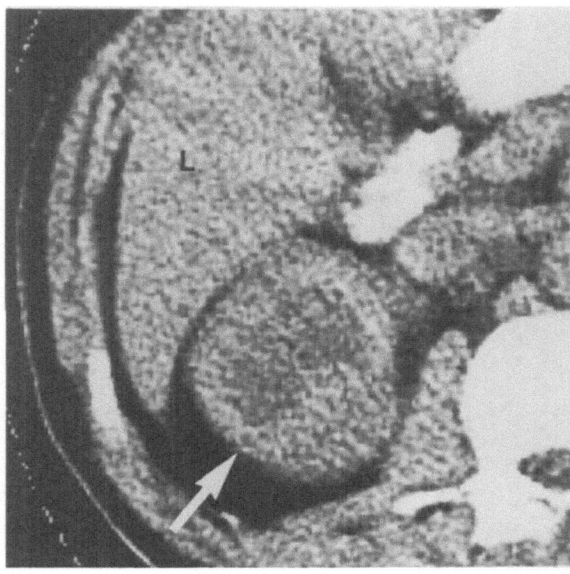

Figure 7.10 Right adrenal phaeochromocytoma (arrowed) showing central area of low density due to haemorrhage. Liver (L)

steroid content (Schaner *et al.*, 1978) (figure 7.11). When small, such tumours may be relatively inconspicuous within the retroperitoneal fat. Tumours may show calcification. They rarely enhance significantly after the injection of intravenous contrast medium, but, occasionally, just the rim enhances.

The different types of adrenal tumour have no characteristic features. For this reason, phaeochromocytomas, adenomas, neuroblastomas and primary and metastatic carcinomas cannot be distinguished on the CT appearances alone. The malignancy of the tumour may be established by the presence of local spread or by the involvement of lymph nodes or by the presence of metastases in the liver or elsewhere. Cysts occur occasionally in the adrenal gland and have the CT appearance of cysts elsewhere.

Metastatic masses in the adrenals are not uncommonly seen as incidental findings in patients having abdominal scans. The commonest sites of origin appear to be the lung and the breast (figure 7.12).

When excluding a tumour, it is important to identify both glands. The identification of two normal glands does not, however, always exclude a tumour. Because the gland extends over several

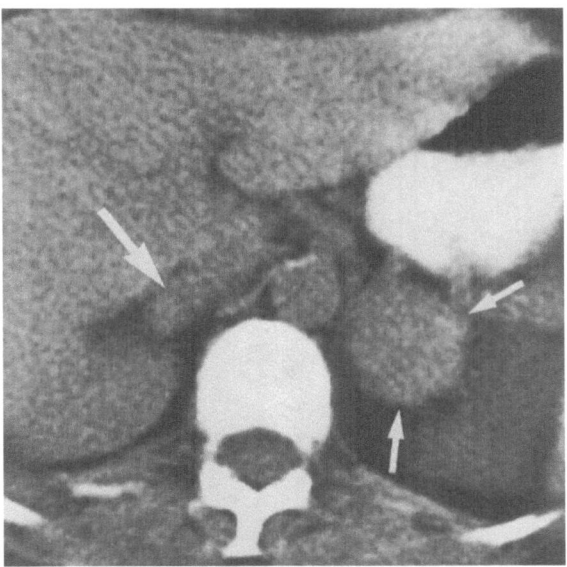

Figure 7.12 Metastasis in left adrenal gland from carcinoma of the breast (arrowed). Smaller metastasis in the gland on the right (larger arrow)

centimetres, a normal gland can be seen in one or two slices when there is a tumour elsewhere in the gland (figure 7.13). This figure also shows how close the upper part of the left gland can be to the stomach, part of which might be mistaken for an adrenal mass unless it is outlined with oral contrast medium (figure 7.14).

Tumours in the adrenals are sometimes difficult to separate from masses in the upper pole of the kidneys. The problem can usually be resolved after injection of intravenous contrast medium. Ultrasound examination in the longitudinal plane can also help to define the planes between the two structures. Tumours in the right adrenal are not likely to be confused with other structures, except the kidney. On the left, a tortuous splenic vessel may be mistaken for an enlarged adrenal but it should be possible to make the distinction by observing the continuity of the vessels in neighbouring slices or by opacifying the vessels with intravenous contrast medium (Montagne *et al.*, 1978). Renal vessels at the hilum are below the level of the normal adrenal but can occasionally cause confusion. Carcinoma of the pancreas can be distinguished from an adrenal mass by the relationship of the splenic vessels, the

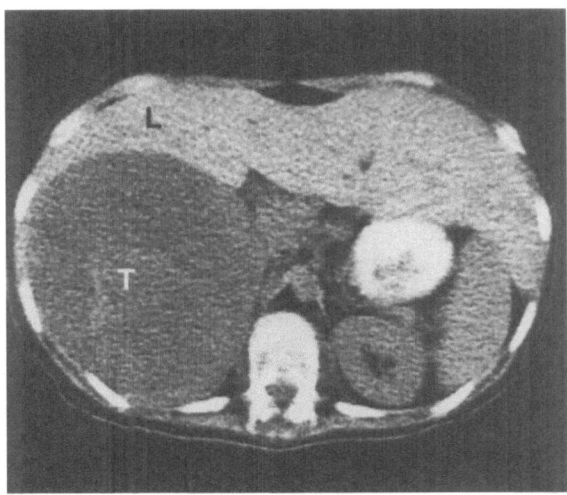

Figure 7.11 Adrenal cortical carcinoma (T) in 22-year-old girl with virilisation. Note that this is another example of a fat-containing tumour much of which has a mean attenuation value close to that of water (+7 EMI units). (See figure 4.17.) Liver (L)

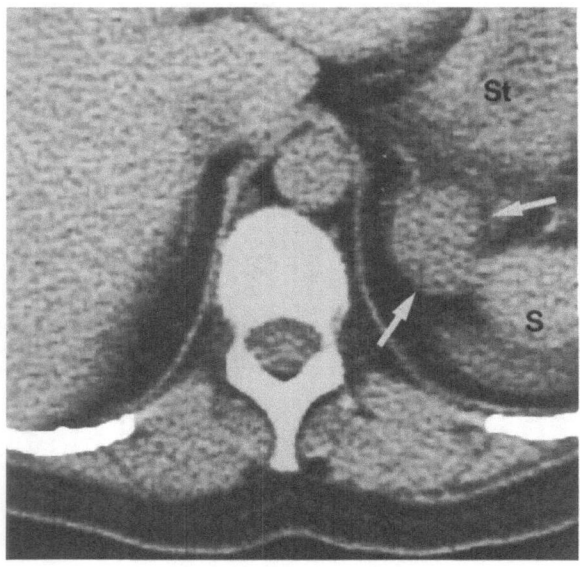

Figure 7.13(a)

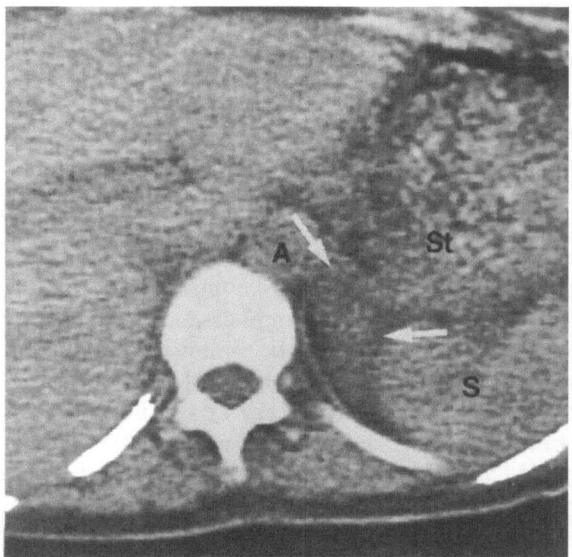

Figure 7.14(a)

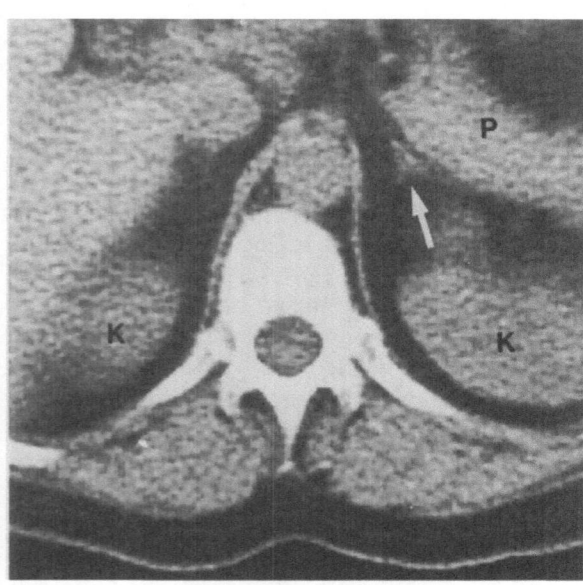

Figure 7.13(b)

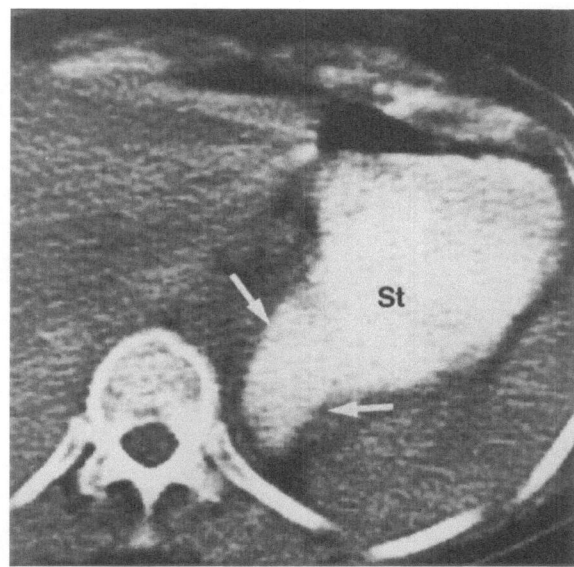

Figure 7.14(b)

Figure 7.13   Tumour in left adrenal involving only part
of the gland. (a) A 3.5 cm tumour in upper part of gland
(arrowed). Stomach (St), spleen (S). (b) Scan 2 cm lower
than (a) showing normal body of gland (arrowed) behind
the pancreas (P). Kidneys (K)

Figure 7.14   Stomach imitating adrenal tumour. (a)
Scan with very little Gastrografin in the stomach (St).
Suspected adrenal mass (arrowed) between the spleen (S)
and the aorta (A). (b) Stomach (St) full of Gastrografin.
'Mass' shown to be the posterior part of the stomach
(arrowed)

pancreatic mass lying anteriorly to the vessels and an adrenal mass lying posteriorly.

CT may be helpful in patients in whom possible adrenal masses have been shown incidentally during other examinations, especially intravenous urography. Not only may normal adrenals be seen but, if there is a mass, the site of its origin is likely to be established.

OTHER ADRENAL LESIONS

In patients with *bilateral adrenal hyperplasia* associated with Cushing's syndrome, the glands may appear rather plump but the normal contours are preserved (figure 7.15). Plump glands are only seen in a proportion of patients with adrenal hyperplasia; in about half, the glands appear normal. A few hyperplastic glands develop hyperplastic nodules which are indistinguishable on CT from small tumours (figure 7.16). *Calcification* in the adrenals is readily seen (figure 7.17).

ACCURACY AND RELATIONSHIP TO OTHER TECHNIQUES

The detection and localisation of adrenal tumours has until recently depended on invasive techniques, such as retroperitoneal pneumography, adrenal arteriography and venography, and venous sampling. In the past few years, isotope scanning techniques have been developed for the diagnosis of adrenal cortical tumours, and grey-scale ultrasound in the best hands has been shown to be capable of visualising the adrenal glands, especially in thin patients.

The great majority of phaeochromocytomas and of adrenal cortical tumours in Cushing's syndrome are larger than 2 cm at the time of presentation, so that it is not surprising that CT is an accurate method of detecting tumours in these conditions. This is particularly so in patients with Cushing's syndrome in whom the glands are very clearly displayed within the excessive amount of retroperitoneal fat. In patients with hyperaldosteronism, tumours are usually less than 2 cm in diameter and

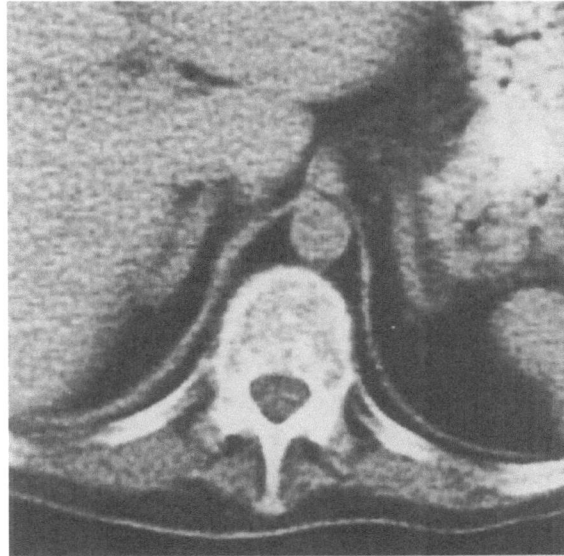

Figure 7.15(a)

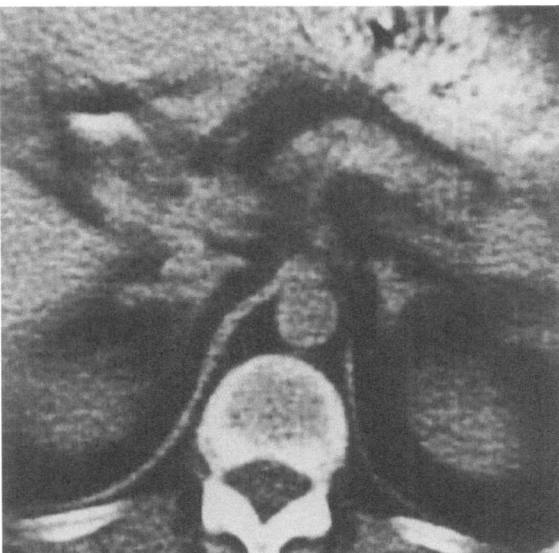

Figure 7.15(b)

Figure 7.15   (a) and (b) Bilateral adrenal hyperplasia. Glands thick but anatomy normal

are likely to be more difficult to detect, especially as they may have a relatively low density (Ganguly *et al.*, 1979). The results of five major studies are summarised in table 7.1 (Karstaedt *et al.*, 1978; Stewart et al., 1978; Dunnick et al., 1979; Korobkin et al., 1979; Eghrari et al., 1980). Combined experience at St Bartholomew's Hospital and the BUPA Medical Centre is in agreement with these findings. Out of 31

Table 7.1   Detection of adrenal tumours by CT. The results of five major studies (see text)

	True positive	False negative
Phaeochromocytomas	31	4
Cushing's syndrome	20	0
Conn's tumours	13	2

patients with Cushing's syndrome, all of 12 tumours in the adrenals were detected. There were no false positives nor false negatives. Five adrenal phaeochromocytomas were detected. There were no false negatives, but, in one patient in whom arteriography had already shown a 4 cm mass in one adrenal and who was being scanned to exclude a lesion on the other side, it was felt that the tumour might have been difficult to diagnose with confidence (figure 7.18). The patient was thin and the tumour was only seen as a low-density area filling the space between the kidneys, the liver and the inferior vena cava. Two patients who had already had phaeochromocytomas removed from one adrenal were scanned in order to exclude recurrence on the opposite side. In both instances, the glands

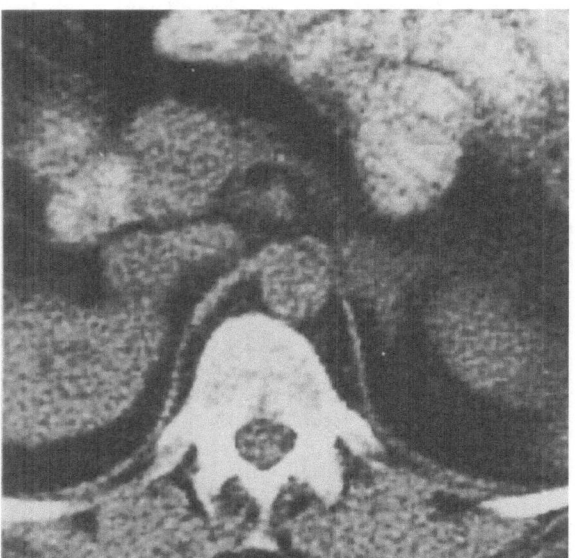

Figure 7.16   Bilateral 2 cm adrenal masses due to hyperplastic nodules in a patient with Cushing's syndrome

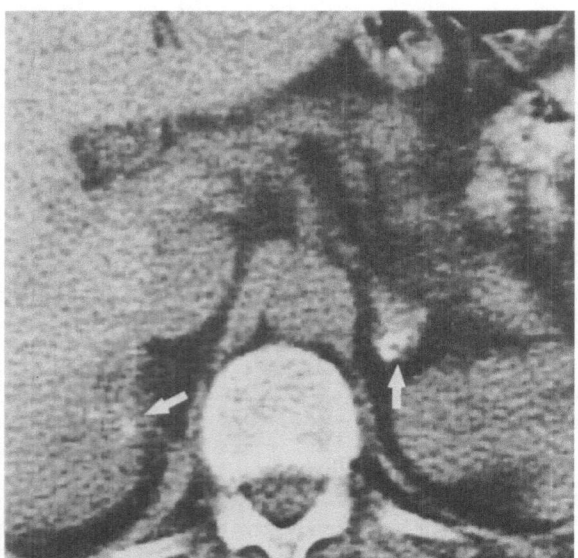

Figure 7.17   Adrenal calcification

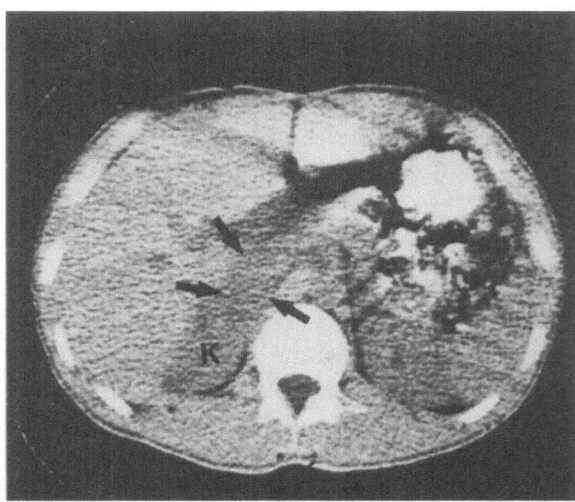

Figure 7.18   A 4 cm phaeochromocytoma (arrowed) in right adrenal gland in front of the right kidney (K) in a thin patient

appeared slightly enlarged and the possibility of recurrence was suggested. In both instances, the glands were found to be simply hypertrophic (figure 7.19). Two out of three Conn's tumours were correctly identified. The tumour that was missed was so small that the gland appeared normal at surgery. Two virilising tumours were correctly identified.

Clearly CT is a highly accurate method of detecting and excluding adrenal tumours in patients with Cushing's syndrome. The great majority of phaeochromocytomas will also be detected but occasional tumours may be difficult to see in thin patients. Many Conn's tumours are small, and it is slightly surprising that the accumulated data suggest that CT detects the great majority. One would expect the detection of Conn's tumours to be less accurate than that of phaeochromocytomas.

Sample and Sarti (1978), who have had a special interest in ultrasound examination of the adrenals (Sample, 1978), compared the accuracy of CT and ultrasound and concluded that CT was much the better technique. Although both types of examination are of comparable accuracy, these workers emphasise the skill required for ultrasound and contrasted it with the relative simplicity of CT. Ultrasound will, however, continue to have a place particularly in the examination of thin patients and in situations where CT is not available.

No comparative studies of isotopic adrenal scanning and CT are available. The delay in diagnosis is the main disadvantage of the isotope technique.

When investigating endocrine-secreting lesions, the precise order of investigation in patients suspected of having adrenal disease will vary according to the available techniques and local circumstances. CT would seem, however, at the present time, to be the logical first choice of investigation for imaging the adrenal glands in patients with Cushing's syndrome and in those who have a suspected phaeochromocytoma.

In Cushing's syndrome, adenomas or carcinomas are readily distinguished from the normal or plump gland of bilateral cortical hyperplasia. If there is suspicion of ectopic adrenocorticotrophic hormone (ACTH) secretion, CT can be used to search the likely areas, such as the pancreas, anterior mediastinum and lungs.

In patients in whom there is clinical or biochemical evidence suggesting the presence of a phaeochromocytoma, a CT scan extending through the adrenal and renal hilar areas down to the aortic bifurcation would seem the logical first step (figure 7.20) (Stewart *et al.*, 1978). Arteriography and venous sampling would seem to be best reserved for those patients in whom CT has failed to show a lesion or in whom further lesions are suspected. If venous sampling locates a lesion to a particular part, this area can be scanned to define the lesion (figure 7.21).

Since CT will only detect larger Conn's tumours, it cannot be used to exclude a tumour, and few tumours will be shown with sufficient confidence to obviate the need for other imaging investigations. Adrenal sampling and venography and isotope scanning are still likely to be needed in the great majority of patients.

Clearly the use of CT is a major advance in the investigation of patients with possible adrenal lesions. It is probably the most effective clinical use of CT outside the brain.

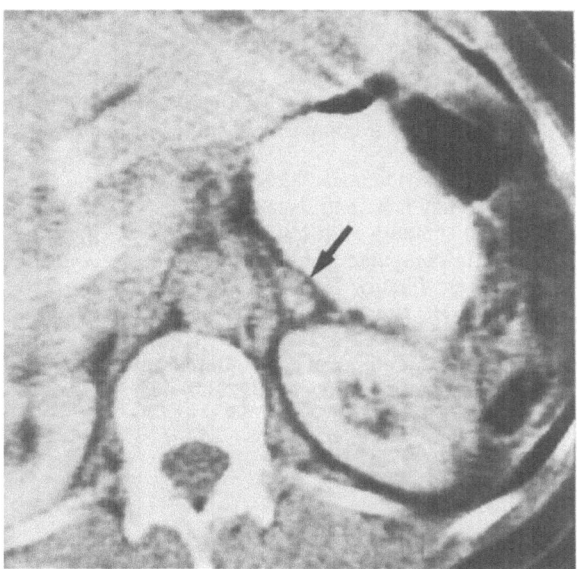

Figure 7.19 Plump left adrenal gland in patient with suspected recurrent phaeochromocytoma. A tumour in the opposite gland had previously been removed

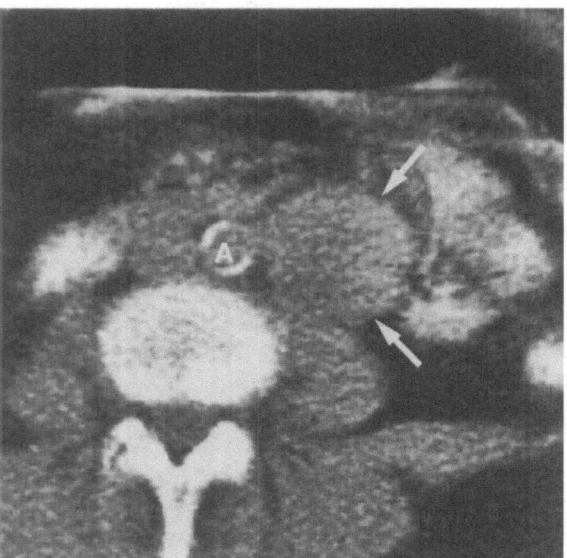

Figure 7.20   A 4.5 cm phaeochromocytoma on left of calcified aorta (A) in a patient in whom arteriography had failed to show a tumour in the adrenal gland

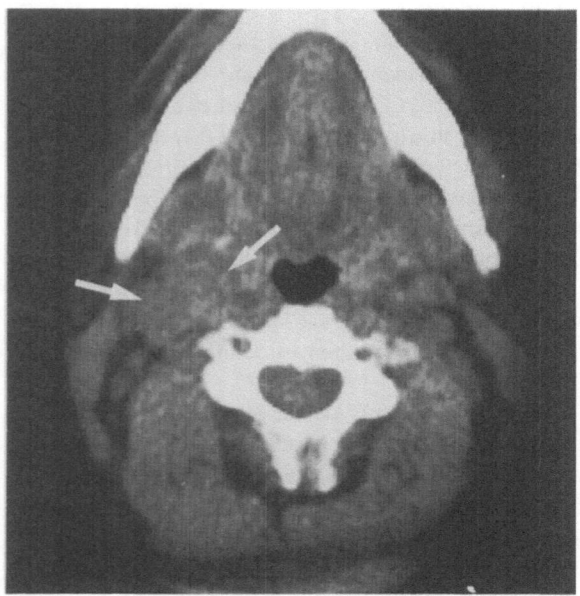

Figure 7.21   Phaeochromocytoma in carotid body in patient in whom venous sampling had shown high levels of catecholamines in the jugular vein

REFERENCES

Brownlie, K. and Kreel, L. (1978). Computer assisted tomography of normal suprarenal glands. *Journal of Computer Assisted Tomography*, **2** (1), 1–10

Dunnick, N. R., Schaner, E. G., Doppman, J. L., Strott, C. A., Gill, J. R. and Javadpour, N. (1979). Computed tomography in adrenal tumours. *American Journal of Roentgenology*, **132**, 43–46

Eghrari, M., McLoughlin, M. J., Rosen, I. E., St Louis, E. L., Wilson, S. R., Wise, D. J. and Yeung, H. P. H. (1980). The role of computed tomography in assessment of tumour pathology of the adrenal glands. *Journal of Computer Assisted Tomography*, **4** (1), 71–77

Ganguly, A., Pratt, J. H., Yune, H. Y., Grin, C. E. and Weinberger, M. H. (1979). Detection of adrenal tumour by computerized tomographic scan in endocrine hypertension. *Archives of Internal Medicine*, **139**, 589–590

Karstaedt, N., Sagel, S. S., Stanley, R. J., Melson, G. L. and Levitt, R. G. (1978). Computed tomography of the adrenal gland. *Radiology*, **129**, 723–730

Korobkin, M., White, E. A., Kressel, H. Y., Moss, A. A. and Montagne, J.-P. (1979). Computed tomography in the diagnosis of adrenal disease. *American Journal of Roentgenology*, **132**, 231–238

Montagne, J.-P., Kressel, H. Y., Korobkin, M. and Moss, A. A. (1978). Computed tomography of the normal adrenal glands. *American Journal of Roentgenology*, **130**, 963–966

Sample, W. F. (1978). Adrenal ultrasonography. *Radiology*, **127**, 461–466

Sample, W. F. and Sarti, D. A. (1978). Computed tomography and gray scale ultrasonography of the adrenal gland: a comparative study. *Radiology*, **128**, 377–383

Schaner, E. G., Dunnick, N. R., Doppman, J. L., Strott, C. A., Gill, J. R. and Javadpour, N. (1978). Adrenal cortical tumours with low attenuation co-efficients: a pitfall in computed tomography diagnosis. *Journal of Computer Assisted Tomography*, **2** (1), 11–15

Stewart, B. H., Bravo, E. L., Haaga, J., Meaney, T. and Tarazi, R. (1978). Localisation of phaeochromocytomas by computed axial tomography. *New England Journal of Medicine*, **299**, 460–461

8

The Abdomen – Liver and Biliary Tract

From its size and generally uniform texture, the liver might be expected, like the brain, to be ideally suited to CT scanning. However, focal lesions frequently have a density very similar to that of the surrounding liver parenchyma and may be difficult to detect even on high-quality scans. For this reason, artefacts are particularly detrimental to CT diagnosis of liver disease, depending, as it does almost entirely, on the detection of differences in density rather than change in size or shape. Unfortunately, streak artefacts from the ribs and from gas in the stomach are common when using slower scanners, and for this reason CT scanning of the liver has until recently been less reliable than might have been hoped. The development of scanners with faster scan times has greatly improved image quality, so much so that this is one of the areas in which faster scanners can be expected to make the most diagnostic impact.

TECHNIQUE OF EXAMINATION

The basic technique is that described for general abdominal scanning. Intervals between scans will vary with the clinical problem, but, when small focal lesions are being sought, scans should be contiguous.

Patients are usually scanned in the supine position. If slight movement produces artefacts and degrades the initial images, scans may be repeated with the patient lying on the right side (Haaga and Reich, 1978). This splints the ribs overlying the liver and lesions may be seen more clearly than in the supine position (figure 8.1). In a study at St Bartholomew's Hospital, there were fewer artefacts over the liver when the patient was lying on the right side in 45 out of 82 consecutive patients scanned with a 20 s scanner (Dixon *et al.*, 1981).

Intravenous contrast medium (e.g. 50 ml Conray 325) should be given if there is doubt about the presence or nature of a lesion on the initial scans or if the liver appears normal in a patient suspected of focal disease. Some lesions are obscured by contrast medium so that the initial scans must always be obtained without enhancement. There is increasing evidence that enhancement of the liver is most effective if scans are obtained immediately after the injection of intravenous contrast medium, especially when using fast scanners. In this way, scans are obtained when the liver parenchyma is opacified but the tumour has not yet taken up the contrast medium (Kreel, 1979; Osteaux *et al.*, 1980).

The biliary tract can be outlined after the administration of an appropriate contrast medium, either calcium ipodate (Solubiloptin) orally or ioglycamate (Biligram) intravenously.

The density of focal lesions, especially metastases, is often only slightly different from that of the surrounding liver parenchyma. To ensure optimum appreciation of minor density differences, the liver must always be viewed with a narrow window width

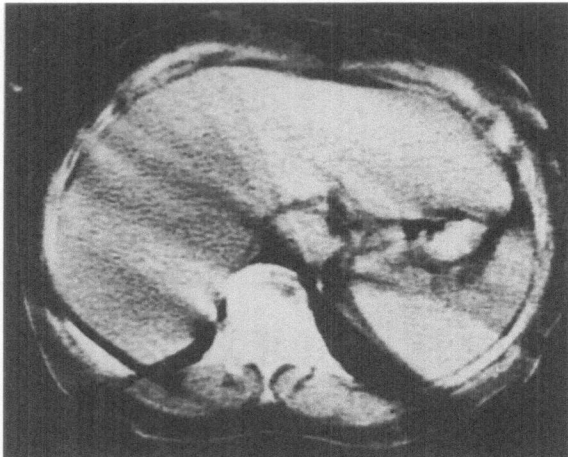

Figure 8.1(a)

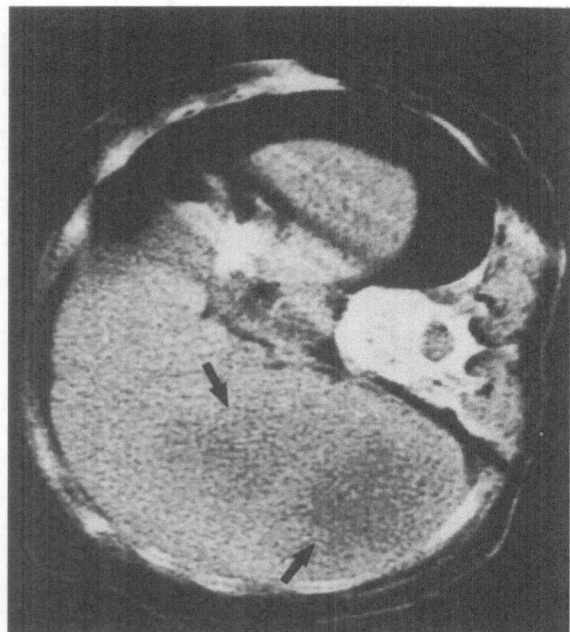

Figure 8.1(b)

Figure 8.1   Effect of decubitus position on artefacts. (a) Streak artefacts across the liver in the supine position. (b) Scan in the right lateral decubitus position. The liver is now free of artefacts and two large metastases (arrowed) are seen in the right lobe which were not identified in the supine position

and at a window level between 25 and 35 EMI units corresponding to the attenuation value of normal liver tissue (*see* chapter 2).

CT ANATOMY

The gross anatomy of the liver is clearly seen in cross section (figure 8.2). The porta hepatis is shown as a horizontal fat-containing cleft entering the hilum of the liver. Running anteriorly from it is another cleft containing the falciform ligament, separating the right and left lobes. The quadrate lobe lies anteriorly between the falciform ligament and the bed of the gall-bladder. At a slightly higher level, the caudate lobe lies above and behind the porta hepatis (figure 8.3) and in front of and lateral to the inferior vena cava. Occasionally the right lobe is prolonged downwards (Reidel's lobe) and may present as a mass lying laterally in the abdomen (figure 8.4).

The porta hepatis is bounded by the left lobe and the quadrate lobe anteriorly and the caudate lobe posteriorly. It contains the portal vein, the hepatic artery and its main branches, the common bile duct, right and left hepatic ducts, nerves and lymph nodes.

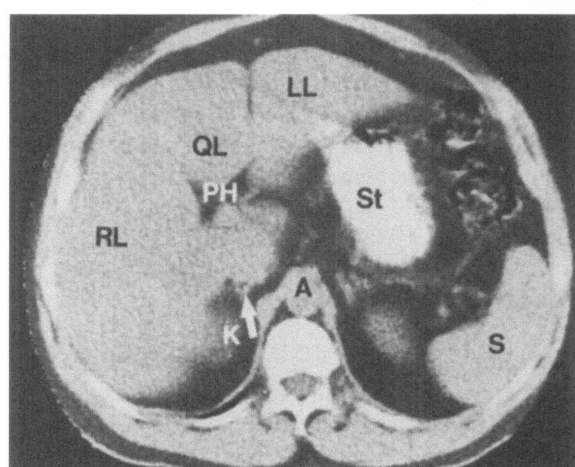

Figure 8.2   Normal liver. Right lobe (RL), left lobe (LL), quadrate lobe (QL), porta hepatis (PH), stomach (St), aorta (A) and spleen (S). Upper pole of right kidney (K), adrenal gland (arrowed)

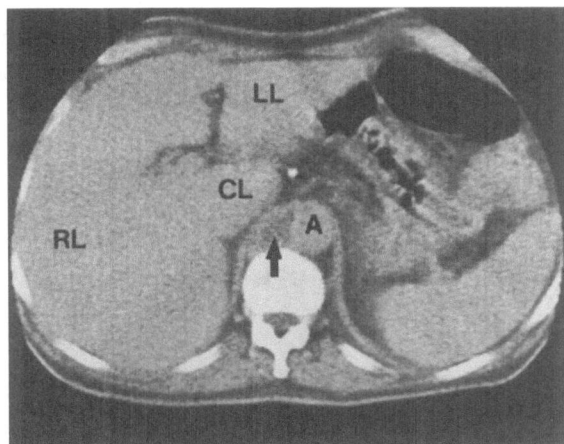

Figure 8.3   Normal liver. Right lobe (RL), left lobe (LL), caudate lobe (CL), aorta (A). Note enlarged retrocrural lymph node (arrowed)

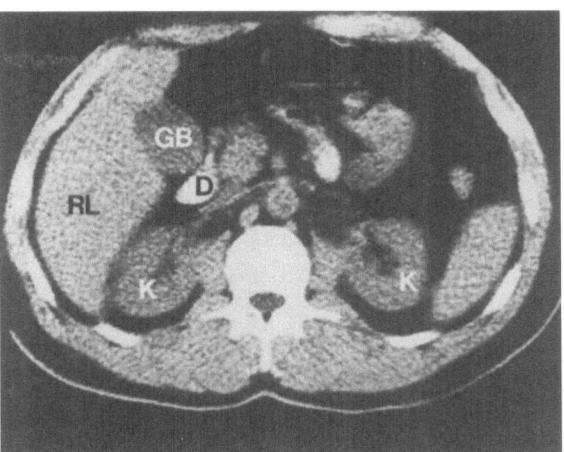

Figure 8.5   Normal liver. Right lobe (RL), kidneys (K), duodenum (D) and gall-bladder (GB)

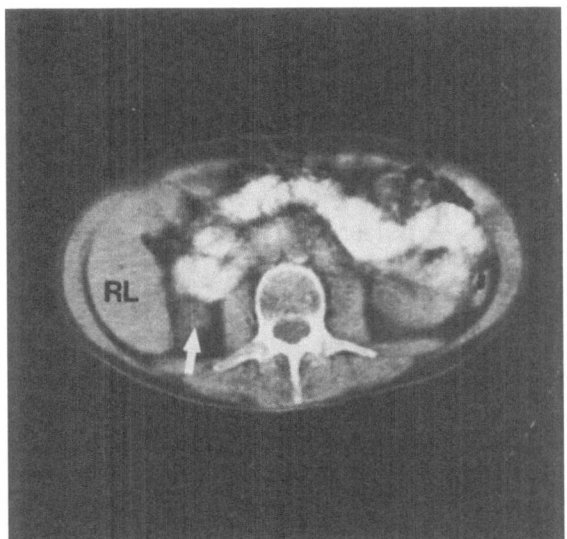

Figure 8.4   Reidel's lobe (RL). The liver extends into the lower abdomen below the right kidney (arrowed)

In patients with sufficient fat, the main vessels and ducts can be identified as separate structures, the common bile duct lying anteriorly to the portal vein and laterally to the hepatic artery.

The convexity of the liver close to the diaphragm is surrounded by lung in the costophrenic recesses. The right lobe is in contact with the adrenal and

kidney posteromedially (figure 8.5, and *see* figure 8.2). At the diaphragmatic hiatus, the right lobe is separated from the aorta only by the crus of the diaphragm. More anteriorly and caudally, the right lobe of the liver is related to the lesser sac and the second part of the duodenum (figure 8.5). The left lobe of the liver is very variable in shape and size, and in its relationship to the stomach. In some patients it extends far to the left, and in others it does not even reach the midline. When it extends to the left, it lies in front of the stomach, which indents it posteriorly (figure 8.6).

The liver is an almost completely intraperitoneal structure and is suspended from the diaphragm by the peritoneal folds bounding the bare area. Medially, the peritoneal cavity extends between the liver and the right kidney, forming Morison's pouch, which may be seen filled with bowel in normal patients (figure 8.7) and which is a common site for the accumulation of ascites or pus.

The gall-bladder is seen as a pear-shaped or circular area of low density situated on the inferomedial aspect of the right lobe (*see* figure 8.5). On upper CT sections it may appear to be completely embedded in liver tissue, emerging to lie medially in the lower cuts, lying on the lateral side of the second part of the duodenum. Occasionally it lies wholly within the liver. The wall is normally no more than 1 or 2 mm thick and is frequently

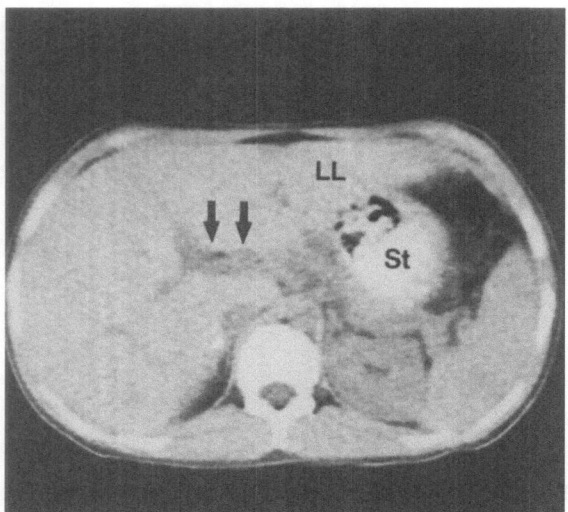

Figure 8.6   Normal liver. The left lobe (LL) lies anterior to the stomach (St). Portal vein (arrowed)

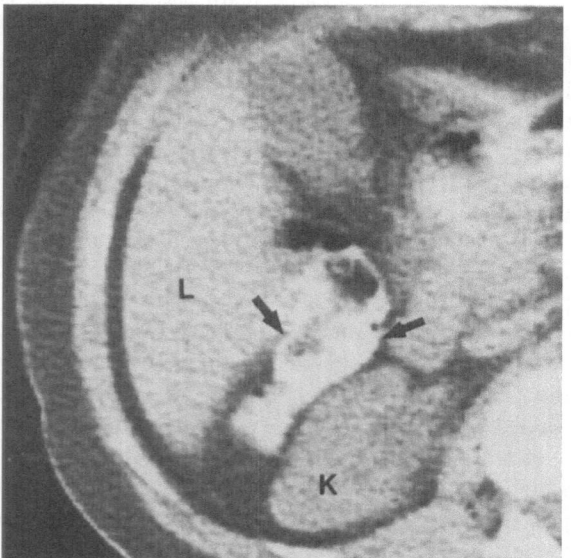

Figure 8.7   Morison's pouch. Bowel in Morison's pouch (arrowed) which lies between the kidney (K) and right lobe of the liver (L)

imperceptible. The intrahepatic bile ducts are not visible within the hepatic parenchyma unless they are dilated or contain air or contrast medium.

Similarly, the undilated common duct cannot usually be identified without contrast medium using

a 20 s scanner, but is visualised in about 50% of cases after Solubiloptin (Kreel, 1979). When dilated, it can be seen as a low-density structure emerging from the porta hepatis and is also seen end-on as it enters the head of the pancreas.

The portal vein lies very close behind the head of the pancreas and is difficult to identify without contrast medium (figure 8.8).

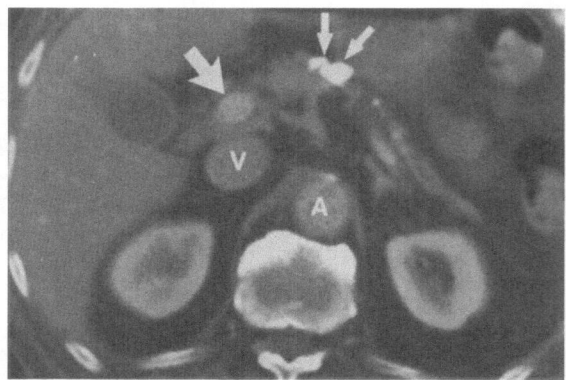

Figure 8.8   Scan   showing   vascular   enhancement immediately   after   injection   of   intravenous   contrast medium using 4.2 s scan time (Philips Tomoscanner 300) showing   portal   vein   (large   arrow)   and   other   major vessels. Note calcification in the pancreas (small arrows). Aorta (A), inferior vena cava (V). (Reproduced by kind permission of Dr Robinson, Leeds General Infirmary)

The density of the liver varies from patient to patient but it is usually slightly denser than other intra-abdominal organs (*see* figures 8.5 and 8.6), its attenuation values in normal subjects ranging from 25 to 40 EMI units. These attenuation values are higher than those expected for blood vessels, so that the major portal radicals and the inferior vena cava can often be identified as areas of relatively low density within the surrounding liver parenchyma (figure 8.9). When the main portal vein runs in the plane of the scan, it appears as a 1 to 2 cm band of relatively low density running almost horizontally into the liver from the porta hepatis (*see* figure 8.6). The intrahepatic portal veins are shown as circular or branching structures converging towards the porta hepatis and may be seen in continuity on contiguous slices (Kressel *et al.*, 1977). The inferior vena cava lies posteromedially just behind or within the caudate lobe (figure 8.9).

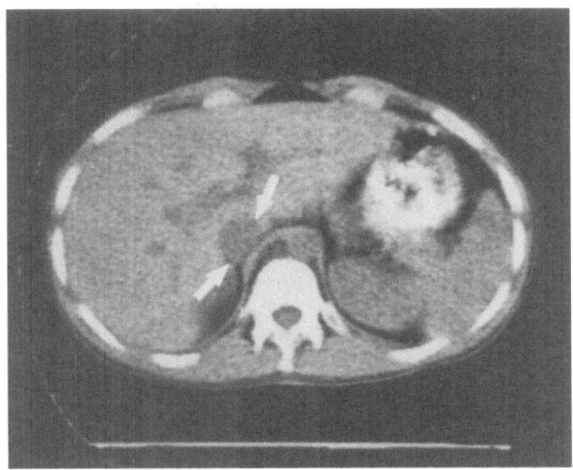

Figure 8.9   Normal liver. The portal vein and its main branches are seen as low-density structures branching through the liver parenchyma. The inferior vena cava has a similar density (arrowed)

Relative attenuation values of liver parenchyma and blood vary widely, so that the intrahepatic vessels are seen much more easily in some patients than in others, and may not be recognised at all when the attenuation value for blood approaches that for the liver parenchyma (New and Aronow,

1976). After injection of contrast medium, the vessels may appear denser than the surrounding liver tissue or isodense with it depending on the rate of injection, the scan time and the time after injection (figures 8.8, 8.9 and 8.10). The vessels can be distinguished from dilated bile ducts because the latter are less dense and do not enhance with intravenous contrast medium.

FOCAL LIVER DISEASE

Primary or Secondary Tumours

These are usually seen as areas of diminished density with attenuation values 10 to 15 EMI units lower than that of normal liver (figure 8.11). Sometimes the lesion will contain a central area of even lower density (figure 8.12). This is often regarded as evidence of necrosis, although *in vitro* studies suggest that central areas of low density can be seen without evidence of necrosis (Scherer *et al.*, 1979). Some tumours appear denser than the normal liver

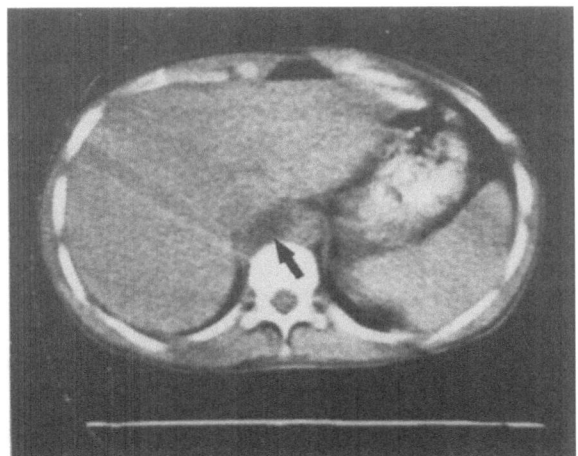

Figure 8.10   CT scan in the same patient as shown in figure 8.9 after injection of intravenous contrast medium. The portal vessels and inferior vena cava are isodense with the normal liver and cannot be identified. Note enlarged retrocrural node mass on the right (arrowed)

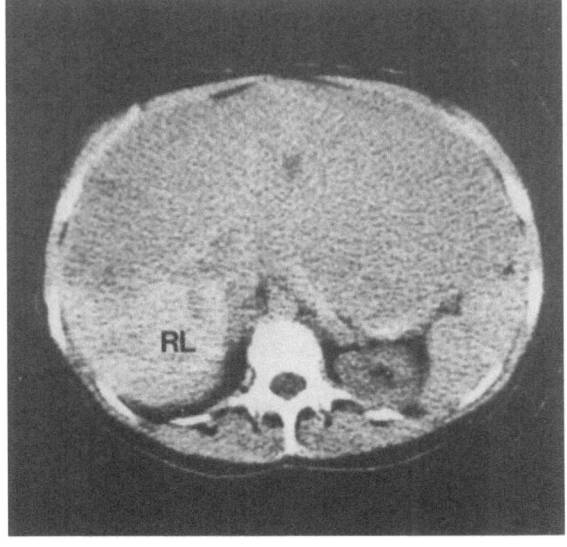

Figure 8.11(a)

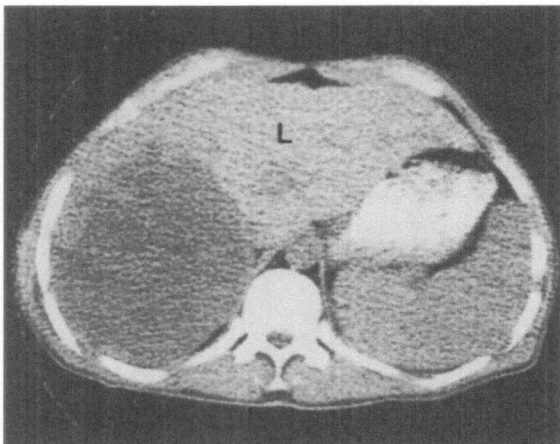

Figure 8.11(b)

Figure 8.11 Liver tumours. (a) Primary hepatoma of the liver. The lesion has a lower density than the normal right lobe (RL). (b) Large solitary metastasis in right lobe of the liver which also has a lower density than the normal liver (L)

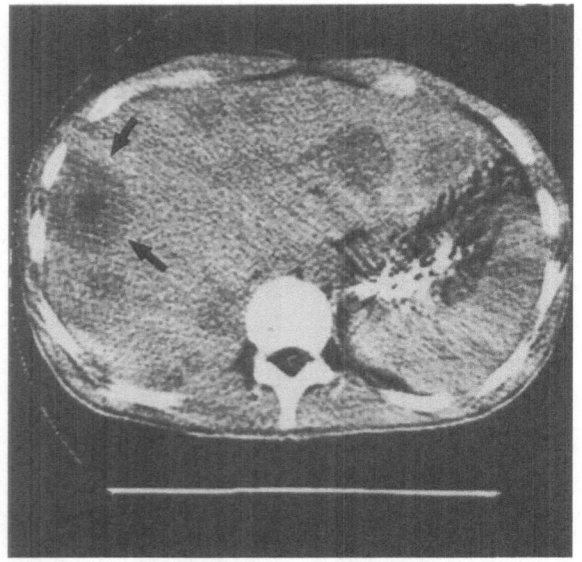

Figure 8.12 Multiple liver metastases. One of these lesions (arrowed) has a central area of low density, presumably due to central necrosis

and some calcify, the calcification being more readily detected by CT than by plain radiography (figure 8.13). Occasionally tumours are isodense

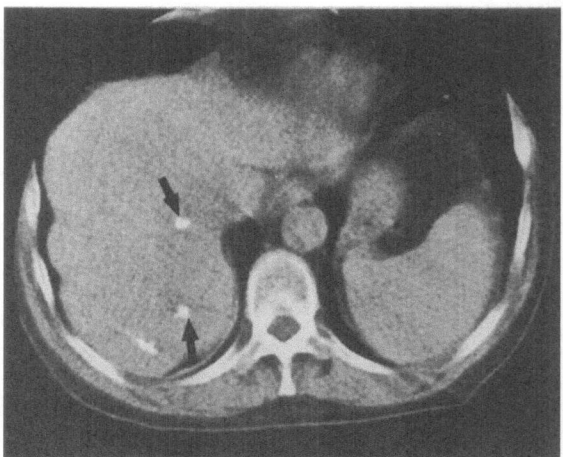

Figure 8.13 Multiple calcified metastases in a patient with carcinoid syndrome (arrowed)

with normal liver tissue. This is particularly likely to be so with the diffusely infiltrating type of hepatoma which merges imperceptibly with the liver parenchyma. In such cases, the scan may appear normal unless there is an alteration of liver contour.

Small metastases may have to be differentiated from portal vein radicals and dilated bile ducts. The distinction can usually be made because these latter structures are more uniform in size and shape than metastases, have a more clearly defined edge, are evenly distributed except for the periphery and may show a branching pattern (Kressel *et al.*, 1977). Examination of adjacent sections will reveal continuity of vascular and biliary channels. In cases of doubt, the injection of intravenous contrast medium will distinguish metastases from veins, but, in the presence of dilated bile ducts, metastases may be impossible to detect unless they lie at the periphery.

Tumours may be seen better after enhancement of the normal parenchyma (figure 8.14) but this is not always so because tumours may themselves enhance with contrast medium (Scherer *et al.*, 1978; Moss *et al.*, 1979). Occasionally tumours which are not visible on the unenhanced scan are revealed after enhancement. In the authors' experience, this is rare when the unenhanced scan is artefact-free and has been viewed at appropriate settings. The main role of enhancement in the detection of focal lesions in the

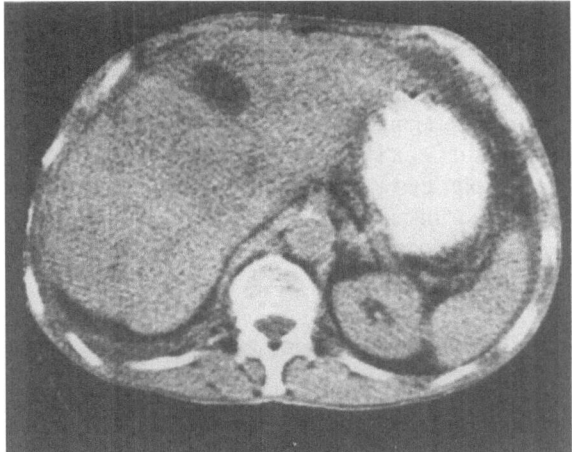

Figure 8.14(a)

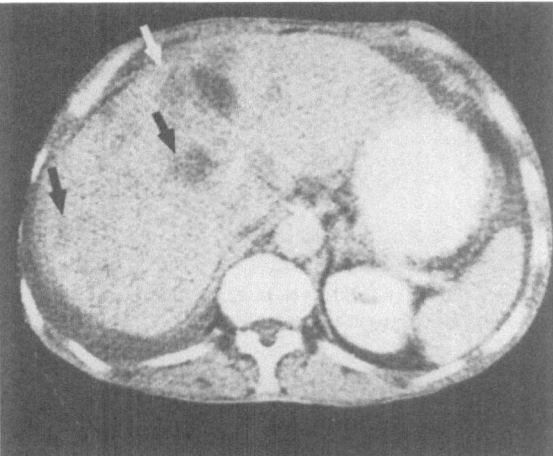

Figure 8.14(b)

Figure 8.14   Liver metastases. (a) Unenhanced scan. (b) Enhanced scan. The lesions (arrowed) are better demonstrated after enhancement

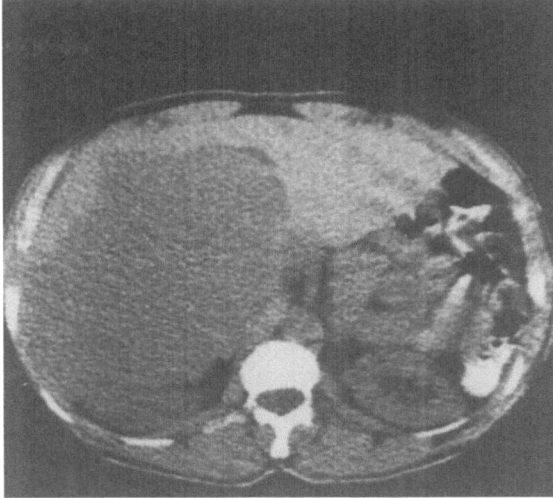

Figure 8.15(a)

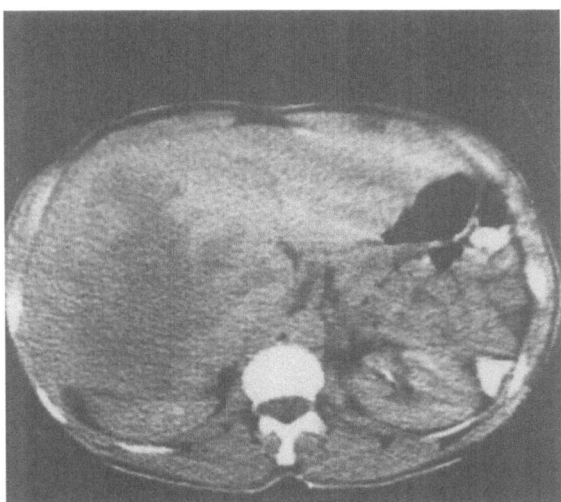

Figure 8.15(b)

Figure 8.15   Cavernous haemangioma of the right lobe of the liver. (a) Unenhanced scan. (b) Enhanced scan. There is irregular opacification of the haemangioma after enhancement

liver is to clarify the situation when there is doubt about the presence or nature of a lesion on the unenhanced scan.

Benign tumours cannot be distinguished from malignant tumours on the basis of CT alone. A possible exception is cavernous haemangioma, which may be suspected if there is obvious irregular opacification after the injection of intravenous contrast medium (figure 8.15).

Cysts

Cysts in the liver can usually be differentiated from solid tumours if they are greater than 1.5 to 2 cm in diameter (figure 8.16). They are seen as areas of lower density than tumours, their attenuation value

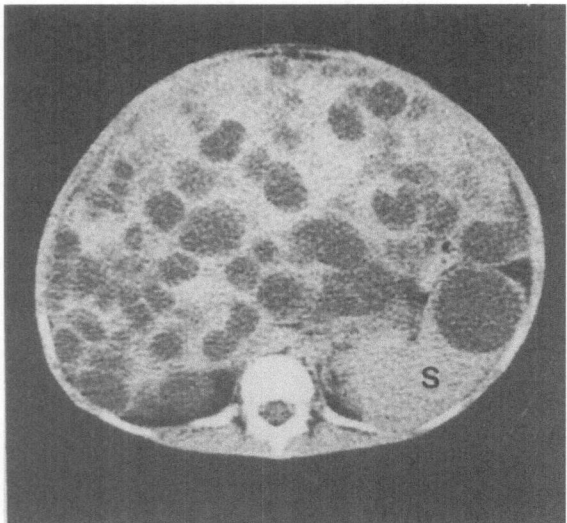

Figure 8.16   Multiple liver cysts. The lesions have a low density and are well defined. Note a solitary cyst in the spleen (S)

approaching that of water (0 to 10 EMI units) and the margins are more sharply defined. The larger the cyst, the easier it is to make a definite diagnosis. Cysts smaller than 2 cm may be affected by partial volume averaging and the attenuation values can be close to that of a solid tumour (figure 8.17).

Multiple cysts may be seen in patients with polycystic disease. Hydatid cysts may show a septate appearance (figure 8.18) and the wall may calcify.

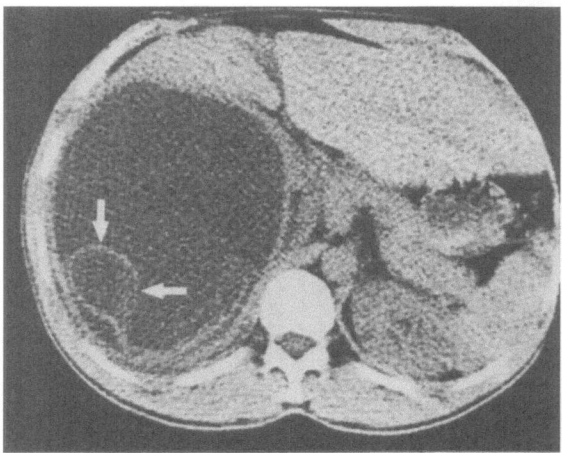

Figure 8.18   Hydatid cyst in the right lobe of the liver. Note possible daughter cyst (arrowed)

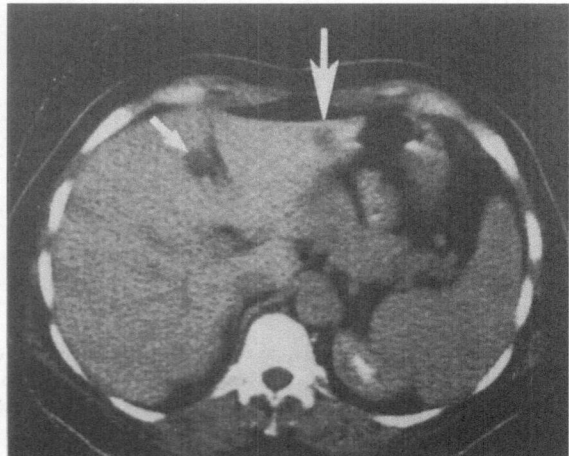

Figure 8.17   Benign liver cysts in a patient with carcinoma of the ovary. The lesion in the left lobe (large arrow) has a density similar to a solid tumour due to partial volume averaging. This lesion was aspirated under CT guidance and found to be a benign cyst. The lesion in the right lobe (small arrow) has a density close to that of water. The patient remains alive and well two years after the CT examination

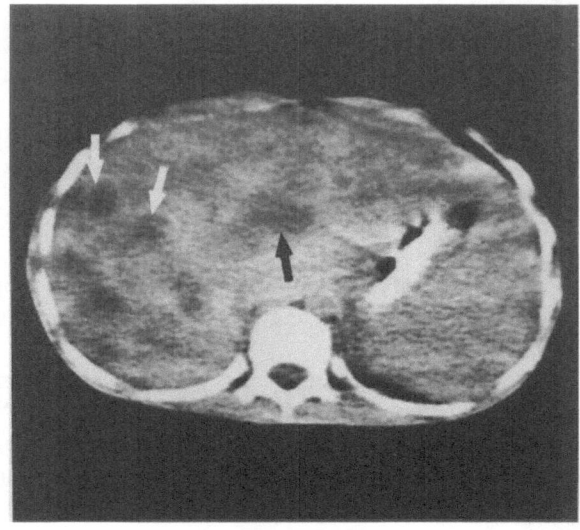

Figure 8.19(a)

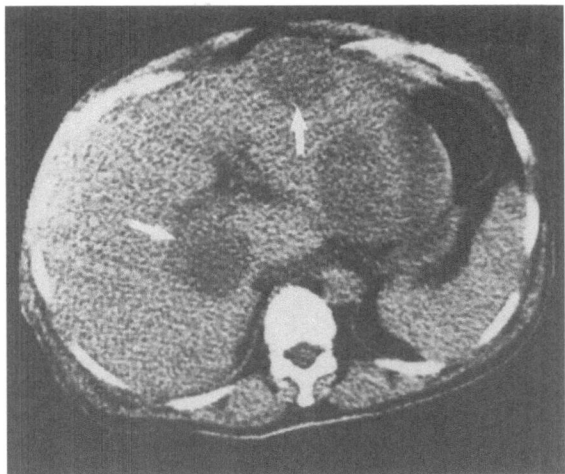

Figure 8.19(b)

Figure 8.19 Liver abscesses. (a) Multiple abscesses, some with a density similar to that of a cyst, others closer to that of soft tissues (arrowed). (b) Abscesses with a low density similar to that of a cyst (arrowed)

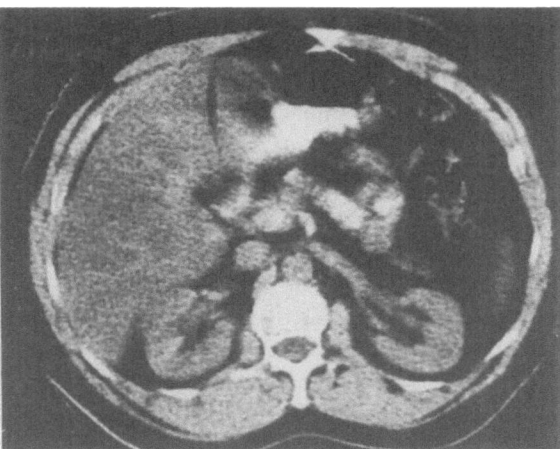

Figure 8.20(a)

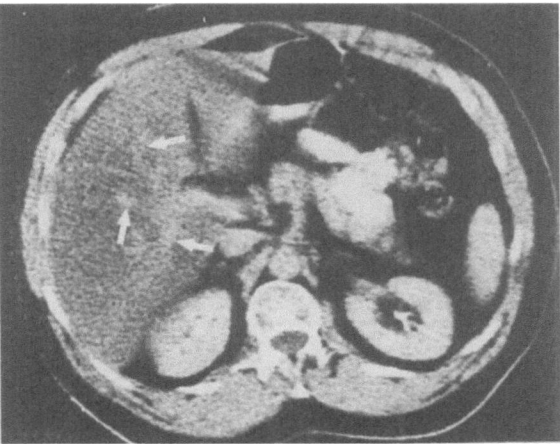

Figure 8.20(b)

Figure 8.20 Localised fatty infiltration in the right lobe of the liver. (a) Unenhanced scan and (b) enhanced scan. The lesion in the right lobe has a lower density than normal liver. After enhancement, vessels are seen passing through the lesion (arrowed) excluding a tumour. Subsequent liver biopsy showed fatty infiltration

Abscesses

Abscesses within the liver usually have an attenuation value less than that of a solid tumour and greater than that of a cyst (Levitt *et al.*, 1977). There is, however, considerable overlap, and it is not possible to make a confident diagnosis of abscess on the CT appearance without an appropriate clinical history (figure 8.19).

Fatty Infiltration (Localised)

This may occasionally be localised and may appear as a well defined focal low-density lesion on CT (figure 8.20). It has the characteristic features associated with generalised fatty infiltration and, once considered, presents little diagnostic difficulty.

Trauma

CT, not being organ-specific, is ideally suited to localising intra-abdominal bleeding. Most patients with severe acute trauma, however, require urgent surgery and are unlikely to be scanned. Sometimes, following less severe trauma, the possibility of

haematoma has to be considered. Intrahepatic and subcapsular haematomas will be clearly seen, the density of the haematoma varying with its age.

DIFFUSE LIVER DISEASE

CT has a very limited role in the diagnosis and management of patients with diffuse liver disease.

The shape of the liver is so variable that only obvious enlargement or shrinkage can be diagnosed with any confidence. CT does, however, allow valid observations about change in size over a period of time.

Cirrhosis

In the early stages of cirrhosis, the liver may be enlarged and may show fatty infiltration. Later, it may become contracted with areas of nodular hyperplasia leading to irregularity of the outline (figure 8.21). Careful analysis of the CT numbers in cirrhotic livers has shown that there is a detectable variation when compared with normal livers (Ritchings *et al.*, 1979). The difference is, however, difficult to detect and is of no clinical significance at the present time. It is, however, of considerable interest as an indication of the way in which CT may develop in the future.

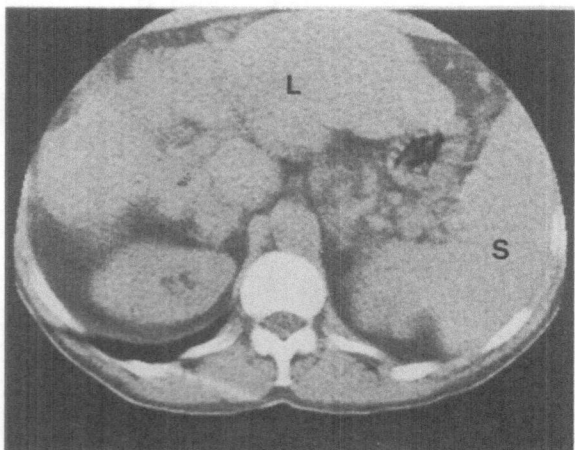

Figure 8.21 Cirrhosis of the liver. There is gross irregularity of the liver contour (L). Note enlarged spleen (S)

Fatty Infiltration

This reduces the density of the liver. The attenuation value approaches that of fat but the precise value depends on the proportion of fat to normal liver tissue. A striking feature is the way in which even unenhanced portal vessels are displayed as higher-density branching structures within the low-density

liver parenchyma (figure 8.22). The fat is usually distributed evenly through the liver but, as already mentioned, is occasionally localised.

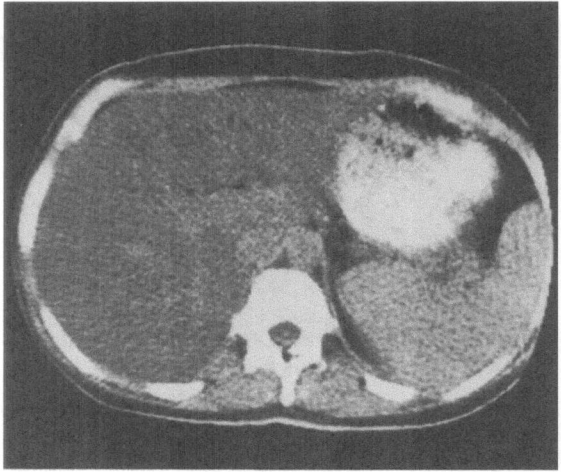

Figure 8.22(a)

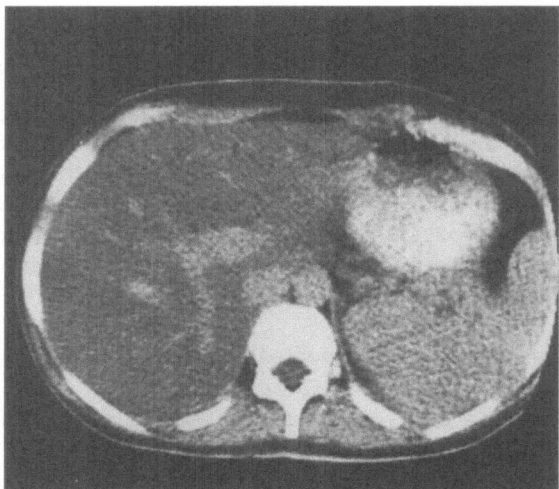

Figure 8.22(b)

Figure 8.22 Diffuse fatty infiltration. (a) Unenhanced scan and (b) enhanced scan. After enhancement, the vessels are seen as high-density structures coursing through the liver

Haemochromatosis

In this and other conditions with iron overload, the liver may appear denser than normal. Changes in the attenuation value of the liver reflect the changes in its iron content (Houang *et al.*, 1979; Chapman *et al.*, 1980).

GALL-BLADDER DISEASE

Calcified gallstones are readily identified with CT (figure 8.23) and may be seen when not visible on plain radiographs. Havrilla *et al.* (1978) report a series of 17 patients in whom gallstones were

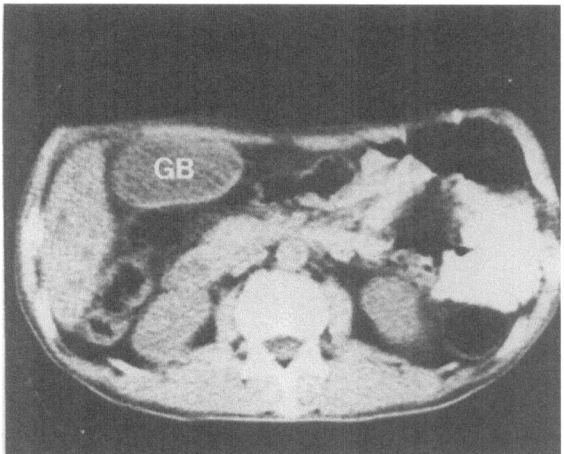

Figure 8.24 **CT scan in a patient with chronic pancreatitis and cholecystitis. The gall-bladder (GB) is dilated and the wall thickened. Note low-density areas in the right lobe of the liver. These represent dilated intrahepatic bile ducts**

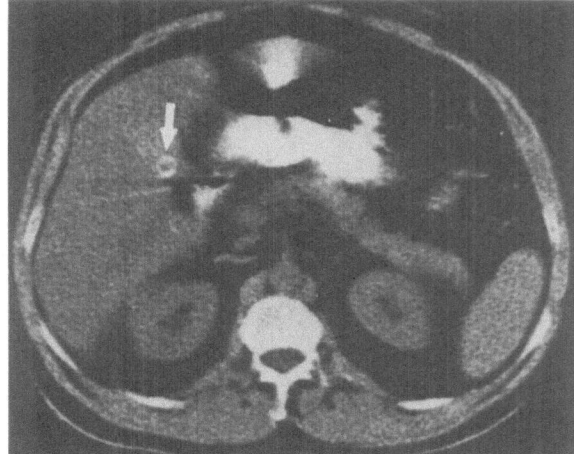

Figure 8.23 **Calcified gallstone (arrowed)**

demonstrated with CT. In only five of these was there evidence of calcification on the plain radiograph. Many gallstones, however, remain 'non-opaque' even with CT because the high cholesterol content makes them virtually isodense with bile.

Extrahepatic Biliary Obstruction

In patients with such an obstruction, the gall-bladder and/or common duct and/or the intrahepatic ducts can be seen to be dilated. A dilated gall-bladder is usually easily identified (figure 8.24). Occasionally, when obstructed, it may become full of biliary sludge. When this occurs, the contents can have a density very close to that of the liver and other soft tissues (figure 8.25).

A dilated common duct can be identified as a low-density structure emerging from the porta hepatis.

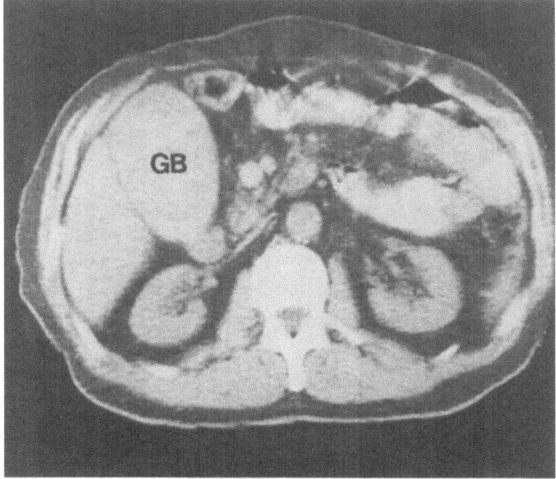

Figure 8.25 **Dilated gall-bladder (GB) containing biliary sludge, the density of which is very similar to that of the liver**

As it enters the head of the pancreas, it may be seen end-on (figure 8.26), particularly after enhancement of the pancreatic tissue which is opacified (Goldberg *et al.*, 1978).

Dilated intrahepatic bile ducts appear as low-density branching structures converging on the

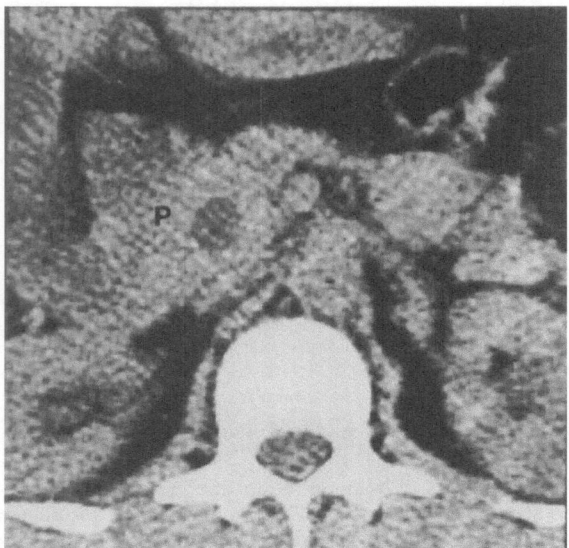

Figure 8.26   Chronic pancreatitis. The dilated common bile duct is seen 'end-on' as it passes through the head of the pancreas (P)

porta hepatis (figure 8.27). They are of lower density than portal venous radicles and are more sharply defined. In cases of doubt, intravenous contrast medium may be injected.

The intrahepatic bile ducts are not always dilated

in patients with obstructive jaundice (Shanser *et al.*, 1978). It is, therefore, important to look for common duct dilatation in jaundice patients when no dilated intrahepatic ducts are seen.

A thickened gall-bladder wall suggests *acute* or *chronic* cholecystitis (*see* figure 8.24). Solomon *et al.*

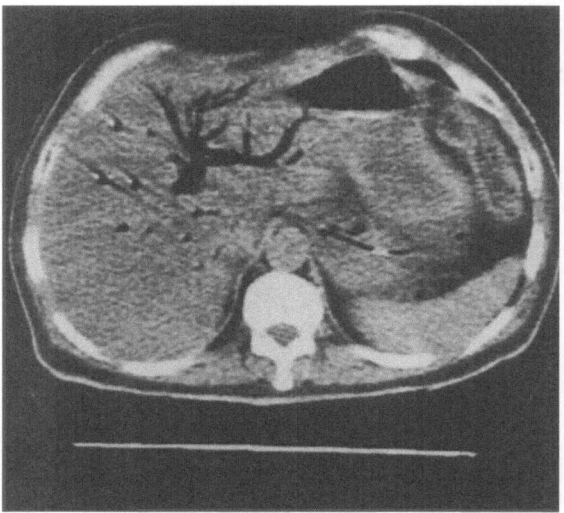

Figure 8.28(a)

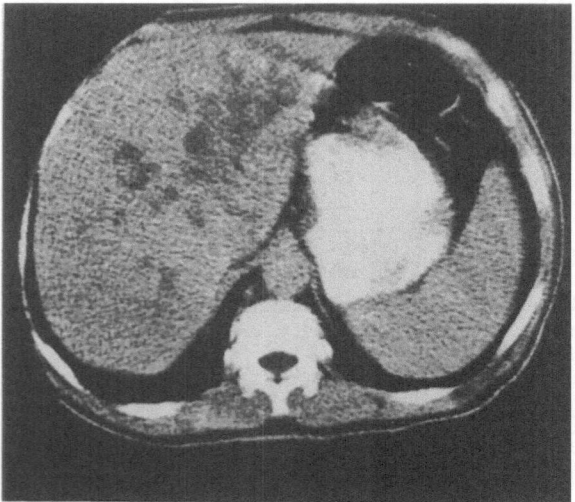

Figure 8.27   Dilated intrahepatic bile ducts. These appear as low-density branching structures within the liver parenchyma

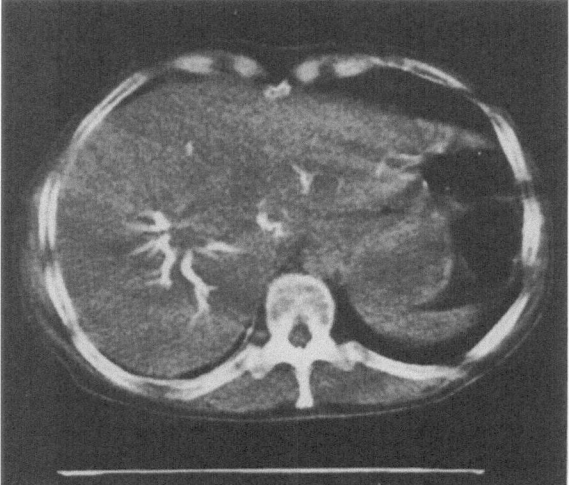

Figure 8.28(b)

Figure 8.28   The intrahepatic biliary tree. (a) Air within the biliary tree in a patient with carcinoma of the head of the pancreas in whom a cholecyst-jejunostomy has been performed. (b) Normal-sized ducts opacified after the administration of Solubiloptin for comparison

(1979) reported patients in whom the demonstration of a thick wall enhancing after intravenous contrast medium in a distended gall-bladder was valuable confirmatory evidence of acute cholecystitis in an appropriate clinical situation.

Air Within the Biliary Tree

This is easily recognised because of the high degree of contrast between it and the surrounding liver; the ducts can be seen extending almost to the periphery (figure 8.28).

USE AND ACCURACY OF COMPUTED TOMOGRAPHY

The main uses of CT in liver disease are the detection and diagnosis of space-occupying lesions and the differential diagnosis of jaundice.

Motion artefacts are the main factors limiting the detection of focal lesions in the liver, especially when using a 20 s scanner. Lesions may be obscured by the artefacts or the artefacts themselves may be mistaken for abnormalities.

Cysts and abscesses can be shown without difficulty because their low density is easily detected within the liver parenchyma. Solid lesions, particularly metastases, are less easily detected. Even with enhancement and with the careful use of appropriate window settings, scans for the presence of metastatic disease are, in the authors' experience, one of the most difficult types of scan to interpret with confidence. Even so, with increasing experience and the development of faster scanners, accuracy rates of about 90% for the detection of focal liver lesions have been reported (Scherer *et al.*, 1978; Snow *et al.*, 1979).

CT will sometimes establish the nature of a focal lesion. Cysts, including hydatid cysts, are usually easily distinguished, but it should be remembered that metastases can occasionally be cystic (figures 8.29 and 8.30). Abscesses are frequently of sufficiently low density to distinguish them from solid lesions. The appearances of solid lesions are, however, usually non-specific, so that a tissue

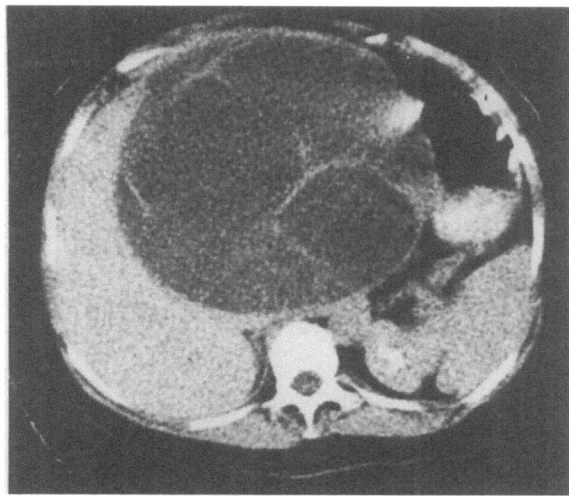

Figure 8.29(a)

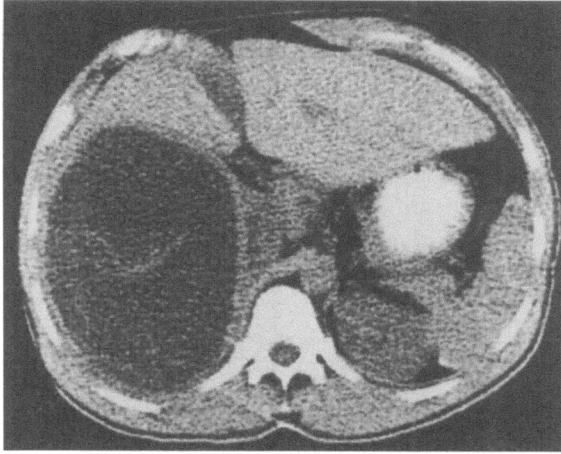

Figure 8.29(b)

Figure 8.29 Two patients with cystic lesions of the liver which have identical appearances. (a) Hydatid cyst. (b) Metastasis from carcinoma of the ovary

diagnosis cannot be established on CT grounds alone. When biopsy is indicated, CT can be useful for guiding a needle, especially when the lesion is small (figure 8.30).

In diffuse liver disease, CT is at present a relatively crude technique and is of very limited value. In a report by Levitt *et al.* (1977), only 10 out of 22 cases of cirrhosis were recognised with CT. Houang *et al.* (1979) and Chapman *et al.* (1980)

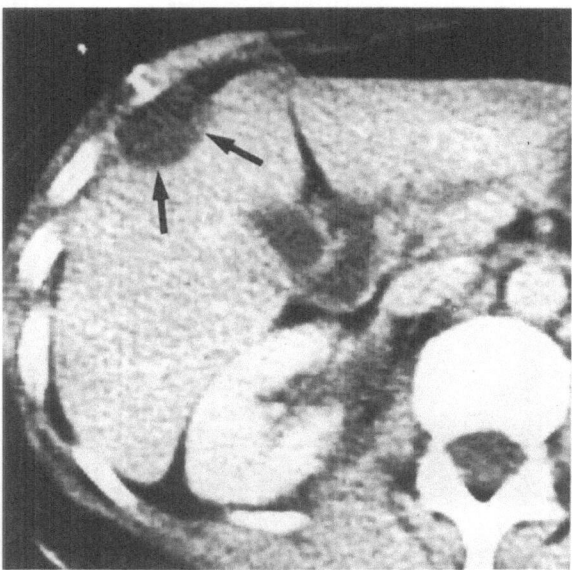

Figure 8.30(a)

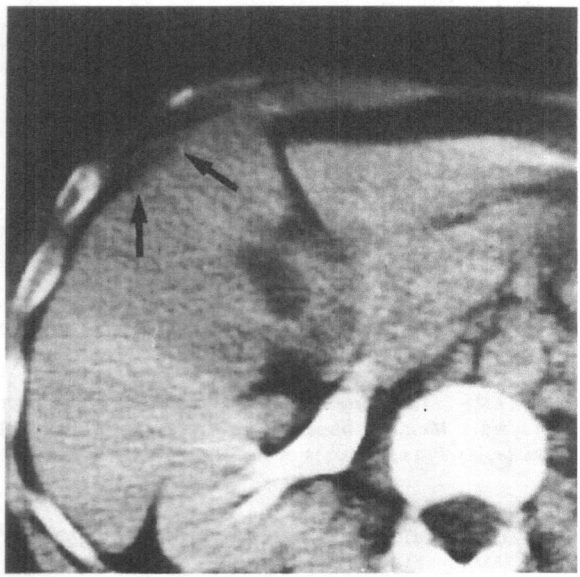

Figure 8.30(b)

Figure 8.30   CT scans in a patient with carcinoma of the ovary. (a) This scan demonstrated a low-density cystic lesion arising from the anterior aspect of the right lobe of the liver (arrowed). CT-guided aspiration of this lesion was performed and cytology revealed malignant cells. (b) Post-aspiration scan showing reduction in size of the lesion (arrowed)

have suggested that CT may have a place in following progress in patients with haemochromatosis and other conditions associated with iron overload.

In patients with suspected extrahepatic biliary obstruction, the detection of dilated bile ducts confirms the diagnosis. Positive identification of dilated ducts is likely to be accurate. When only the common duct is dilated, diagnosis may not be so easy to establish. Thus, Goldberg *et al.* (1978) initially identified obstruction in only 15 out of 18 patients with extrahepatic biliary obstruction. On review, however, they were able to identify dilatation of the common duct in two of the remaining three patients.

Not only may a diagnosis of extrahepatic biliary obstruction be substantiated by CT but the cause of the obstruction can also frequently be identified (Stanley *et al.*, 1977; Levitt *et al.*, 1977). Haaga and Reich (1978) reported an accuracy of 77% in determining the underlying cause of obstruction in a series of 44 patients.

There is considerable overlap of information provided by CT, ultrasound and isotope techniques. The main limitation of ultrasound examination of the liver is that about 10% of examinations are technically unsuccessful. The accuracy of successful investigations is very similar to that reported for CT (Cosgrove and McCready, 1978).

Radionuclide imaging identifies most lesions greater than 3 cm. A major disadvantage is that no information is obtained regarding the composition of a 'cold' area and it may be difficult to distinguish a genuine focal lesion from anatomical variations (figure 8.31). Single focal lesions in problem areas, such as the porta hepatis or gall-bladder fossa, may be impossible to elucidate with radionuclide imaging alone.

As might be expected, reports of comparative assessments of the three techniques provide inconsistent results (Grossman *et al.*, 1977; Biello *et al.*, 1978; Snow *et al.*, 1979). Taking into account general availability, comfort, lack of hazard and cost, it would seem appropriate at the present time to use isotope techniques and ultrasound as initial screening procedures when seeking evidence of focal lesions, particularly metastatic disease, reserving CT for those patients in whom the results are equivocal.

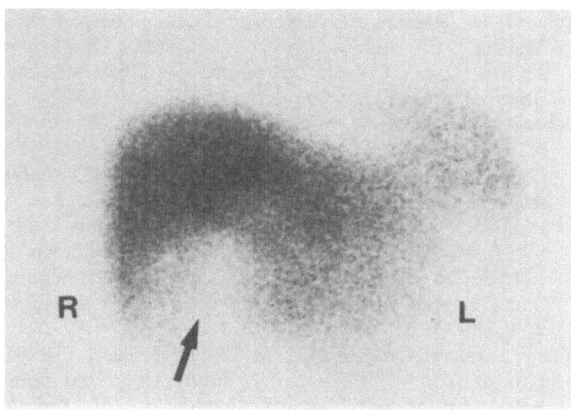

Figure 8.31(a)

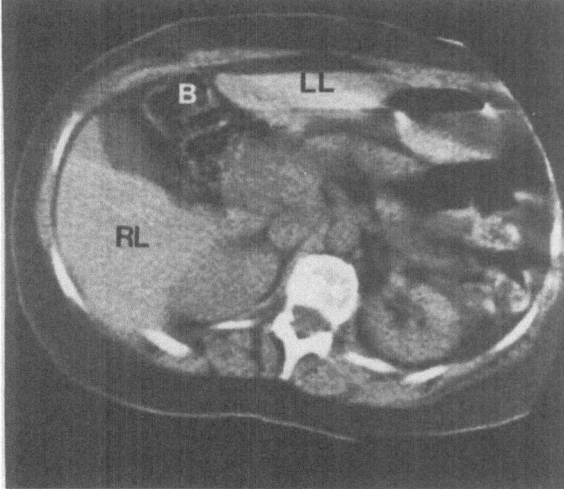

Figure 8.31(b)

Figure 8.31 (a) Radionuclide scan and (b) CT scan in a patient with carcinoma of the breast. The radionuclide scan suggested a large focal lesion in the anterior aspect of the right lobe of the liver (arrowed). A CT examination was therefore performed and showed that the right lobe (RL) is separate from the left lobe. The space between the lobes is occupied by bowel (B) and fat

Isotope studies provide no information about the nature of a focal lesion. Ultrasound and CT are complementary in this respect.

Evaluation of obstructive jaundice appears to be equally successful with CT and ultrasound. Both achieve accuracy rates of over 90% in detecting extrahepatic biliary obstruction (Taylor and McCready, 1976; Havrilla *et al.*, 1978; Goldberg *et al.*, 1978). Ultrasound is, therefore, the imaging investigation of first choice in this situation when the appropriate expertise is available, CT being reserved for those patients in whom the ultrasound is unsuccessful or the findings are equivocal.

REFERENCES

Biello, D. R., Levitt, R. G., Siegel, B. A., Sagel, S. S. and Stanley, R. J. (1978). Computed tomography and radionuclide imaging of the liver: a comparative evaluation. *Radiology*, **127**, 159–163

Chapman, R. W. G., Williams, G., Bydder, G., Dick, R., Sherlock, S. and Kreel, L. (1980). Computed tomography for determining liver iron content in primary haemochromatosis. *British Medical Journal*, **1**, 440–442

Cosgrove, D. O. and McCready, V. R. (1978). Diagnosis of liver metastases using ultrasound and isotope scanning techniques. *Journal of Royal Society of Medicine*, **71**, 652–657

Dixon, A. K., Stringer, D. A., Hallett, M. G. and Fry, I. K. (1981). The use of the right decubitus position in computerised tomography of the liver and pancreas. *Clinical Radiology*, **132**, 113–116

Goldberg, H. I., Filly, R. A., Korobkin, M., Moss, A. A., Kressel, H. Y. and Callen, P. W. (1978). Capability of CT body scanning and ultrasonography to demonstrate the status of the biliary ductal system in patients with jaundice. *Radiology*, **129**, 731–737

Grossman, Z. D., Wisto, B. W., Bryan, P. J., Dinn, W. M., McAfee, J. G. and Kieffer, S. A. (1977). Radionuclide imaging, computed tomography and gray-scale ultrasonography of the liver: a comparative study. *Journal of Nuclear Medicine*, **18**, 327–332

Haaga, J. and Reich, N. E. (1978). In *Computed Tomography of Abdominal Abnormalities*, Mosby, St Louis, pp. 39–85

Havrilla, T. R., Reich, N. E., Haaga, J. R., Seidelmann, F. E., Cooperman, A. M. and Alfidi, R. J. (1978). Computed tomography of the gallbladder. *American Journal of Roentgenology*, **130**, 1059–1067

Houang, M. T. W., Aruzena, Z., Skalicka, A., Huehns, E. R. and Shaw, D. G. (1979). Correlation between computed tomographic values and liver iron content in thalassaemia major with iron overload. *Lancet*, **i**, 1322–1323

Kreel, L. (1979). In *Medical Imaging*, ed. L. Kreel, H M & M Publishers, Aylesbury

Kressel, H. Y., Korobkin, M., Goldberg, H. I. and Moss, A. A. (1977). The portal venous tree simulating dilated biliary ducts on computed tomography of the liver. *Journal of Computer Assisted Tomography*, 1, 169–175

Levitt, R. G., Sagel, S. S., Stanley, R. J. and Jost, R. G. (1977). Accuracy of computed tomography of the liver and biliary tract. *Radiology*, 124, 123–128

Moss, A. A., Schrumpf, J., Schynder, P., Korobkin, M. and Shimshak, R. R. (1979). Computed tomography of focal hepatic lesions: a blind clinical evaluation of the effect of contrast enhancement. *Radiology*, 131, 427–430

New, P. F. J. and Aronow, S. (1976). Attenuation measurements of whole blood and blood fractions in computed tomography. *Radiology*, 121, 635–640

Osteaux, M., Peetrons, P., Shita-Hayer, F., Matelart, A. L. and Jeanmart, L. (1980). Appearance and disappearance of hepatic metastases in contrasted CT: a better comprehension by anatomical and microangiographic confrontations. Presented at the *International Symposium on Whole Body Computed Tomography, 5th CARVAT*, Rome, May 1980

Ritchings, R. T., Pullan, B. P., Lucas, S. B., Fawcitt, R. A., Best, J. F. K., Isherwood, I. and Morris, I. A. (1979). An analysis of the spatial distribution of attenuation values in computed tomographic scans of the liver and spleen. *Journal of Computer Assisted Tomography*, 3 (1), 36–39

Scherer, U., Rainier, R., Eisenburg, J., Schildberg, F. W., Meister, P. and Lissner, J. (1978). Diagnostic accuracy of CT in circumscript liver disease. *American Journal of Roentgenology*, 130, 711–714

Scherer, U., Santos, M. and Lissner, J. (1979). CT studies of the liver *in vitro*: a report on 82 cases with pathological correlation. *Journal of Computer Assisted Tomography*, 3, 589–595

Shanser, J. D., Korobkin, M., Goldberg, H. I. and Rohlfing, B. M. (1978). Computed tomographic diagnosis of obstructive jaundice in the absence of intrahepatic ductal dilatation. *American Journal of Roentgenology*, 131, 389–392

Snow, J. H., Jr, Goldstein, H. M. and Wallace, S. (1979). Comparison of scintigraphy, sonography and computed tomography in the evaluation of hepatic neoplasms. *American Journal of Roentgenology*, 132, 915–918

Solomon, A., Kreel, L. and Pinto, D. (1979). Contrast computed tomography in the diagnosis of acute cholecystitis. *Journal of Computer Assisted Tomography*, 3, 585–589

Stanley, R. J., Sagel, S. S. and Levitt, R. G. (1977). Computed tomography of the liver. *Radiologic Clinics of North America*, 15, 331–348

Taylor, K. J. W. and McCready, V. R. (1976). A clinical evaluation of grey-scale ultrasonography. *British Journal of Radiology*, 49, 244–252

9

The Abdomen – Pancreas

CT would seem particularly well suited to delineating an organ lying, like the pancreas, mainly in the transverse axial plane. In practice, it has definite limitations, particularly in thin patients. Even so, it seems to be the most effective technique currently available.

TECHNIQUE OF EXAMINATION

The CT appearances vary so much from patient to patient and the interpretation of scans in the region of the pancreas needs so much care that examination of this area requires meticulous supervision by the radiologist.

Oral contrast medium and an anticholinergic agent are given as already described for the general examination of the abdomen. The patient should lie on his/her right side after the last dose of oral contrast medium to ensure filling of the second part of the duodenum. Scans are initially obtained at 1 cm intervals through the gland but intervening slices may be required. The number of sections needed to

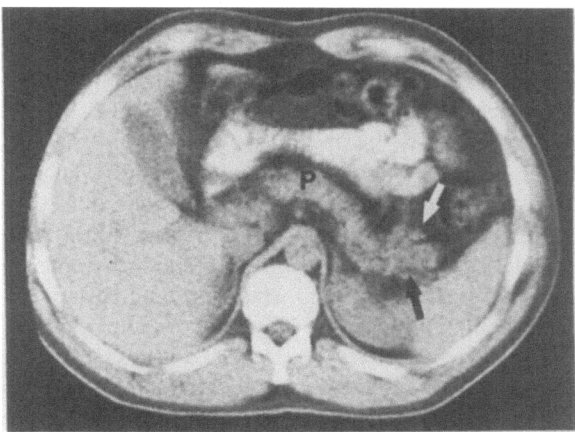

Figure 9.1(a)

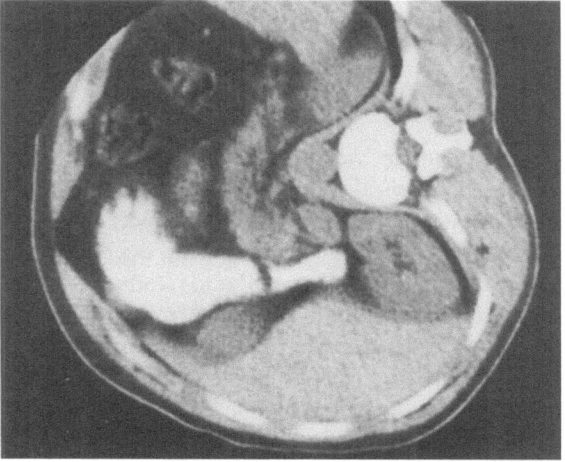

Figure 9.1(b)

Figure 9.1 Normal pancreas (P). (a) A loop of jejunum overlies the pancreatic tail (arrowed). (b) The right lateral decubitus position. The head of the pancreas is clearly separated from the second part of the duodenum. The pancreatic tail is not obscured

define the normal gland will vary according to its obliquity in the abdomen.

The patient is examined first in the supine position. If the pancreas is not clearly defined, it is worth repeating the examination in the right lateral decubitus position after further oral contrast medium. Not only does this ensure that the duodenal loop is outlined, so that the head is clearly defined, but it also results in the bowel moving anteriorly and caudally, so that the body and tail are not obscured (Haaga and Reich, 1978) (figure 9.1).

When densities are observed in or close to the pancreas, it may be difficult to determine whether these are due to calcification in the pancreas or contrast medium in the bowel. When this occurs, the patient should be re-examined omitting the oral contrast medium.

When using a 20 s scanner, we have not found the administration of intravenous contrast medium necessary as a routine procedure in the examination of patients with possible pancreatic disease. Parenchymal enhancement may, however, help in the detection of a dilated main pancreatic duct or a dilated common bile duct within the head of the pancreas (Lee *et al.*, 1979). Vascular enhancement will show the position of the portal or splenic veins when these cannot be seen to be separate from the pancreas and when there is anxiety about the size of the gland. In patients with suspected or established pancreatic carcinoma, enhancement may be indicated to identify metastases in the liver or dilated intrahepatic bile ducts.

CT ANATOMY

The pancreas is clearly seen in the majority of patients because it is surrounded by a layer of retroperitoneal fat. It lies obliquely in the retroperitoneal space, extending from the duodenum behind the transverse colon and stomach to the hilum of the spleen. It is bowed forwards in the midline over the superior mesenteric artery, aorta and vertebra (figure 9.2a). The body thus lies in front of the mid-coronal plane, more anteriorly than is generally expected. In thin patients, it may be very close to the anterior abdominal wall (figure 9.2b).

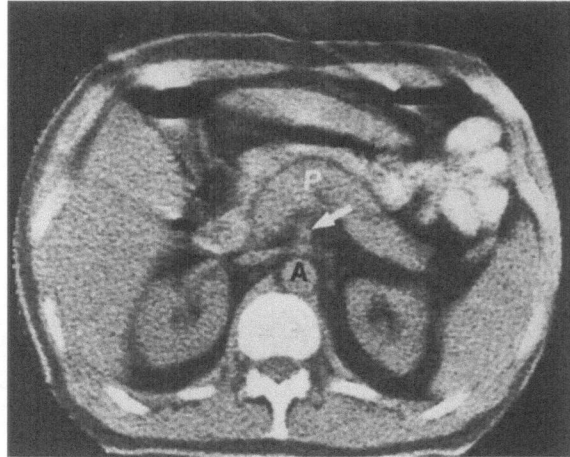

Figure 9.2(a)

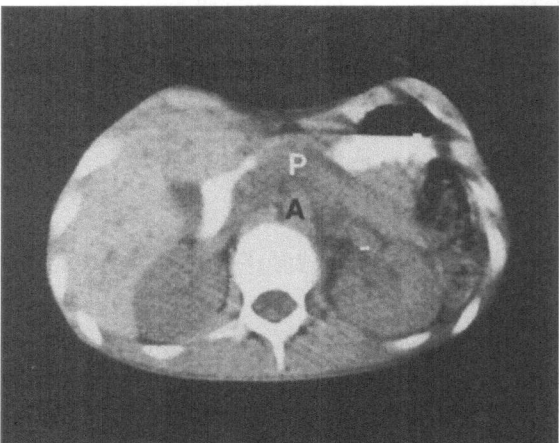

Figure 9.2(b)

Figure 9.2 **Normal pancreas (P). (a) Patient with plenty of intra-abdominal fat. (b) Thin patient. Aorta (A), superior mesenteric artery (arrowed)**

The *head* of the pancreas lies within the curve of the duodenum, behind the antrum of the stomach and first part of the duodenum; it is related posteriorly to the inferior vena cava (figure 9.3a). The left renal vein joins the inferior vena cava just behind the pancreatic head and this is a useful landmark (Kuhns *et al.*, 1978). The uncinate process projects upwards and to the left of the pancreatic head and lies behind the superior mesenteric vein (figure 9.3b).

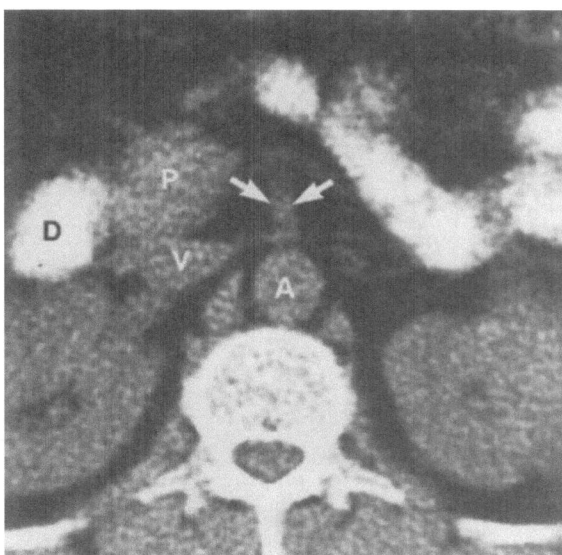

Figure 9.3(a)

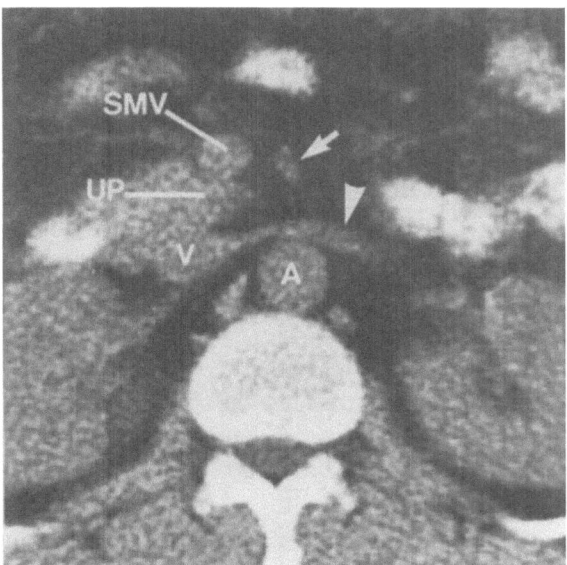

Figure 9.3(b)

Figure 9.3 Normal scans through the pancreas. (a) Head of pancreas (P), duodenum (D), inferior vena cava (V), aorta (A). Superior mesenteric artery (arrowed). (b) Uncinate process (UP), superior mesenteric vein (SMV), superior mesenteric artery (arrowed), left renal vein (arrowhead)

The *neck* of the pancreas joins the head of the gland to the body and lies in front of the portal vein at the junction of the splenic and superior mesenteric veins.

The *body* is situated immediately in front of the aorta and the origin of the superior mesenteric artery (figure 9.4). The latter runs forwards for approximately 1 to 2 cm before turning caudally and is a most important landmark for identifying the position of the pancreas, especially in patients with little perivisceral fat. The third part of the duodenum

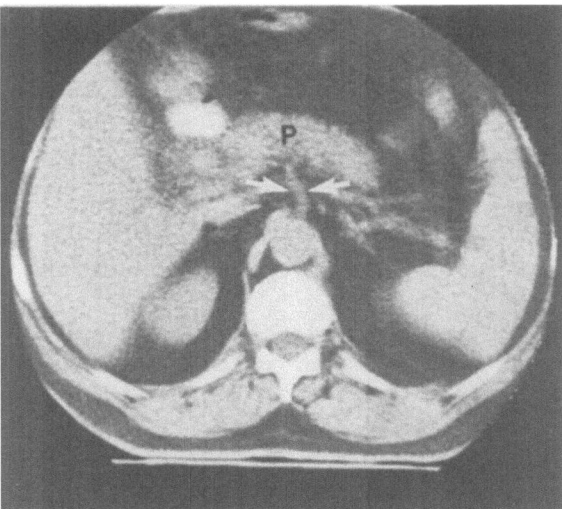

Figure 9.4 Normal scan showing the body of the pancreas (P). Superior mesenteric artery (arrowed)

may sometimes resemble the body of the pancreas as it crosses the midline but can be distinguished because it is found at a lower level and lies behind the mesenteric vessels (figure 9.5)

The *tail* of the pancreas passes in front of the left adrenal gland and left kidney and behind the stomach to reach the hilum of the spleen (figure 9.6). The splenic vein is closely related to the posterior aspect of the tail and body, separating them from the left kidney, superior mesenteric artery and aorta (figure 9.7). The pancreatic duct runs through the centre of the gland and can sometimes be seen on contrast-enhanced scans even when not dilated.

Some glands appear as structures of uniform soft-tissue density with a smooth outline, whereas others

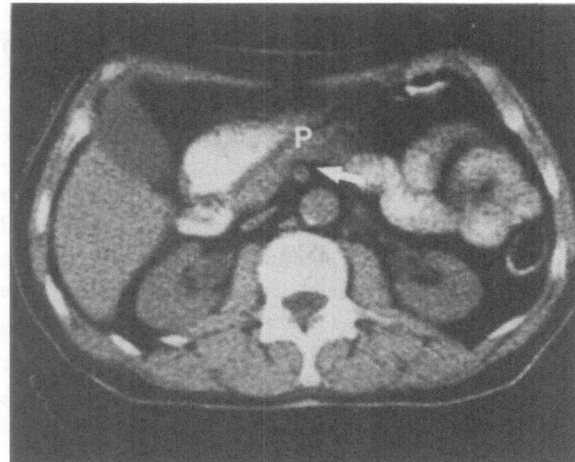

Figure 9.5(a)

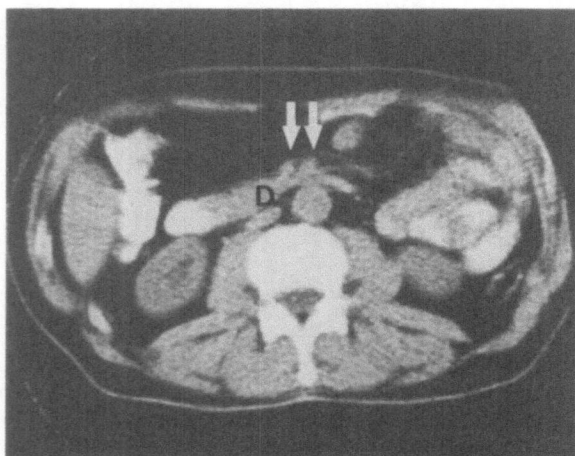

Figure 9.5(b)

Figure 9.5 (a) Normal scan showing the body of the pancreas (P); superior mesenteric artery (arrowed) lies behind the pancreas. (b) Scan 2 cm lower. The duodenum (D) may be mistaken for the pancreas, but the superior mesenteric vessels (arrowed) lie anterior to the duodenum

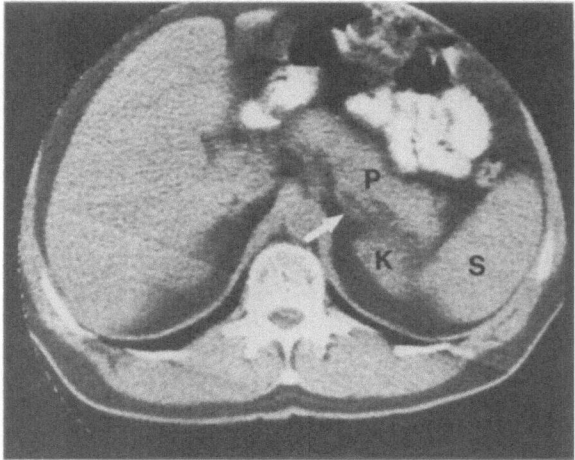

Figure 9.6 Normal tail of pancreas (P). Left adrenal gland (arrowed), upper pole of left kidney (K), spleen (S)

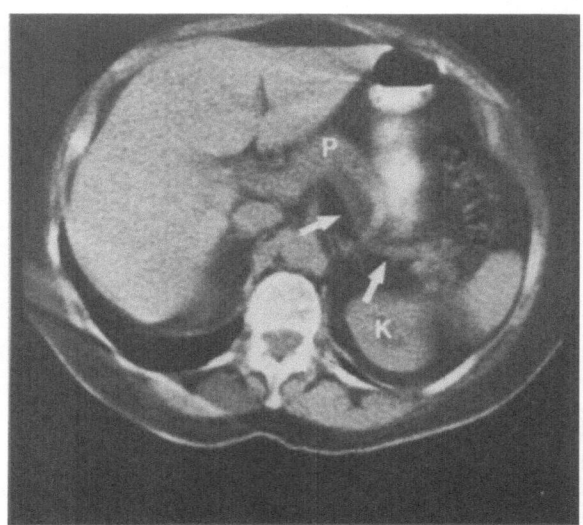

Figure 9.7 Normal scan showing the splenic vein (arrowed). Pancreas (P), left kidney (K)

are lobulated and have a mottled appearance, particularly in obese patients (figure 9.8). The gland tends to be relatively large in young patients, becoming smaller with increasing age (figure 9.9). Normal measurements of the pancreas have been made by several workers. Haaga *et al.* (1976) related the width of the pancreas to the transverse diameter of the vertebral body on the same section. They concluded that the width of the head should not be larger than the full diameter of the vertebral body and that the width of the body and tail should be no greater than two-thirds of this measurement. Although these values were useful guidelines in the early days of CT scanning, experience has shown that they overestimated the size of the normal pan-

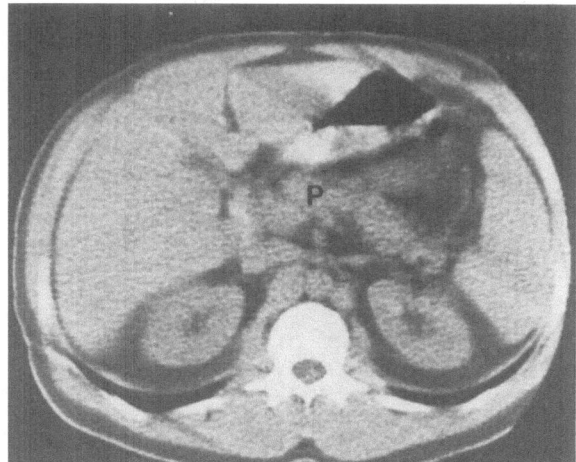

Figure 9.8   Normal scan showing mottled appearance of pancreas (P)

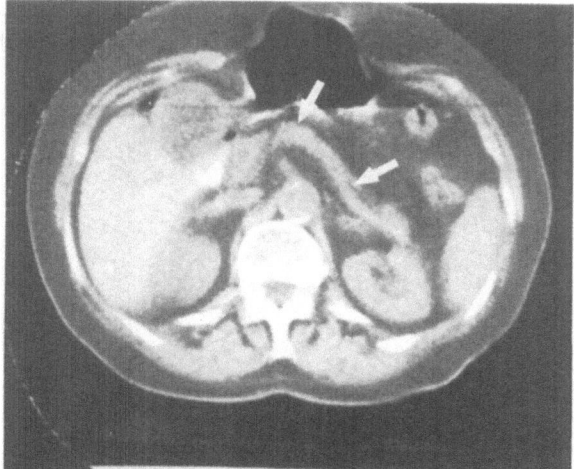

Figure 9.9   Atrophic pancreas (arrowed) in a 78-year-old female

considerable normal variations. More important than the absolute size is the fact that the size of different parts of the gland should be in proportion. Disproportionate enlargement, especially in the head, is an important factor when attempting to determine whether the pancreas is normal (figure 9.10).

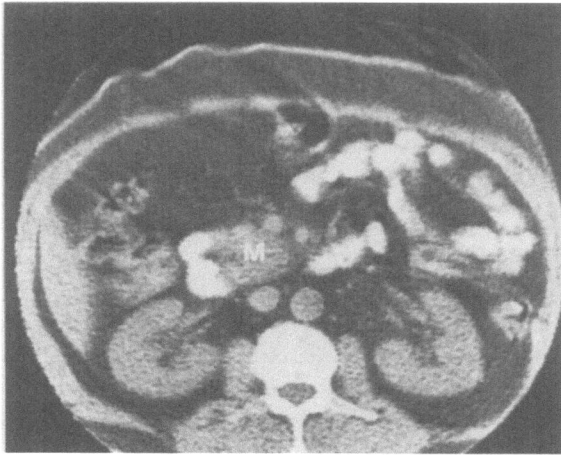

Figure 9.10(a)

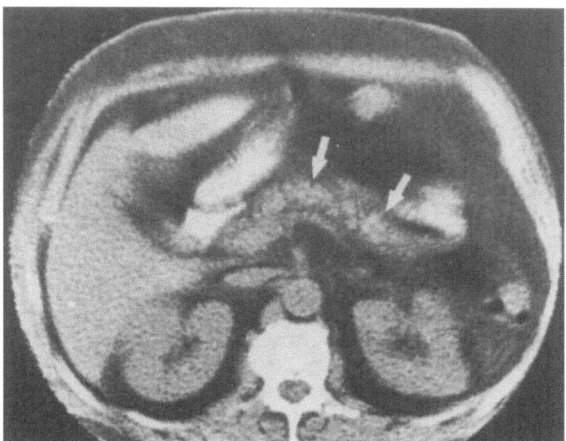

Figure 9.10(b)

Figure 9.10   Mass (M) in the head of the pancreas. In (a) there is disproportionate enlargement of the head compared with the body and tail (arrowed) shown in (b). Chronic pancreatitis found at surgery

creas, even taking into account that the measurements included the portal and splenic vessels. We have found that the measurements reported by Kreel *et al.* (1977) are more accurate. Their normal values for the width at right angles to the surface of the gland excluding vascular structures were: for the head, 3 cm; for the body, 2.5 cm; and for the tail, 2 cm. Although such measurements are a reasonable guideline, it is clear, as in other organs, that there are

SIGNS OF PANCREATIC DISEASE

The *primary* signs are

(a) enlargement,
(b) alteration of density,
(c) loss of peripancreatic fat planes,
(d) calcification,
(e) atrophy, and
(f) dilatation of pancreatic duct;

and *secondary* signs are

(a) dilatation of the extrahepatic or intrahepat
      biliary tree, and
(b) metastases, especially in the liver.

Enlargement

Enlargement of the gland is the most important sign
in the diagnosis of pancreatic disease. Generalised
enlargement may be seen in acute or chronic pancreatitis and is usually easy to detect (figure 9.11).
Localised masses, which may be inflammatory or
neoplastic, are commonest in the head of the gland
where lesions 4 cm or more in size can be recognised
without difficulty (figure 9.12). Masses smaller than
this may not be large enough to distort the outline
and may be difficult to detect unless they produce

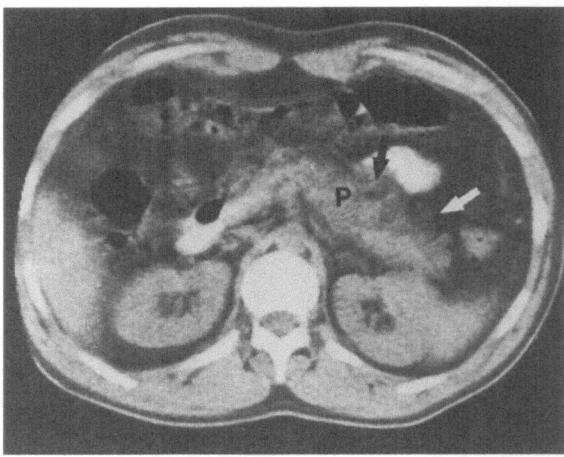

Figure 9.11(b)

Figure 9.11   Pancreatitis. (a) There is diffuse enlargement of the pancreatic body and tail (P). Note loss of
clarity of the retropancreatic fat. (b) Scan in the same
patient 1.5 cm lower. The pancreatic outline is ill-defined
due to inflammation of the peripancreatic tissue (arrowed)

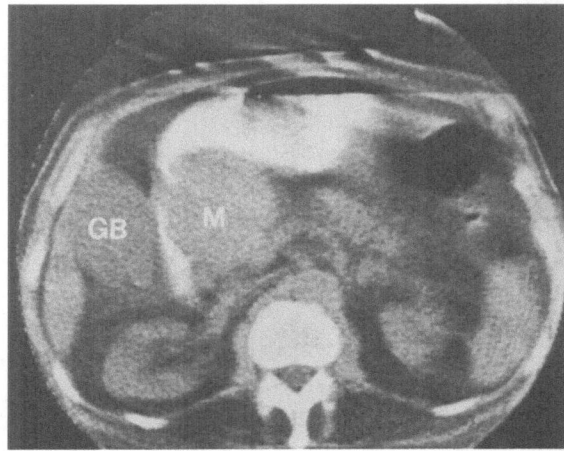

Figure 9.12   Large mass (M) in the head of the pancreas.
This is a carcinoma. The gall-bladder (GB) is dilated

secondary changes such as dilatation of the biliary
tree. Masses in the body and tail are more easily
shown (figure 9.13). Sometimes a mass appears as a
localised bulge on one surface of the gland, and,
when this occurs, quite small tumours can be recognised (Husband *et al.*, 1977) (figure 9.14).

Certain normal structures may simulate areas of

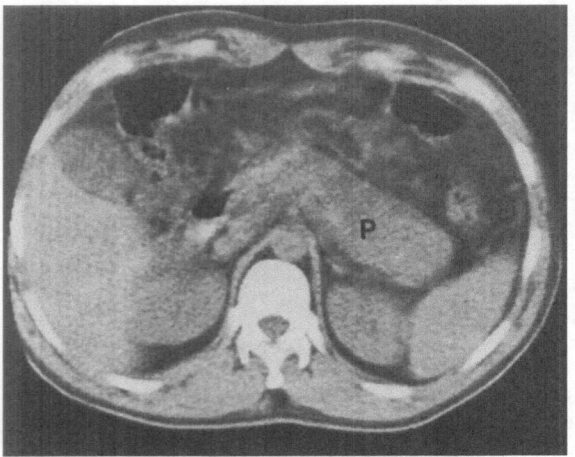

Figure 9.11(a)

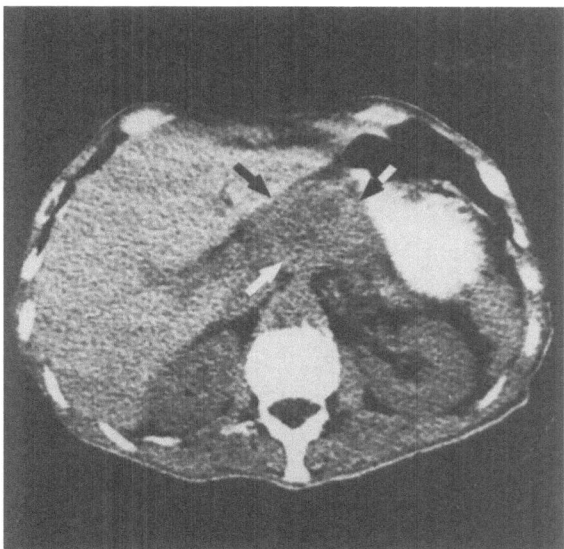

Figure 9.13(a)

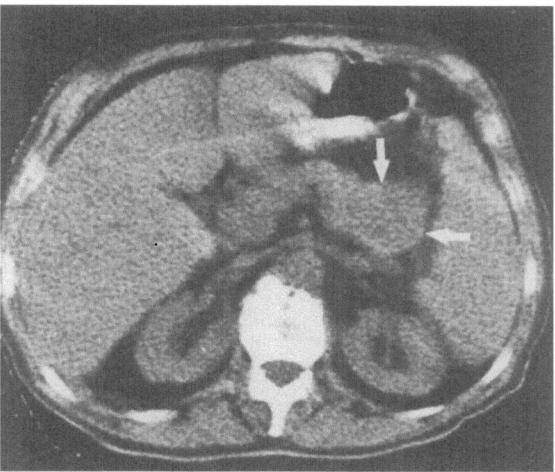

Figure 9.14 Carcinoma of the tail of the pancreas (arrowed). This tumour is approximately 3 cm in diameter and is recognised because it has produced a bulge on the anterior surface of the gland

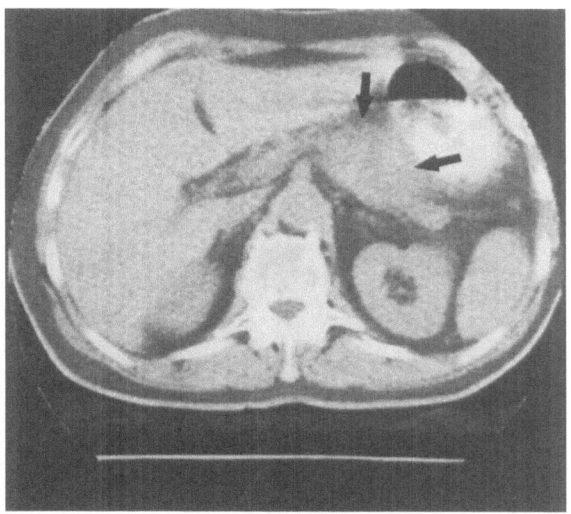

Figure 9.13(b)

Figure 9.13 Carcinoma of the pancreas: (a) in the body (arrowed) and (b) in the tail (arrowed)

focal pancreatic enlargement. The duodenum lies immediately adjacent to the pancreas and, if it contains fluid, may be misinterpreted as a pancreatic mass arising from the head (figure 9.15). Loops of jejunum in the vicinity of the tail of the pancreas

may also mimic a tumour (Husband and Kreel, 1977) (*see* figure 9.1). The importance of ensuring that contrast reaches these parts of the bowel cannot be overstressed. Other structures which may cause difficulty in interpretation by simulating tumours are the fundus of the stomach and the splenic vessels. Awareness of these pitfalls and the judicious use of contrast medium should reduce such errors to a minimum.

Masses lying close to but not involving the pancreas may be mistaken for enlargement of the pancreas. These include lymphadenopathy involving coeliac and other peripancreatic nodes (figures 9.16 and 9.17), tumours of the biliary system, metastases in the mesentery, aneurysms of visceral vessels, and tumours of the stomach, duodenum or colon (figure 9.18). The most common of these lesions to be confused with a carcinoma is lymphadenopathy. An example of an extrinsic lesion involving the pancreas and producing enlargement is illustrated in figure 9.19. This 72-year-old female patient presented with weight loss and typical pancreatic pain. The CT scan showed focal enlargement of the pancreas which contained two specks of calcification. In spite of the areas of calcification, a diagnosis of

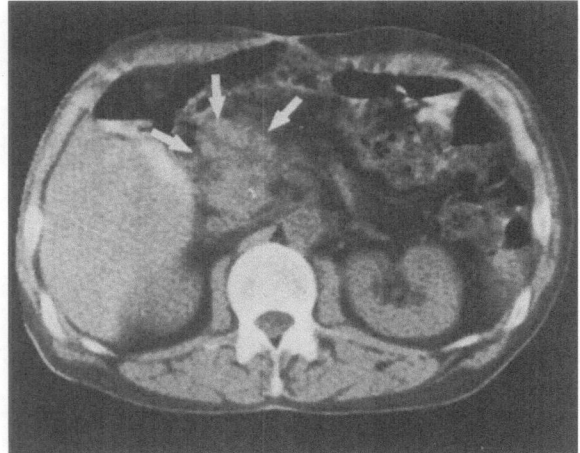

Figure 9.15(a)

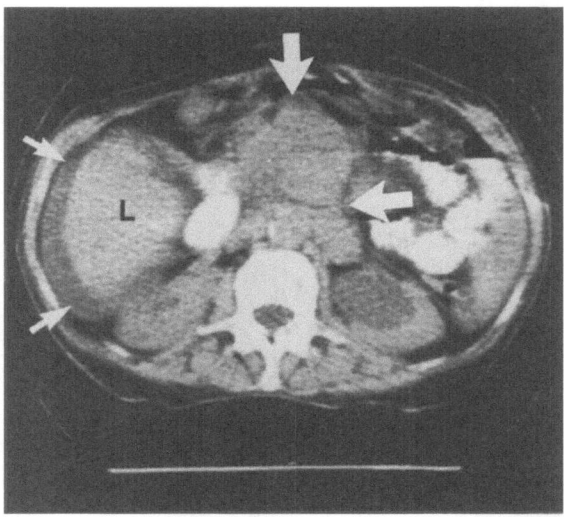

Figure 9.16 A 45-year-old female patient was referred for CT examination with suspected carcinoma of the pancreas. The scan shows enlarged para-aortic and peripancreatic lymph nodes (large arrows). Note ascites (small arrows) lateral to the right lobe of the liver (L). The left kidney is hydronephrotic. Enlarged lymph nodes were demonstrated throughout the para-aortic region. A diagnosis of lymphoma was made and confirmed at laparotomy

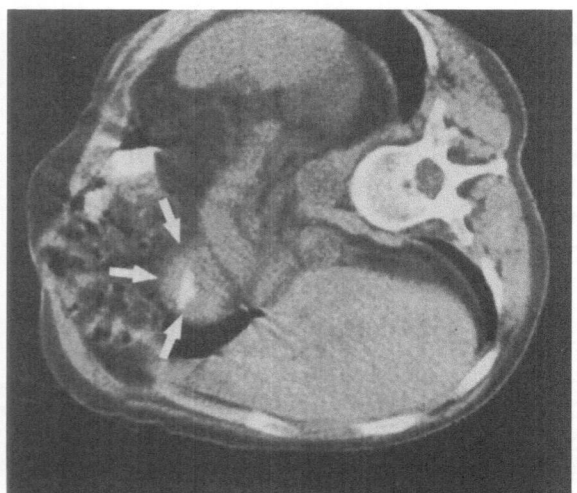

Figure 9.15(b)

Figure 9.15 Bowel simulating pancreatic mass. (a) In the supine position, the appearances suggest a large mass in the pancreatic head (arrowed). (b) Scans were repeated in the right lateral decubitus position after a further dose of oral Gastrografin had been given. The soft tissue opacity simulating a mass in scan (a) is now seen to contain Gastrografin (arrowed). It lies anterior and separate from the pancreas. This opacity represents the fluid-filled duodenum following gastroenterostomy

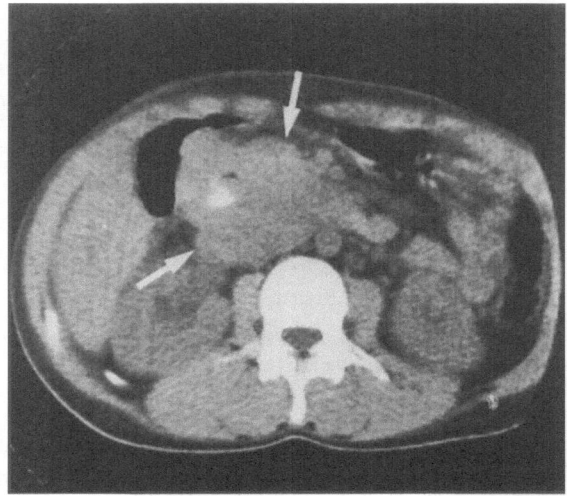

Figure 9.17 Non-Hodgkin's lymphoma. Large peripancreatic nodes simulating a tumour at the head of the pancreas (arrowed)

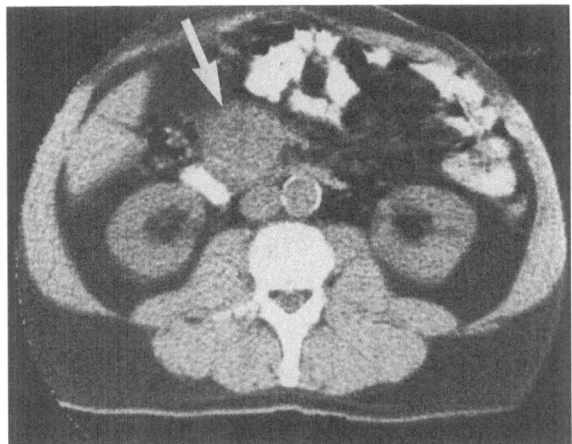

Figure 9.18 Leiomyoma of the duodenum (arrowed). This mass is indistinguishable from tumour arising in the pancreatic head

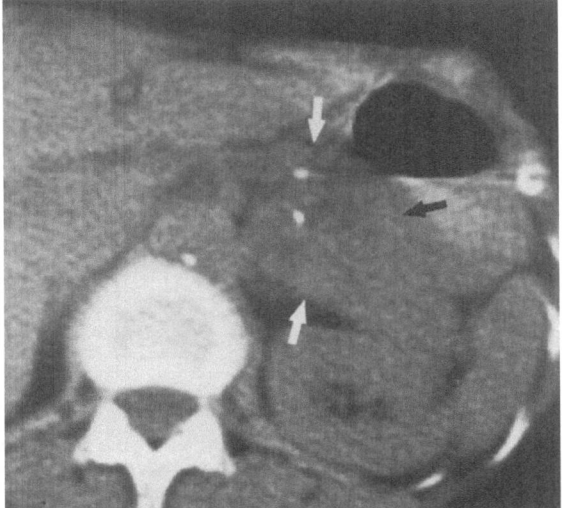

Figure 9.19 CT scan showing a mass in the tail of the pancreas (arrowed) considered to be due to a pancreatic carcinoma. Note flecks of calcification within the mass not visible on the plain abdominal radiograph. Fine-needle aspiration under CT control demonstrated inflammatory cells only. At laparotomy, a benign gastric ulcer was found. It had eroded into the pancreas producing pancreatitis

pancreatic carcinoma was thought most likely. At laparotomy, a benign gastric ulcer was found penetrating the pancreas, producing pancreatitis.

Alteration of Density

The most obvious alteration of density in the pancreas occurs with pseudocysts. These are usually recognised without difficulty, being seen as encapsulated lesions with well defined margins, the density of the contents being near to that of water (0–10 EMI units) (figure 9.20). Bleeding within a pseudocyst causes an increase in density.

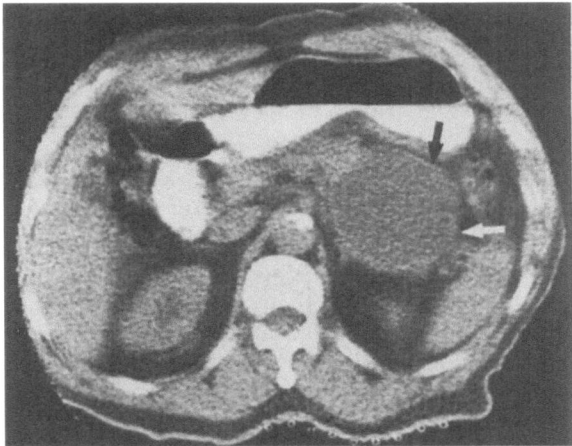

Figure 9.20 Pseudocyst of the tail of the pancreas (arrowed). The wall of the cyst has a higher density than the contents

Abscesses may also contain areas of low density. They usually appear as areas of focal enlargement with an irregular outline and a thick wall with a low-density centre (figure 9.21). The density can vary between that of a pseudocyst and that of a solid tumour, but it is usually somewhere between the two. If the abscess contains gas-forming organisms, pockets of gas with or without a fluid level may be seen.

The majority of pancreatic tumours are isodense with normal pancreatic tissue, but occasionally necrosis produces a central area of low density within the mass.

Cystadenocarcinoma of the pancreas can also present as a mass with areas of low density within it due to mucin-containing cystic areas.

Pseudocysts, abscesses and necrotic tumours have to be distinguished from localised low-density

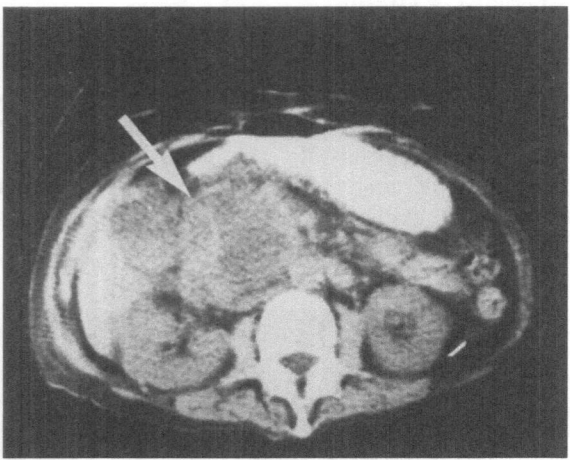

Figure 9.21   **Large abscess in the head of the pancreas (arrowed). This mass has an ill-defined edge and a low-density centre**

masses in neighbouring tissues. For instance, a fluid-filled loop of bowel or an abscess in the lesser sac may easily be mistaken for a pancreatic lesion.

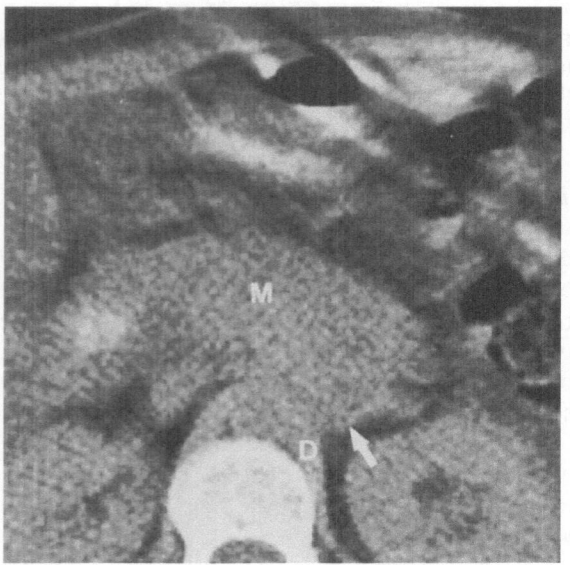

Figure 9.22   **Carcinoma (M) of the body of the pancreas. The tumour extends posteriorly into the peripancreatic fat (arrowed) and has obscured the margins of the superior mesenteric artery and the left crus of the diaphragm (D)**

Loss of Peripancreatic Fat Planes

Like enlargement, loss of peripancreatic fat planes occurs in both neoplastic and inflammatory disease of the pancreas. It is easiest to appreciate when the tumour infiltrates posteriorly, obliterating the margins of the superior mesenteric vessels, aorta and inferior vena cava (figure 9.22). It is a more difficult sign to assess than enlargement, especially in patients with a limited amount of fat.

Calcification

Calcification in the pancreas has to be distinguished not only from contrast medium in the bowel but also from calcification in neighbouring structures, such as lymph nodes and the superior mesenteric or splenic arteries (figure 9.23). Calcification may be

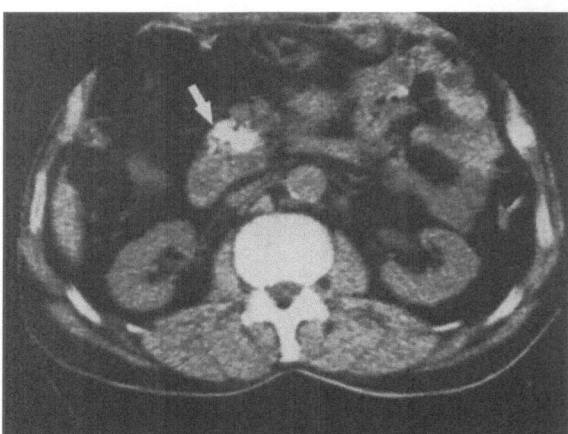

Figure 9.23   **Calcification in the uncinate process due to chronic pancreatitis (arrowed). This calcification could easily have been confused for contrast medium in the duodenum**

seen in the pancreas on CT when none can be seen on the plain abdominal radiograph (*see* figure 9.19). Thus, Ferrucci *et al.* (1979) observed calcification on CT which was not visible on the plain abdominal films in nine out of 50 patients with proven chronic pancreatitis. In advanced cases the whole pancreas may appear to be calcified (figure 9.24).

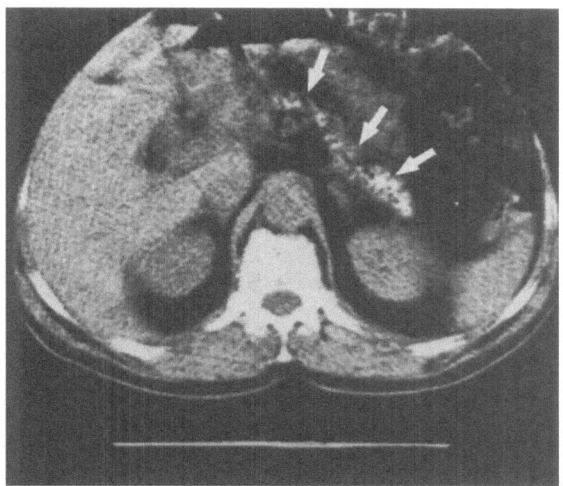

Figure 9.24   Chronic pancreatitis. There is extensive calcification throughout the body and tail (arrowed)

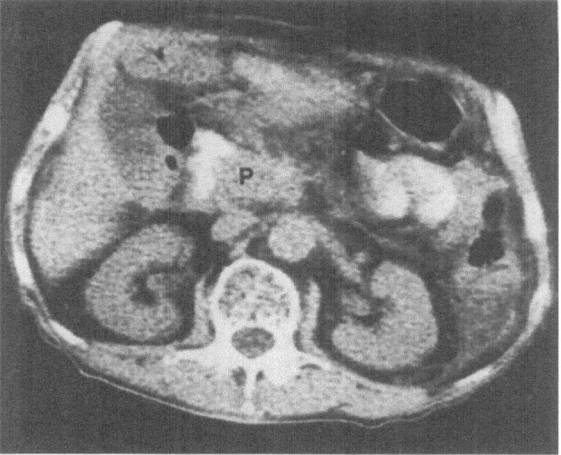

Figure 9.25(a)

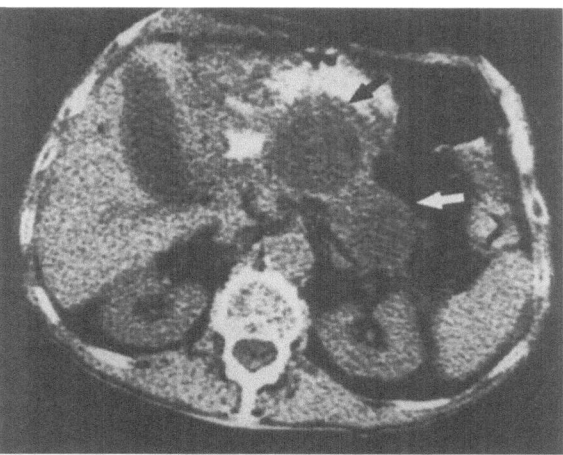

Figure 9.25(b)

Figure 9.25   Carcinoma of the pancreas. (a) The tumour lies in the head of the pancreas (P) but is difficult to identify with CT because there is little enlargement. (b) A scan at a higher level shows cysts in the body and tail (arrowed) which were considered to have resulted from obstruction to the pancreatic duct

Atrophy

Generalised atrophy of the pancreas occurs in chronic pancreatitis. It reflects the end stage of repeated episodes of inflammation and scarring and is likely to be associated with some calcification.

Localised atrophy in the body and tail has been reported in association with neoplasms in the head of the pancreas, sometimes when the tumour is too small to be seen (Ferrucci *et al.*, 1979).

Dilatation of Pancreatic Duct

Dilatation of the pancreatic duct due to obstruction occurs in some patients with chronic pancreatitis and occasionally in those with a carcinoma of the head of the pancreas. The CT appearance of a dilated duct has to be distinguished from the fat plane between the pancreas and the normal splenic vein seen in some normal patients. An unusual sign associated with duct obstruction is the demonstration of *'para-ductal'* cysts (Fawcitt *et al.*, 1978) (figure 9.25)

Dilatation of the Biliary Tree

This reflects an obstructing lesion in the head of the pancreas, usually a carcinoma but sometimes pancreatitis. The dilated common duct may be seen coursing upwards through the pancreatic head (see p. 92).

Metastases

Metastases in the liver and regional lymph nodes are valuable secondary evidence of malignant disease.

DIFFERENTIAL DIAGNOSIS AND THE USE OF COMPUTED TOMOGRAPHY IN PANCREATIC DISEASE

As usual, it is easier to show an abnormality with CT than to determine its nature.

A *solid mass* may be due to a neoplasm, benign or malignant, or to pancreatitis, acute or chronic. Calcification, duct dilatation or cyst formation may be taken as evidence of pancreatitis, but it is important to recognise that pancreatitis and carcinoma may coexist and that the presence of calcification within the gland does not rule out carcinoma (figure 9.26). It may be possible to reach a definite diagnosis of carcinoma if there is local extension of tumour, lymph node enlargement

(figure 9.27), liver metastases or bile duct obstruction. In the absence of such signs, the distinction between a solid pancreatic neoplasm and pancreatitis cannot be made on CT evidence alone. If the clinical evidence and the results of other tests are equivocal, and if laparotomy is to be avoided, then

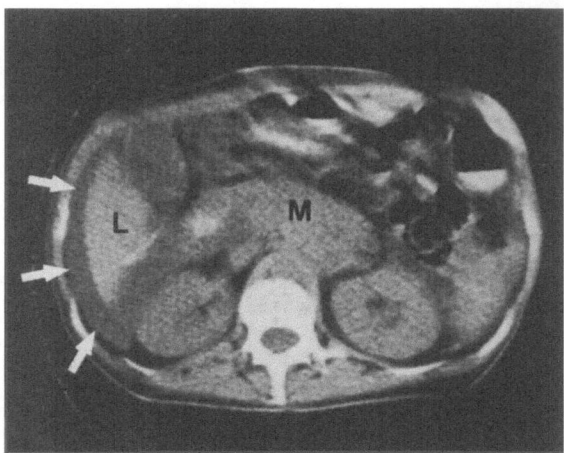

Figure 9.27(a)

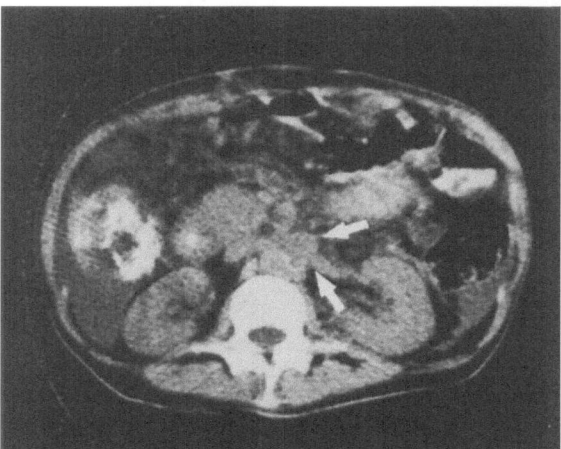

Figure 9.27(b)

Figure 9.27   Carcinoma of the body of the pancreas. (a) Tumour (M) extends posteriorly into the peripancreatic fat. Ascites (arrowed), right lobe of liver (L). (b) The scan through the head of the pancreas shows large para-aortic lymph nodes (arrowed). These findings were confirmed at post-mortem. (Scan (a) reproduced by kind permission of Pitman Press)

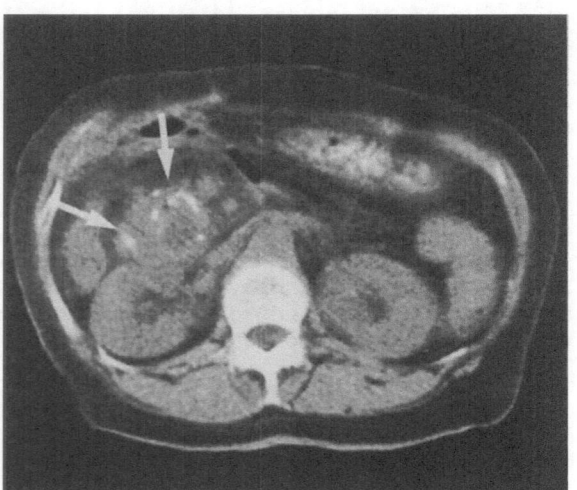

Figure 9.26   CT scan of a patient with histologically proven carcinoma of the head of the pancreas. There is a mass in the head of the pancreas (arrowed) which contains speckled calcification

percutaneous biopsy may be indicated using either CT or ultrasound for guidance.

As with solid masses, the nature of a *low-density mass* may not be clear from the CT evidence alone. If the lesion has the characteristic appearances of a

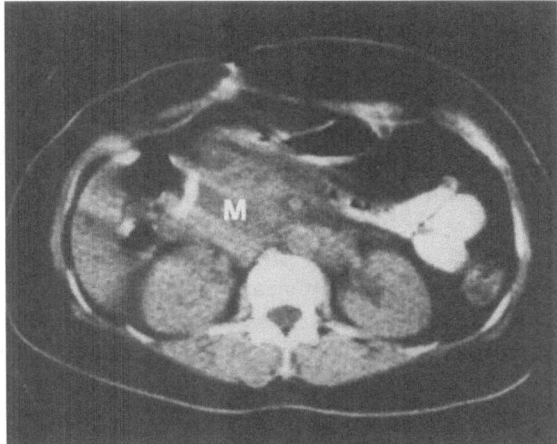

Figure 9.28(a)

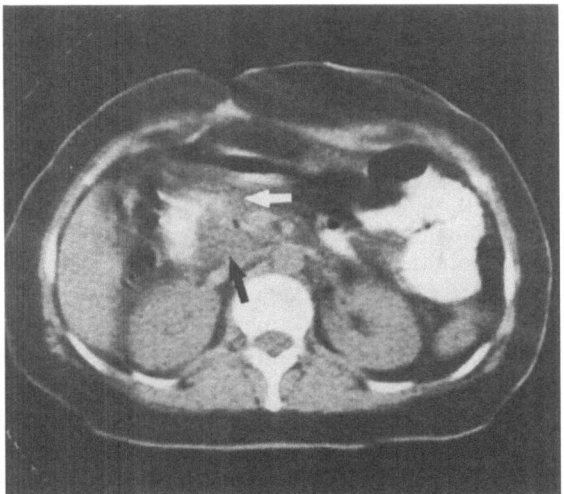

Figure 9.28(b)

Figure 9.28 **Carcinoma of the head of the pancreas in a 39-year-old female patient. (a) The scan at presentation shows a large ill-defined mass (M) in the pancreatic head. (b) The examination was repeated eight weeks later after chemotherapy. There has been considerable reduction in the size of the pancreatic mass**

pseudocyst and the clinical picture is appropriate, diagnosis usually presents no problem. However, if the wall is not well defined and smooth, and if the density of the contents are not absolutely characteristic of a cyst, the distinction between pseudocyst, abscess or neoplasm with a large area of central necrosis may not be possible. Under these circumstances, diagnosis will depend as much on the clinical features as on the CT appearances.

Generalised enlargement of the pancreas can be taken as evidence of pancreatitis. *Generalised atrophy* indicates chronic pancreatitis, except in old age.

It must be emphasised that a normal gland on CT does not exclude pancreatitis or a carcinoma, even when there is plenty of retroperitoneal fat and the pancreas is clearly seen.

The main diagnostic uses of CT in relation to pancreatic disease are in the investigation of patients presenting with a palpable mass which might be arising from the pancreas or in the investigation of patients without a mass in whom the symptoms and signs suggest pancreatic disease. It is also useful in the investigation of patients with known pancreatic disease in whom a complication is suspected. In patients with proven pancreatic carcinoma in whom non-surgical treatment is indicated, CT has a place both for radiotherapy treatment planning and for monitoring the response after radiotherapy or chemotherapy (figure 9.28).

It might be thought that CT would be an ideal method for detecting islet cell tumours of the pancreas. However, few are large enough to distort the outline of the gland and the majority are not recognised on CT even after enhancement (Haaga *et al.*, 1977; Husband and Kreel, 1977).

ACCURACY OF COMPUTED TOMOGRAPHY AND RELATIONSHIP TO OTHER TECHNIQUES

CT provides an excellent method of visualising the pancreas, provided that there is sufficient perivisceral fat. Problems in identifying the gland occur in thin patients, but, even in patients with very little fat, the origin of the superior mesenteric artery can be used to locate the body and surrounding contrast-filled bowel may outline the gland sufficiently to show that there is no room for a mass. A review of patients presenting with possible pancreatic disease over a two-year period at the Royal Marsden Hospital indicates that failure to visualise the gland sufficiently for diagnostic purposes occurs in not more than 2% of adults. Errors of CT in the evaluation of pancreatic disease are, therefore, mainly due to errors of interpretation. False positive examinations in which normal structures are mistaken for pancreatic masses decrease with experience but are difficult to eliminate entirely. False negative examinations occur when lesions are too small to be recognised with CT or are overlooked. It is also important to recognise the lack of tissue specificity of CT, so that, as already discussed, an inflammatory mass may be indistinguishable from a neoplasm.

Despite the limitations of pancreatic imaging with CT, the accuracy of diagnosis is high. As early as 1977, Sheedy *et al.* (1977) were able to report an accuracy of 83% in 331 patients referred for possible pancreatic disease. Accuracy rose to 88% if technically unsatisfactory examinations were excluded. Similar figures have been reported by other workers (Stanley *et al.*, 1977; Haaga *et al.*, 1977; Husband *et al.*, 1977; Wittenberg and Ferrucci, 1979).

False positive diagnoses account for most of the errors. These are of two sorts: those in which a normal structure, such as a fluid-filled loop of bowel, is mistaken for a pancreatic lesion, and those in which an extrinsic mass is mistaken for a mass in the pancreas. Greater awareness of the manner in which normal structures may mimic pancreatic masses has undoubtedly reduced the number of false positive examinations, although some errors still occur.

False negative examinations are less common in carcinoma of the pancreas than in chronic pancreatitis. Thus, Sheedy *et al.* (1977) reported only 5% negative reports in 56 patients with carcinoma of the pancreas who had technically satisfactory scans, whereas 19% of their patients with pancreatitis had normal scans. Likewise, Ferrucci *et al.* (1979) showed no abnormality in 16% of the patients with chronic pancreatitis.

The latter study also illustrates the difficulty of distinguishing the nature of a pancreatic mass on CT. Although 28 of the 50 patients with chronic pancreatitis showed specific signs, i.e. pseudocyst/abscess, calcification, atrophy or duct dilatation, 12 showed only non-specific diffuse or focal pancreatic enlargement indistinguishable from carcinoma. In two patients, chronic pancreatitis and carcinoma coexisted and the carcinoma could not be diagnosed on the scan.

The results of CT in pancreatic disease compare favourably with those of ultrasound. Wittenberg and Ferrucci (1979) have reported an overall accuracy of 86% with CT and 71% with ultrasound in pancreatic disease. The same group, comparing CT and ultrasound in patients with chronic pancreatitis, found ultrasound less informative than CT (Ferrucci *et al.*, 1979). When technically successful, ultrasound was almost as good as CT in demonstrating enlargement of the pancreas and pseudocyst/abscess. It was, however, not so effective in demonstrating atrophy, calcification or duct dilatation. In a study at Northwick Park Hospital, ultrasound and CT were compared in 50 patients with suspected pancreatic disease (Husband *et al.*, 1977). The diagnostic accuracy of CT was 94% compared with 64% using ultrasound. The difference was mainly due to the number of unsuccessful examinations with ultrasound (15%). When the findings were compared in patients in whom both examinations were technically satisfactory, the accuracy was similar for both techniques.

There are two main reasons why ultrasound may be unsuccessful when examining the pancreas. First, bowel gas is a problem, especially when examining the region of the tail. Secondly, the pancreas may be difficult to demonstrate by ultrasound in fat patients.

In general, the advantages of using ultrasound are such that when both techniques are available, ultrasound is likely to be used initially, especially in thin patients. If the examination is unsuccessful or the results are equivocal or disagree with the clinical findings, then CT will be indicated. CT is likely to be the investigation of first choice in obese patients.

Isotope techniques are generally considered unreliable in the demonstration of pancreatic disease. However, there may still be a place for pancreatic isotope scanning as a screening test (Braganza *et al.*, 1978).

CT has reduced the need for endoscopic pancreatography (ERCP) (Sheedy *et al.*, 1977; Stanley *et al.*, 1977; Wittenberg *et al.*, 1978). ERCP has the advantage that it can demonstrate changes in the duct system, indicating disease processes which may not be appreciated with ultrasound or CT.

Since the advent of CT and effective ultrasound, arteriography of the pancreas is rarely required. It remains, however, the best method of demonstrating islet cell tumours.

The number of techniques available for imaging the pancreas illustrates one of the central problems of modern diagnosis. A blunderbuss approach is undesirable, especially since some of the techniques are uncomfortable for the patient and carry some risk, while others are costly. In what order should tests be done? Which should be done first and in what clinical circumstances?

The diagnostic strategy will vary according to the techniques which are available and the experience and expertise which accompany them. An example of a scheme which relates the role of CT to other techniques in the investigation of pancreatic disease and which takes into account the merits and limitations of each technique is illustrated in table 9.1 (Wittenberg and Ferrucci, 1979). Individual problems will be approached differently in different centres, but this scheme illustrates the sort of approach that is required if CT is to be used to best advantage.

REFERENCES

Braganza, J. N., Fawcitt, R. A. Forbes, W. St C., Isherwood, I., Russell, J. J. B., Prescott, M., Testa, H. J., Torrance, H. B. and Howat, H. T. (1978). A clinical evaluation of isotope scanning, ultrasonography and computed tomography in pancreatic disease. *Clinical Radiology*, **29** (6), 639–647

Fawcitt, R. A., Forbes, W. St C., Isherwood, I., Braganza, J. N. and Howat, H. T. (1978). Computed tomography in pancreatic disease. *British Journal of Radiology*, **51** (601), 1–4

Ferrucci, J. T., Wittenberg, J., Black, E. B., Kirkpatrick, R. H. and Hall, D. A. (1979). Computed body tomography in chronic pancreatitis. *Radiology*, **130**, 175–182

Haaga, J. R., Alfidi, R. J., Havrilla, T. R., Tubbs, R., Gonzalez, L., Meaney, T. and Corsi, M. (1977). Definitive role of CT scanning of the pancreas. *Radiology*, **124**, 723–730

Haaga, J. R., Alfidi, R. J., Zelch, M. G., Meaney, T. F., Boller, M., Gonzalez, L. and Jelden, G. (1976). Computed tomography of the pancreas. *Radiology*, **120**, 589–596

Haaga, J. and Reich, N. E. (1978). In *Computed Tomography of Abdominal Abnormalities*, Mosby, St Louis, chapter 3, pp. 86–127

Husband, J. E. and Kreel, L. (1977). Computerised axial tomography of the pancreas. In *First European Seiminar in Computed Tomography in Clinical Practice*, eds. G. H. du Boulay and I. F. Moseley, Springer-Verlag, Berlin, pp. 372–381

Husband, J. E., Meire, H. B. and Kreel, L. (1977). Comparison of ultrasound and computer-assisted tomography in pancreatic diagnosis. *British Journal of Radiology*, **50**, 855–862

Kreel, L., Haertel, M. and Katz, D. (1977). Computed tomography of the normal pancreas. *Journal of Computer Assisted Tomography*, **1** (3), 290–299

Kuhns, L. R., Borlaza, G. S., Seigel, R. and Cho, K. J. (1978). Localization of the head of the pancreas using the junction of the left renal vein and inferior vena cava. *Journal of Computer Assisted Tomography*, **2**, 170–172

Table 9.1 A radiological approach to pancreatic disease incorporating computed tomography (after Wittenberg and Ferrucci, 1979)

Pancreatic problem	First investigation	Supplemental investigation
Acute pancreatitis, uncomplicated	US	CT
Acute pancreatitis with suspected phlegmon, abscess or necrosis	CT	US
Pseudocyst	US	CT
Chronic pancreatitis	CT	ERCP
Carcinoma, head and body without jaundice	US/CT (Thin/Fat)	ERCP
Obstructive jaundice	US	PTC
Carcinoma of the tail	CT	ERCP
Functional islet cell tumours	ANG	CT

US = ultrasound; CT = computed tomography; ERCP = endoscopic retrograde cholangio-pancreatography; PTC = percutaneous transhepatic cholangiography; ANG = angiography.

Lee, J. K. T., Stanley, R. J., Melson, G. L. and Sagel, S. S. (1979). Pancreatic imaging by ultrasound and body tomography. *Radiologic Clinics of North America*, **16**, 105–117

Sheedy, P. F., II, Stephens, D. H., Hattery, R. R., MacCarty, R. L. and Williamson, B. (1977). Computed tomography of the pancreas. *Radiologic Clinics of North America*, **XV** (3), 349–366

Stanley, R. J., Sagel, S. S. and Levitt, R. G. (1977). Computed tomographic evaluation of the pancreas. *Radiology*, **124**, 715–722

Wittenberg, J. and Ferrucci, J. (1979). A radiological approach to pancreatic disease incorporating computed tomography. Presented at the *International Symposium and Course of Computed Tomography*, Las Vegas, April 1979. Abstract in *Journal of Computer Assisted Tomography*, **3** (4), 558

Wittenberg, J., Fineberg, H. V., Black, E. B., Kirkpatrick, R. H., Schaffer, D. L., Ikeda, M. K. and Ferrucci, J. T. (1978). Clinical efficacy of computed body tomography, *American Journal of Roentgenology*, **131**, 5–14

10

The Abdomen – Miscellaneous Topics

There are several abdominal conditions which are not organ-specific because they primarily involve the intra-abdominal spaces. These lesions are considered in this chapter and include retroperitoneal space masses (excluding lymphadenopathy), intra-abdominal abscesses and ascites. CT-guided aspiration techniques are also discussed. Finally, the spleen is included here because CT examinations are rarely undertaken primarily for the investigation of this organ.

THE RETROPERITONEAL AND PERITONEAL SPACES

Technique of Examination

There is no routine procedure for examination of the retroperitoneal and intraperitoneal spaces. The number of CT scans and slice intervals and the need for intravenous contrast medium depend on the clinical problem and on the anatomical site.

Anatomy

The Retroperitoneal Space

The retroperitoneal space extends from the diaphragm superiorly to the pelvic brim inferiorly. It is bounded by the posterior parietal peritoneum anteriorly and the transversalis fascia posteriorly (figure 10.1). Laterally, the space is limited by the lateroconal fascia (the lateroconal fascia is formed by fusion of the anterior and posterior renal fascia, Gerota's fascia (Meyers, 1976)). The major organs and structures within the retroperitoneal space are the adrenal glands, kidneys, ureters, the pancreas, aorta and inferior vena cava. The duodenum and ascending and descending colon are also retroperitoneal structures.

The retroperitoneal space is divided into three distinct regions – the anterior pararenal space, the perirenal space and the posterior pararenal space (Meyers, 1976). The anterior pararenal space contains the duodenum, the pancreas and the extraperitoneal part of the colon. Collections of fluid, pus or blood in this space tend to accumulate on one side of the abdomen or the other, although the space is continuous across the midline. The perirenal space, however, is separated into right and left compartments by the connective tissue surrounding the aorta and inferior vena cava. The posterior pararenal space is limited medially by fusion of the transversalis fascia with the lumbar muscles but laterally it is continuous with the properitoneal fat of the abdominal wall.

The aorta and inferior vena cava have a constant relationship to each other throughout the retroperitoneal space, except in the upper part where the inferior vena cava passes forwards to enter the posterior aspect of the right lobe of the liver. These

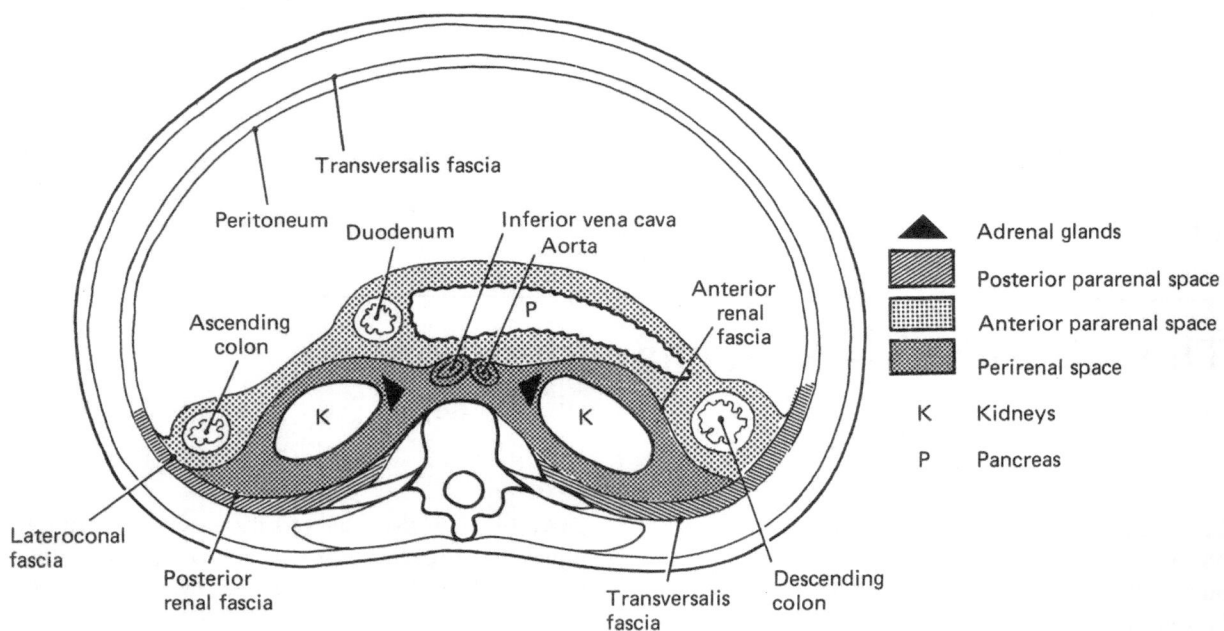

Figure 10.1 Diagram to show the compartments of the retroperitoneal space

vessels have attenuation values similar to other soft tissues but are surrounded by retroperitoneal fat (figure 10.2) and can almost always be identified even in very thin patients and children. The complete contour of the aorta is seen in the majority of normal patients, and soft tissue obscuring any part of the margin is thus a useful abnormal sign except in extremely thin patients. The inferior vena cava is

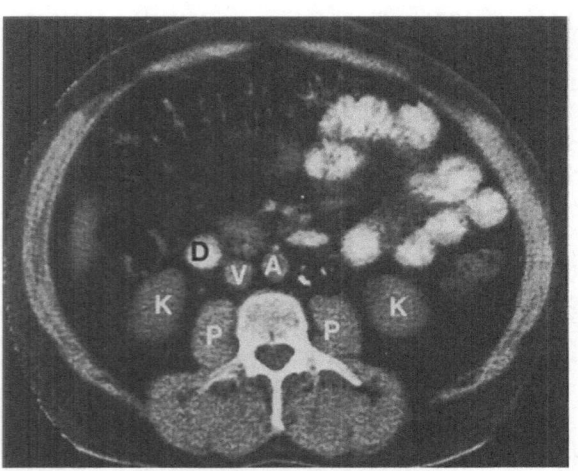

Figure 10.2 Normal retroperitoneum showing the aorta (A), the inferior vena cava (V), lower poles of kidneys (K), duodenum (D), psoas muscles (P)

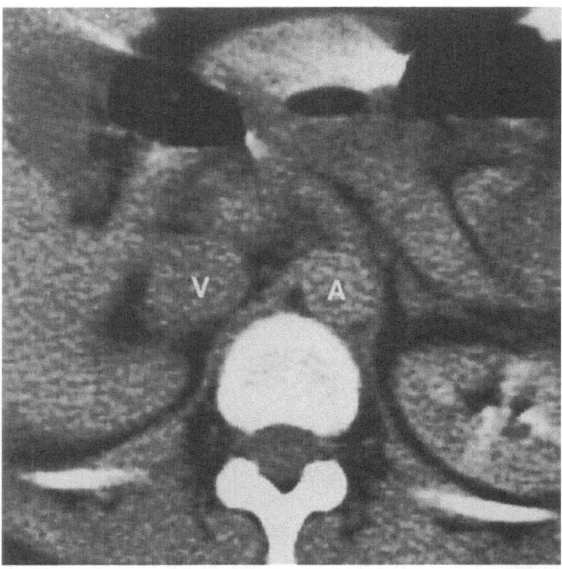

Figure 10.3(a)

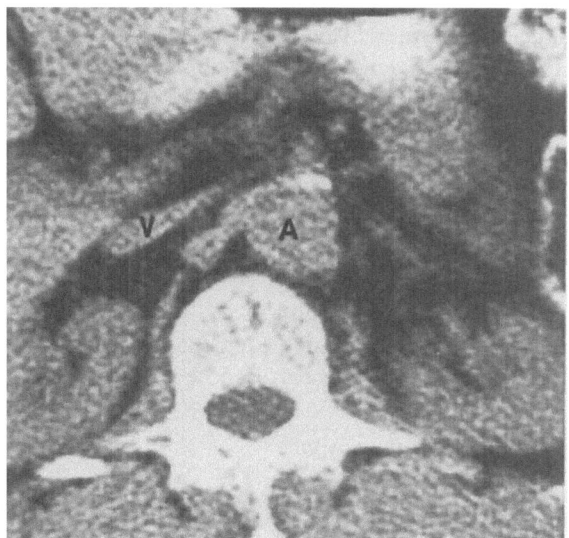

Figure 10.3(b)

Figure 10.3   Normal inferior vena cava. (a) The inferior vena cava (V) is larger than the aorta. (b) The inferior vena cava (V) appears collapsed. Aorta (A)

not so well demarcated and its shape varies enormously. It may appear as a globular structure, sometimes larger than the aorta, or as a flattened, somewhat triangular-shaped, vessel (figure 10.3). Its shape depends partly on the phase of respiration.

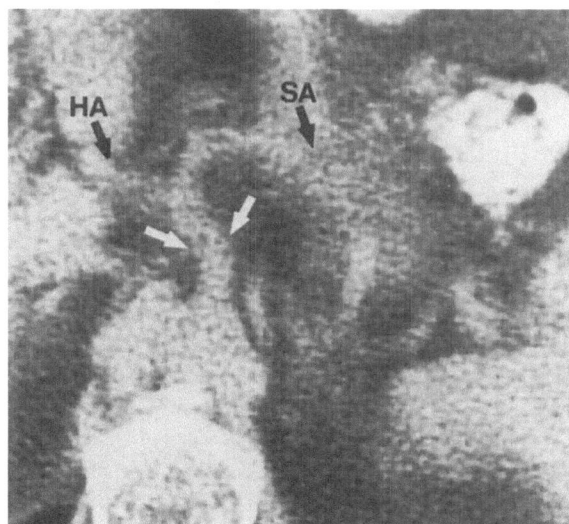

Figure 10.4(a)

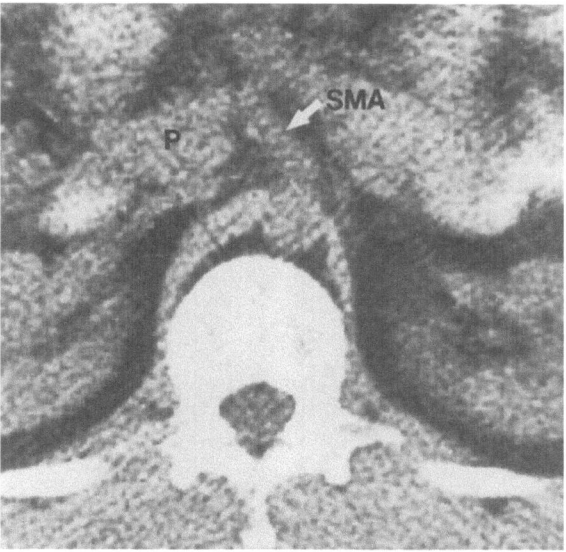

Figure 10.4(b)

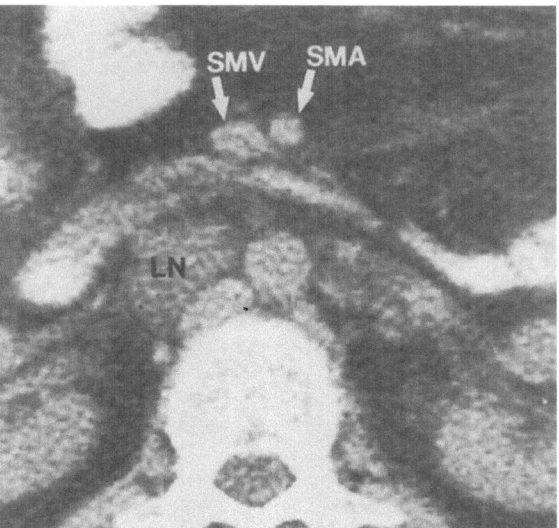

Figure 10.4(c)

Figure 10.4   Major branches of the aorta. (a) Coeliac axis (arrowed), splenic artery (SA), hepatic artery (HA). (b) At its origin, the superior mesenteric artery (SMA) passes anteriorly for 1 to 2 cm and is a useful landmark for identifying the pancreas (P). (c) At a slightly lower level, the superior mesenteric artery (SMA) and superior mesenteric vein (SMV) are seen lying adjacent to each other near the midline as they run caudally. The vein is larger than the artery. Note lymph node mass (LN) in this patient

The major branches of the aorta recognised with CT are the coeliac trunk (figure 10.4a), superior mesenteric and renal arteries. Of these, the superior mesenteric artery is most often identified because it passes anteriorly for approximately 1 to 2 cm before turning caudally to enter the small bowel mesentery (figure 10.4b). At a slightly lower level the artery is seen as a circular structure lying to the left of the superior mesenteric vein (figure 10.4c).

The renal veins are seen in the majority of patients. The left renal vein courses anteromedially to pass in front of the aorta before joining the inferior vena cava, whereas the right renal vein has a shorter course (figure 10.5).

The region of the aortic bifurcation is the most difficult retroperitoneal site to assess because the diverging common iliac arteries and the converging veins take a variable course (figure 10.6). Here it may be difficult to exclude a retroperitoneal mass.

The retrocrural space is discussed in chapter 11.

The Intraperitoneal Space

The peritoneal cavity is divided into two major compartments by the transverse mesocolon (the supra- and inframesocolic compartments) and into a number of smaller compartments by other peritoneal reflections. These include the right and left infracolic space, the paracolic gutters and the subphrenic space (figure 10.7). They communicate freely with

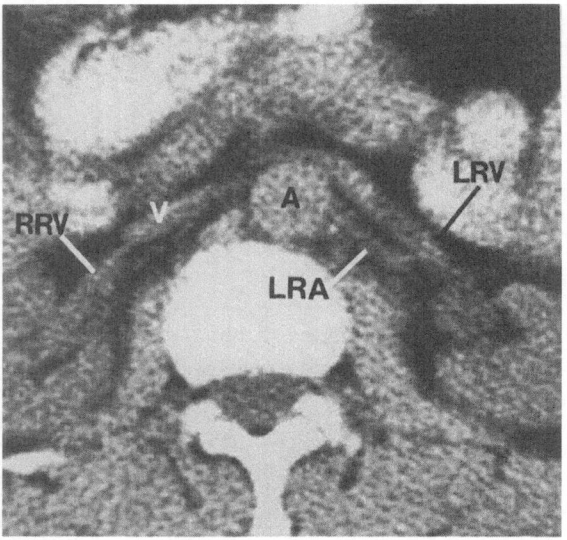

Figure 10.5   Renal vessels. Left renal vein (LRV), right renal vein (RRV), inferior vena cava (V), left renal artery (LRA), aorta (A)

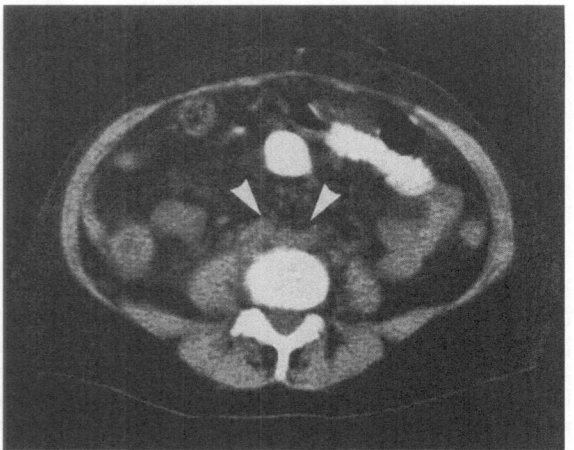

Figure 10.6   Normal scan just below the aortic bifurcation in a fat patient. Common iliac vessels (arrowheads)

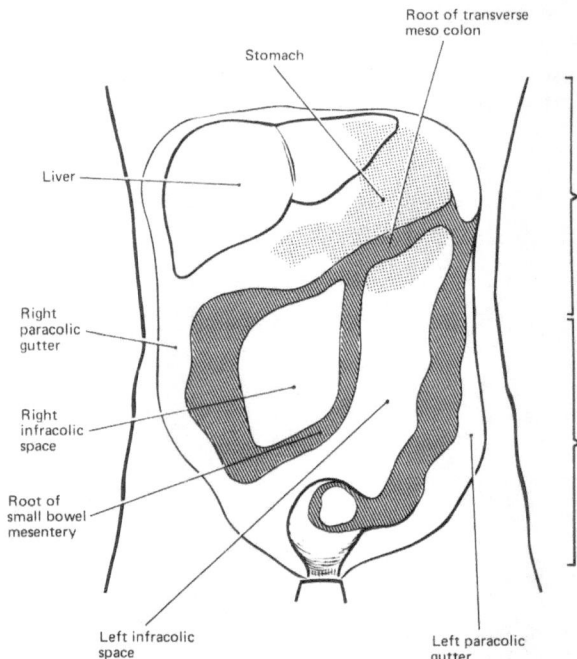

Figure 10.7   Diagram to show the major compartments of the peritoneal cavity

each other, influencing the spread of malignant and infectious processes. For example, fluid collecting in the pelvis first lies in the pouch of Douglas, extends into the paravesical recesses and then spreads preferentially up into the abdomen along the right paracolic gutter to the right subhepatic and subphrenic spaces (figure 10.8, and *see also* figure 6.3).

The lesser sac lies behind the stomach and duodenal bulb and posteriorly is related mainly to the pancreas. Although this space communicates freely with the remainder of the peritoneal cavity, effusion and abscesses in this space are most likely to result from pancreatitis or duodenal ulceration.

Masses of the Retroperitoneal and Intraperitoneal Spaces

Primary Tumours These have similar attenuation values to other soft tissues (figure 10.9) although areas of lower density may sometimes be seen within

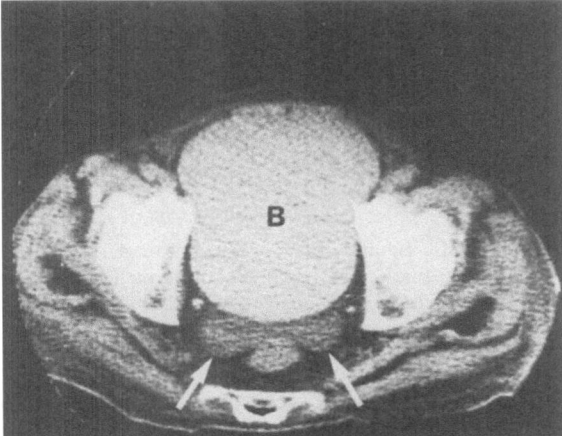

Figure 10.8(a)

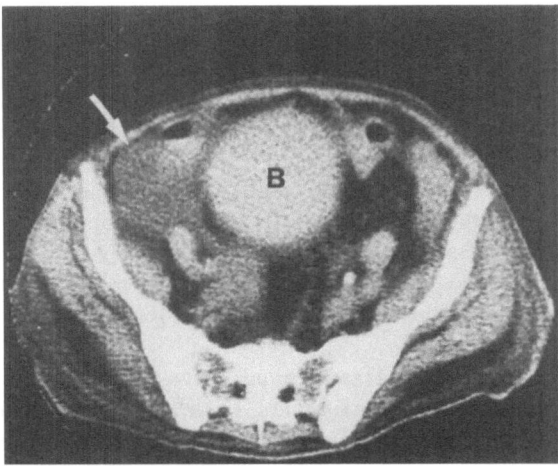

Figure 10.8(b)

Figure 10.8 Distribution of intraperitoneal fluid. (a) Fluid in the pouch of Douglas (arrowed). Contrast-filled bladder (B). (b) At a higher level in the same patient, the fluid is seen to have spread into the right paracolic gutter (arrowed)

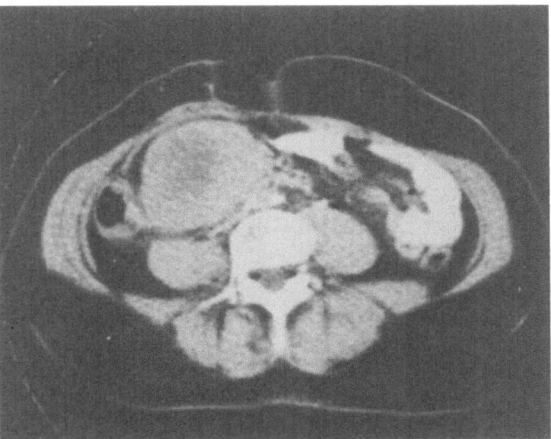

Figure 10.9 Fibrosarcoma of the retroperitoneum. The mass has a low-density centre and a clear fat plane around it

the mass. It is usually impossible to provide any information regarding tumour type unless the mass contains a significant amount of fat, such as a liposarcoma. The precise attenuation values recorded depend on the amount of fat present; the higher the proportion of fat the lower the density (Mendez *et al.*, 1980) (figure 10.10). Occasionally the fat content may be so great that the lesion may be difficult to separate from the surrounding intra-abdominal fat (figure 10.10b).

A clear fat plane may be seen round the tumour (*see* figure 10.9) or it may be inseparable from adjacent normal structures such as the psoas

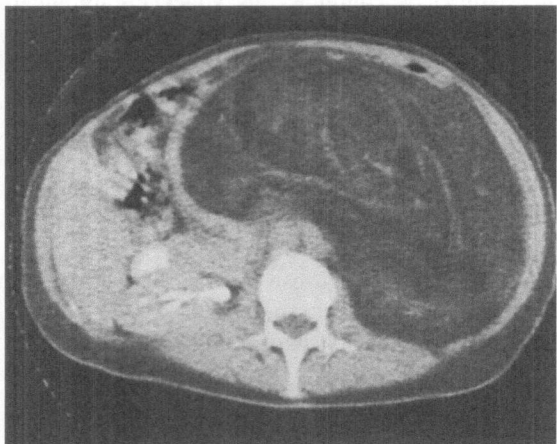

Figure 10.10(a)

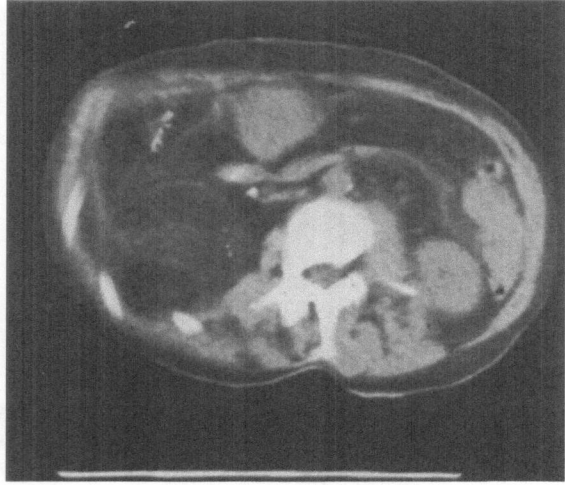

Figure 10.10(b)

Figure 10.10 Two patients with retroperitoneal liposarcoma. (a) The tumour contains some areas of higher attenuation value than fat, presumably due to soft tissue within the tumour. (b) Recurrent liposarcoma on the right side of the abdomen. The tumour is difficult to differentiate from the normal intraperitoneal fat

muscle. Such loss of intervening fat does not necessarily indicate tumour invasion (Mendez *et al.*, 1980) and thus, in general, benign tumours cannot be distinguished from malignant ones (figure 10.11).

There is usually no difficulty in separating primary tumours from metastatic lymph node disease. First, several lymph nodes may be involved,

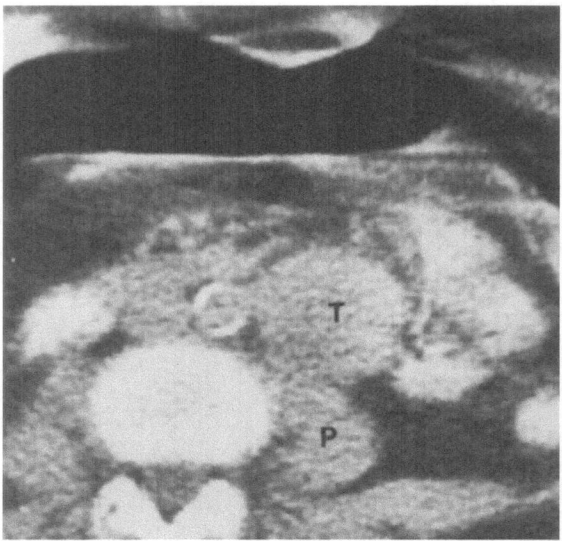

Figure 10.11 Benign phaeochromocytoma at the level of the fourth lumbar vertebra. This tumour (T) is closely applied to the left psoas muscle (P) so that the intervening fat plane is not seen

so that a number of separate masses are seen. Secondly, large nodes may be present throughout the para-aortic chain, so that abnormal masses are demonstrated at all levels. Abdominal nodal metastases from testicular teratoma are an exception to this rule. This tumour frequently produces a solitary lymph node mass which may be indistinguishable from primary tumour (*see* chapter 11). Thirdly, a primary tumour tends to arise on one side of the retroperitoneum and, even if it does extend across the midline, it does not usually obliterate the great vessels, whereas a conglomerate lymph node mass frequently presents in the midline and obliterates the major vessels (figure 10.12).

Haematomas Haematomas have many features similar to primary tumours. In the retroperitoneum, they are seen as localised masses which obliterate the normal margins of adjacent structures (figure 10.13a). Within the peritoneal cavity, the mass usually displaces the surrounding loops of bowel (figure 10.13b). The CT numbers of the haematoma may be higher or lower than those of the surrounding tissue depending upon the length of time between

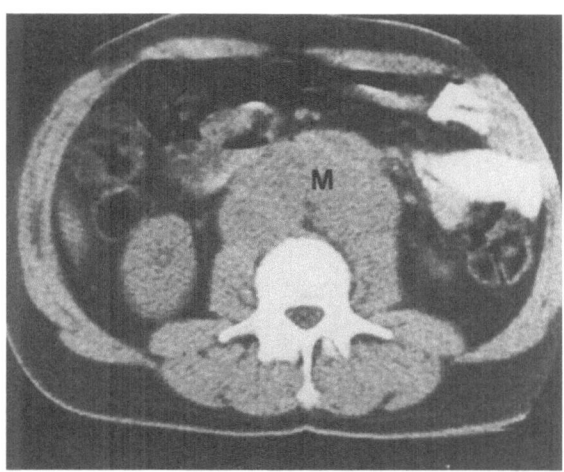

Figure 10.12 Conglomerate mass (M) of enlarged nodes in a patient with testicular teratoma. The mass lies centrally in the retroperitoneal space completely obliterating the aorta and inferior vena cava

the bleed and the CT scan (Sagel *et al.*, 1977). As the haematoma ages, the attenuation values fall, so that a chronic lesion may appear cystic. However, Amendola *et al.* (1979) were unable to demonstrate decrease in attenuation values in 20 patients with retroperitoneal haemorrhage following translumbar aortography. They conclude that this was due to the small size and rapid resolution of the haematomas in the majority of patients.

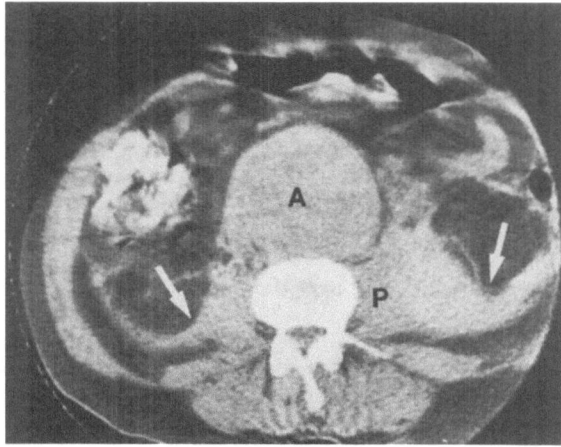

Figure 10.13(a)

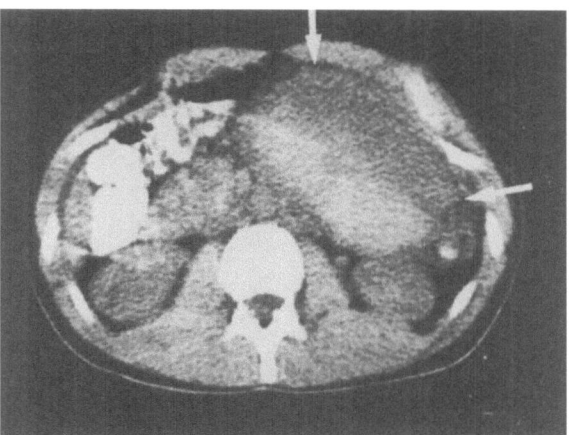

Figure 10.13(b)

Figure 10.13 Intra-abdominal haemorrhage. (a) Retroperitoneal haemorrhage from an aortic aneurysm (A). The density of the blood (arrowed) is higher than the adjacent psoas muscle (P). This is more noticeable on the left. (b) Localised intramesenteric haemorrhage (arrowed). The mass contains areas of low density due to liquefaction of the haematoma and areas of higher density

Abscesses The demonstration of retroperitoneal abscesses is one of the most rewarding uses of CT in the abdomen and pelvis. Here, as elsewhere, abscesses have attenuation values which overlap with those of other processes, such as tumours and haematomas (Callen, 1979) (figure 10.14). Abscesses tend to collect close to the diseased organ or in dependent sites such as the pelvis or around the liver. The pathognomonic sign of an abscess is the presence of pockets of extraluminal gas within the mass and this occurs in up to 40% of patients (Callen, 1979; Daffner *et al.*, 1979). Although pockets of gas within the mass may indicate an abscess, the appearances may easily be confused with unopacified bowel if the abscess is not large (figure 10.15).

'Rim enhancement' after injection of intravenous contrast medium may be shown (*see* figure 10.14a). This simply reflects the vascularity of the wall of the abscess and may also occur in tumours (Wolverson *et al.*, 1979).

CT is particularly effective in demonstrating

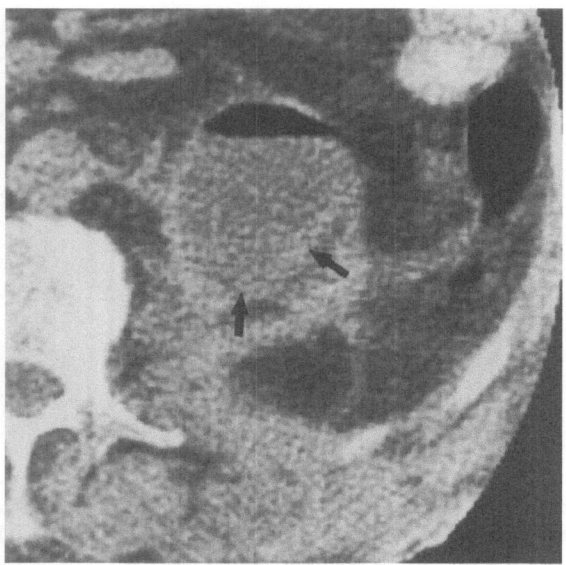

Figure 10.14(a)

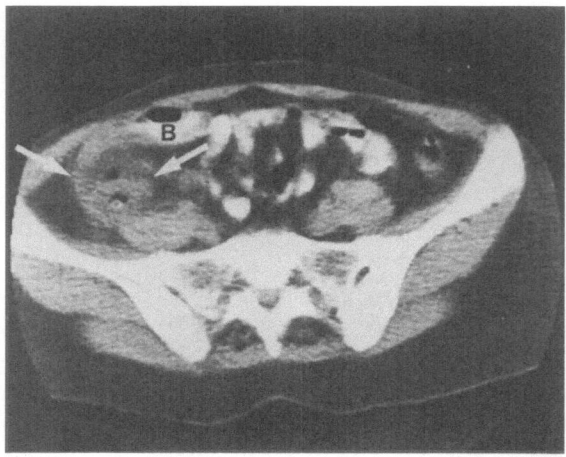

Figure 10.15(a)

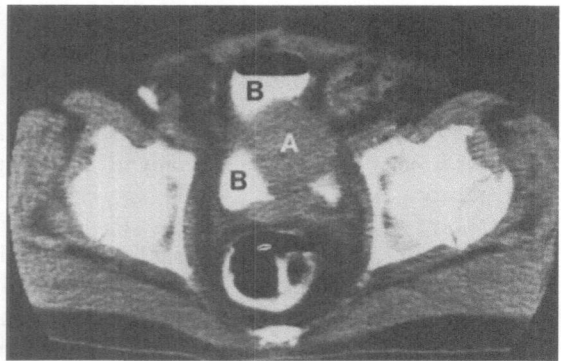

Figure 10.14(b)

Figure 10.14 Abdominal abscesses. (a) Left renal bed
abscess following nephrectomy. The rim has enhanced
following an injection of intravenous contrast medium
(arrowed). Note fluid level within the abscess. (b) Pelvic
abscess (A) from diverticular disease. The mass com-
presses the bladder (B) which has been opacified with
contrast medium. There is no gas in this abscess and its
density is indistinguishable from that of a tumour

psoas abscesses which are difficult to diagnose by
other means (figure 10.16a). Such abscesses are
usually seen as collections of low attenuation within
the muscle, extending from the upper lumbar region

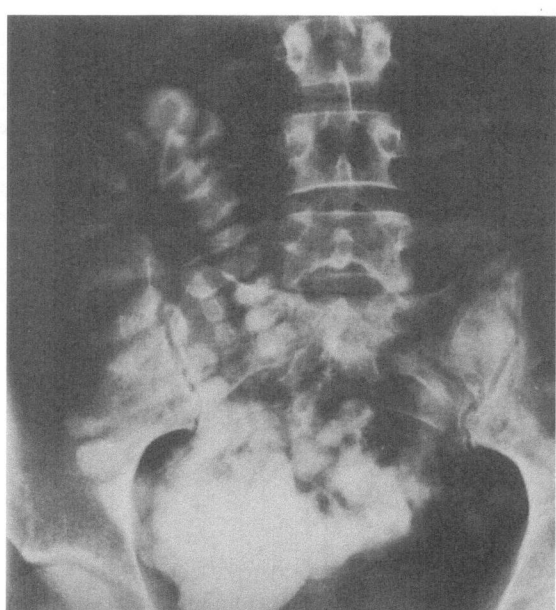

Figure 10.15(b)

Figure 10.15 Abscess in right iliac fossa. (a) CT scan
shows small pockets of air within a mass. Although there
is contrast medium in some of the bowel (B), this mass
could easily be confused with caecum. (b) Plain radiograph taken at the time of the scan to ensure that the
oral contrast medium had filled the caecum

towards the inguinal canal (figure 10.16b and c) (Ralls *et al.*, 1980).

Fibrosis Retroperitoneal fibrosis also presents as a mass (figure 10.17). The mass may be indistinguishable from enlarged lymph nodes, as it has a soft-tissue density and obscures the margins of the great vessels and psoas muscles (Sterzer *et al.*, 1979).

It is clear that it is frequently difficult to distinguish retroperitoneal tumours from haematomas, abscesses or fibrosis. However, the clinical features

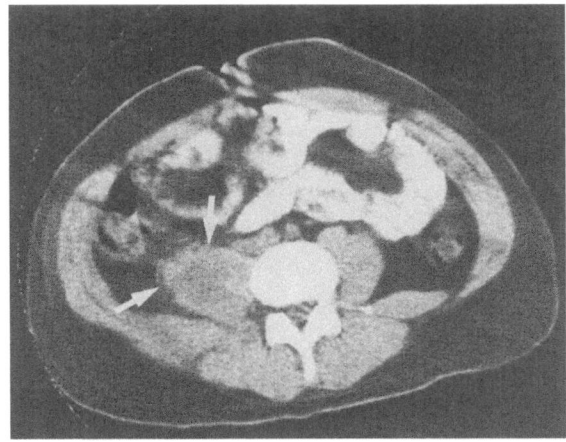

Figure 10.16(c)

Figure 10.16   Psoas abscesses. (a) Tuberculous psoas abscess (arrowed). Note the abscess has a lower density than the adjacent psoas muscle (P). (b) and (c) Two scans from patient with psoas abscess due to actinomytosis (arrowed). The abscess has a low-density centre which extends laterally into the iliopsoas muscle

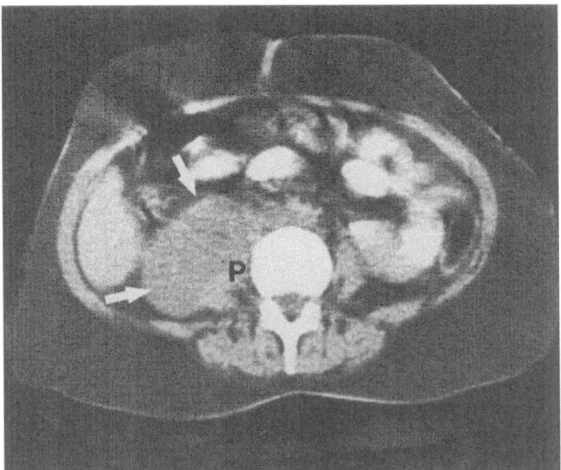

Figure 10.16(a)

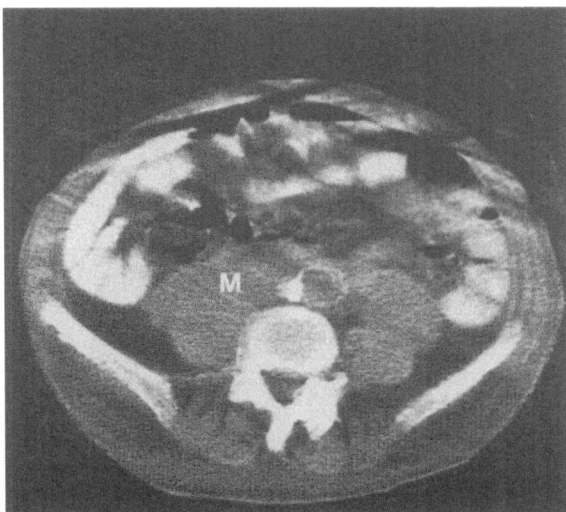

Figure 10.17   Retroperitoneal fibrosis. The mass (M) has similar appearance to enlarged nodes. The margins of adjacent structures are obscured

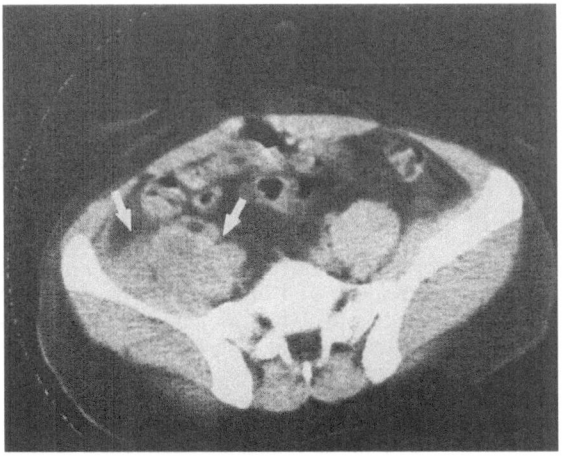

Figure 10.16(b)

usually permit the correct diagnosis to be made, but, if there is doubt, CT-guided aspiration/biopsy can be readily carried out.

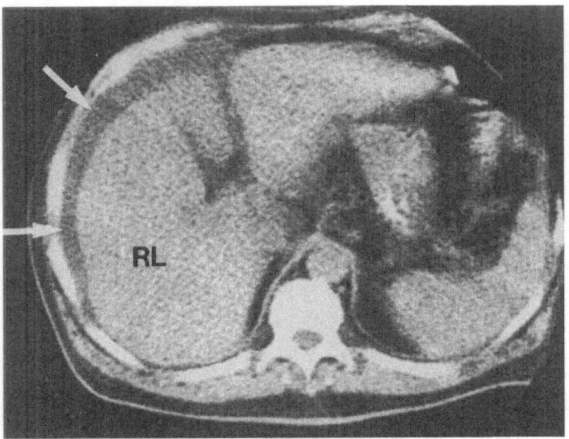

Figure 10.18(a)

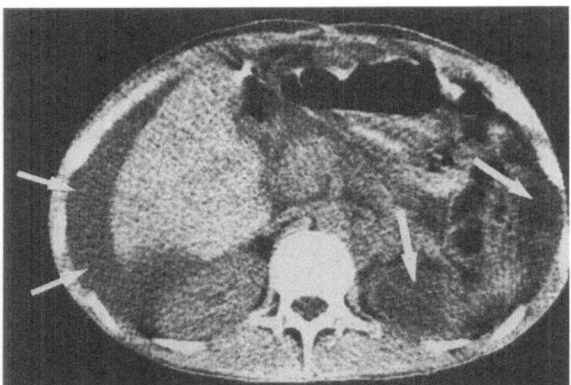

Figure 10.18(b)

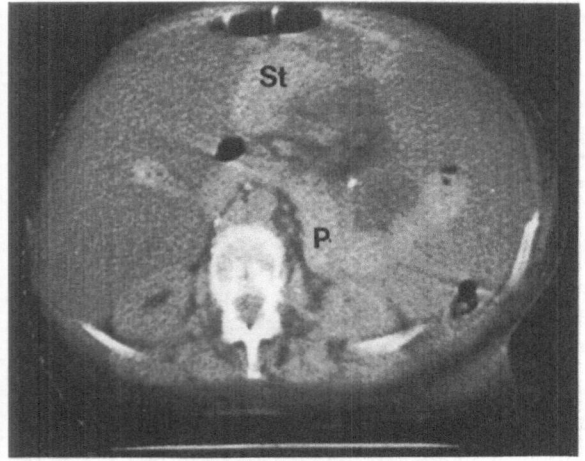

Figure 10.18(c)

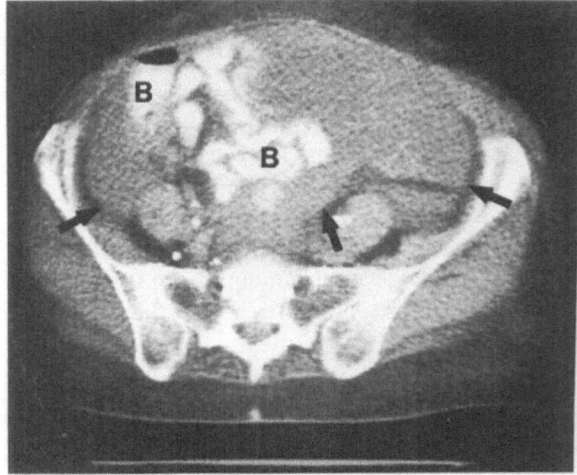

Figure 10.18(d)

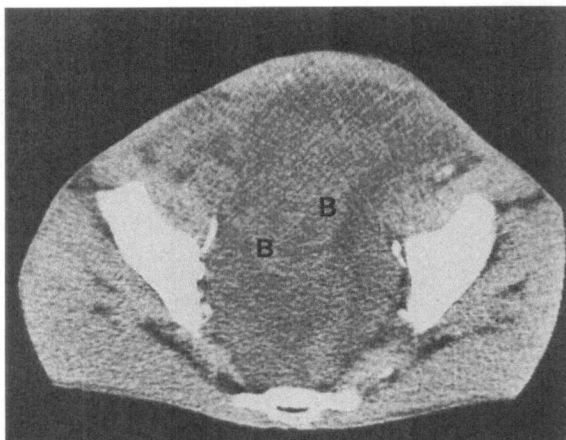

Figure 10.18(e)

Figure 10.18 Ascites. (a) Minimal ascites (arrowed). There is accumulation of fluid around the anterolateral aspect of the right lobe of the liver (RL). There is no evidence of fluid on the left side of the abdomen. (b) Moderate ascites. Fluid (arrowed) can be seen around the right lobe of the liver and also on the left side of the abdomen (arrowed). (c) Gross ascites. The pancreas (P) and stomach (St) are seen as high-density structures surrounded by fluid. (d) Gross ascites showing loops of small bowel opacified with contrast medium (B). Note the line of the posterior peritoneum (arrowed). (e) Gross ascites. Bowel loops have not been opacified and interpretation is difficult (B)

ASCITES

Ascites spreads along well defined pathways, as described by Meyers (1976). Fluid produced in the inframesocolic compartment (*see* figure 10.7) accumulates first in the pouch of Douglas (*see* figure 10.8) and then ascends along both paracolic gutters but more on the right than on the left. It then passes deep to the inferior edge of the liver into the right subhepatic space, Morison's pouch. Fluid produced in the right supramesocolic compartment also flows into the right subphrenic space and thence to the pelvis. It is for this reason that ascites is often seen around the right lobe of the liver on CT (figure 10.18a) when none is demonstrated on the left. Fluid collections on the left side of the abdomen (figure 10.18b) do not move so freely, and any large amount of fluid spreads to the pelvis. In gross ascites, all the compartments of the abdomen and pelvis are occupied by fluid (figure 10.18c).

Ascites in the upper abdomen is clearly shown with CT because the liver and other soft tissues have a higher density than does the surrounding fluid. The fluid is limited posteriorly by the peritoneal reflection giving a characteristic appearance (figure 10.18a). If there is only a small amount of ascites, the appearances may be confused with a subphrenic abscess.

Ascites lower down in the abdomen or pelvis shows the normal structures bathed in fluid (figure 10.18c). However, if bowel loops are unopacified, then the appearances may be confusing (figure 10.18d and e). The appearance of a small amount of ascites in the pelvis is illustrated elsewhere in figure 10.8a.

Ascites may be demonstrated with CT when there is no clinical indication of its presence.

AORTA

Aortic aneurysms are elegantly demonstrated with CT because their margins are well defined. An aneurysm has a uniform soft-tissue density on the unenhanced scan (figure 10.19a), but after the injection of intravenous contrast medium the effective lumen can be seen separated from the wall by low-density thrombus (figure 10.19b). CT is an accurate

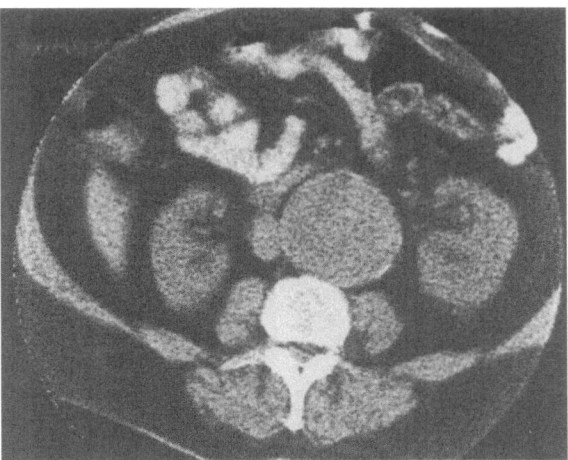

Figure 10.19(a)

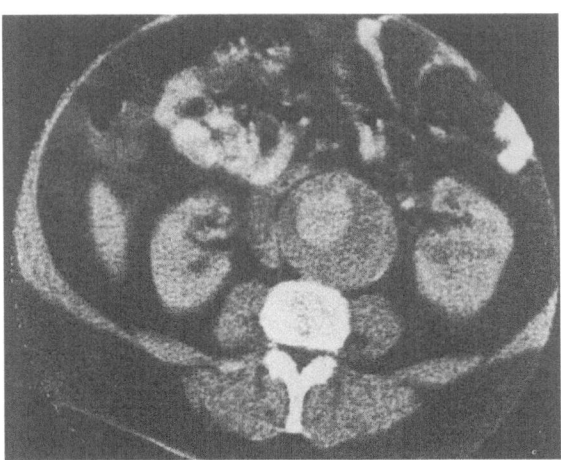

Figure 10.19(b)

Figure 10.19 Aortic aneurysm. (a) Before injection of intravenous contrast medium, the aneurysm has a homogeneous density. Note calcification in the wall. (b) After injection of intravenous contrast medium, the effective lumen is demonstrated

method of measuring the dimensions of the aneurysm and its relationship to the renal vessels (Gomes, 1978; Dixon *et al.*, 1981). Bleeding from an aortic aneurysm is seen as an irregular soft-tissue mass around the enlarged aorta (figure 10.20, and *see* figure 10.13a). Dissection of the aorta can only

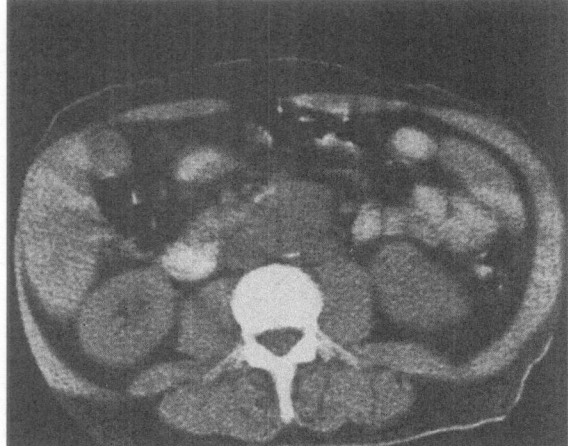

Figure 10.20(a)

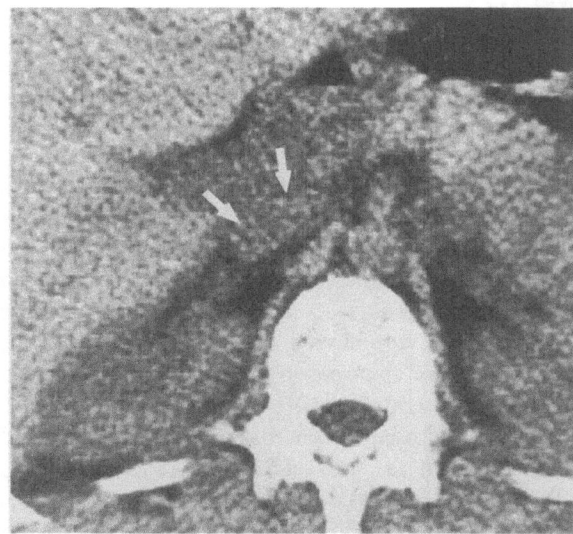

Figure 10.21(a)

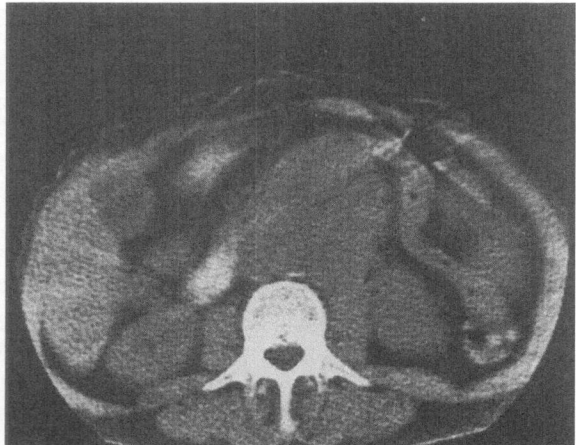

Figure 10.20(b)

Figure 10.20   Bleeding aortic aneurysm. (a) Scan shows the aneurysm before the haemorrhage. (b) Scan three months later shows the aneurysm immediately after an acute bleed

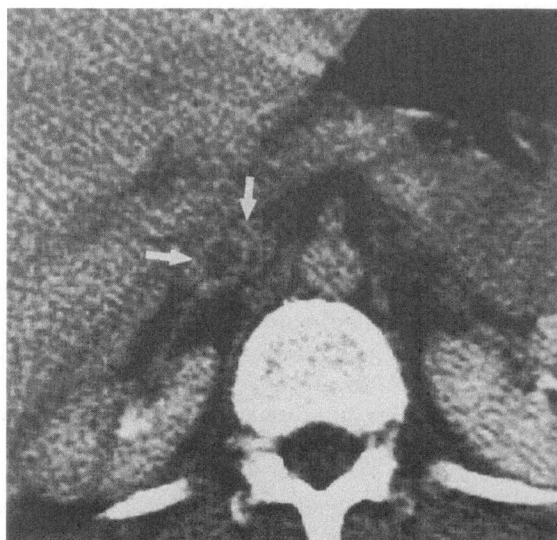

Figure 10.21(b)

Figure 10.21   Thrombus in the inferior vena cava. (a) No abnormality is seen before the injection of contrast medium. Inferior vena cava (arrowed). (b) After the injection of intravenous contrast medium into a vein in the foot, a well-defined lucency is seen lying centrally in the inferior vena cava (arrowed)

be diagnosed with confidence if both lumina can be demonstrated after the injection of contrast medium.

INFERIOR VENA CAVA

Filling defects within the inferior vena cava are demonstrated with CT after injection of intravenous contrast medium (figure 10.21). If the inferior vena cava is not enlarged, it is impossible to distinguish

thrombus from tumour invasion. However, Marks *et al.* (1978) considered that enlargement of the inferior vena cava together with dilatation of the contiguous renal vein indicated tumour thrombus in patients with renal cell carcinomas (figure 10.22).

CT may also be used to evaluate anomalies of the inferior vena cava and renal veins (Royal and Callen, 1979).

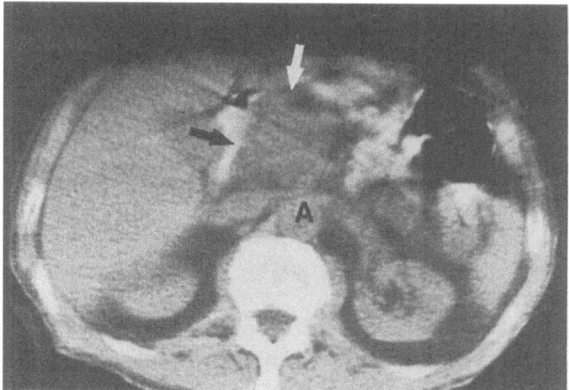

Figure 10.23(a)

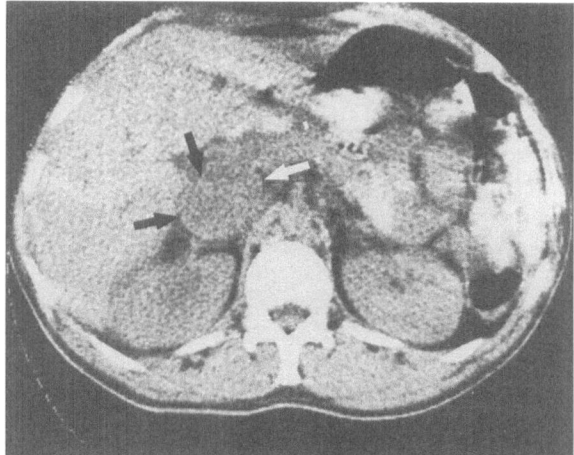

Figure 10.22 **Enlarged inferior vena cava (arrowed) due to tumour thrombus**

USE OF COMPUTED TOMOGRAPHY IN ASSESSMENT OF INTRA-ABDOMINAL MASSES

CT is making an important impact in the investigation of patients with abdominal masses. It can confirm the presence of a mass and can indicate its site and sometimes its nature. Even more important, normal scans showing no evidence of a mass may preclude further investigation (figure 10.23). CT is particularly valuable for the elucidation of possible masses in the left upper quadrant, an area which is frequently difficult to assess by other means.

CT is also very helpful in the diagnosis of intra-abdominal abscess. The accuracy of reported series is well over 90% (Daffner *et al.*, 1979; Wolverton *et al.*, 1979). Gerzof *et al.* (1978) emphasised that surgical incision and drainage may be replaced by CT-guided percutaneous catheter drainage in many patients.

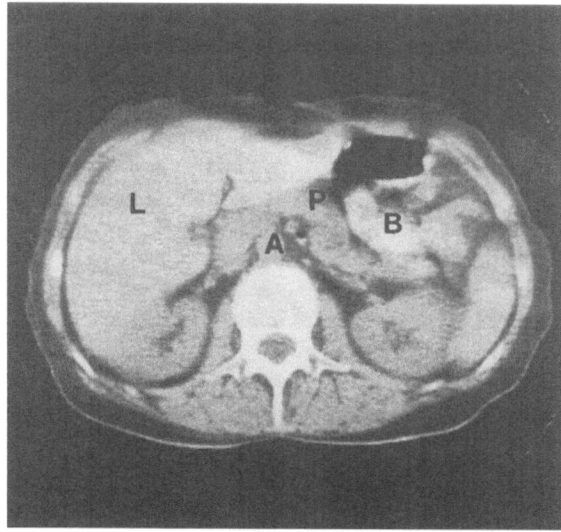

Figure 10.23(b)

Figure 10.23 **Two patients with pulsatile epigastric masses. (a) The scan shows a large mass lying anteriorly in the head of the pancreas (arrowed) due to a carcinoma. The aorta (A) appears normal. (b) In this thin elderly female patient, the scan shows a normal aorta (A) and no evidence of an abnormal mass. Pancreas (P), liver (L), bowel (B)**

CT appears to be the best method available for the assessment of aortic aneurysms, because it is more effective than ultrasound for demonstrating the relationship of the aneurysm to the renal vessels, and is not hampered by overlying bowel gas.

Callen *et al.* (1979) also point out that CT is

better than ultrasound for examination of the retroperitoneum in patients with ascites. In the presence of ascites, the retroperitoneal structures are often obscured when using ultrasound, but good visualisation is obtained with CT.

SPLEEN

The spleen is invariably demonstrated as a well defined soft-tissue structure in the left upper quadrant (figure 10.24a). It has a similar density to that of the liver. The splenic vein passes behind the tail and body of the pancreas and is more commonly identified than the splenic artery. In some patients, the spleen has a prominent bulge medially when seen in cross section (figure 10.24b). Unless recognised, this can be confused with a mass in the upper pole of the kidney. The size of the spleen is variable but is generally considered to be enlarged if it extends below the costal margin. Moderate and gross splenic enlargement is easily identified with CT but minimal alteration in size is difficult to appreciate.

Splenic abnormalities demonstrated with CT include cysts, haematomas, calcification and occasionally tumours.

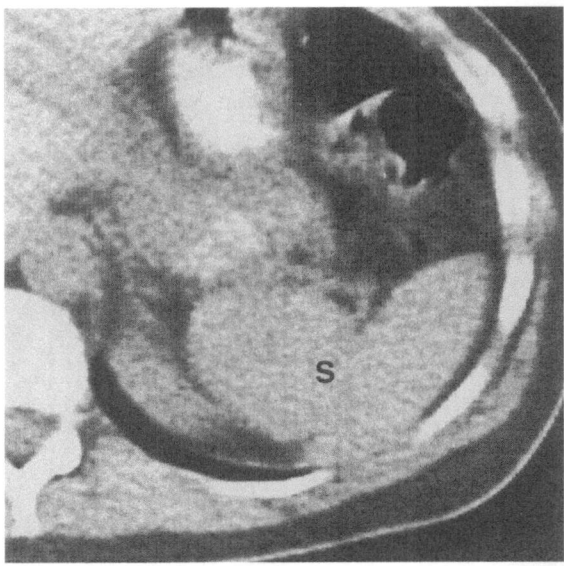

Figure 10.24(b)

Figure 10.24   Normal spleen (S): (a) showing vessels (arrowed), and (b) showing medial bulge. This normal appearance can be confused with an abnormality of the upper side of the kidney

Figure 10.25a illustrates a *splenic cyst*. The lesion has a low density similar to other cysts in the body and a well defined margin. The body of the spleen and the stomach are displaced medially by the mass.

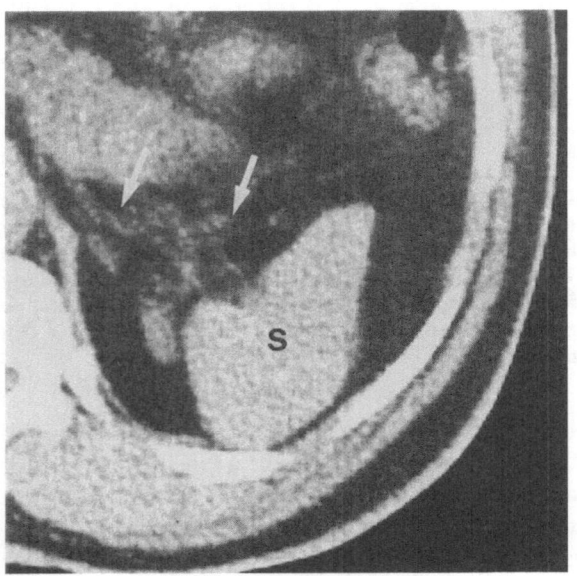

Figure 10.24(a)

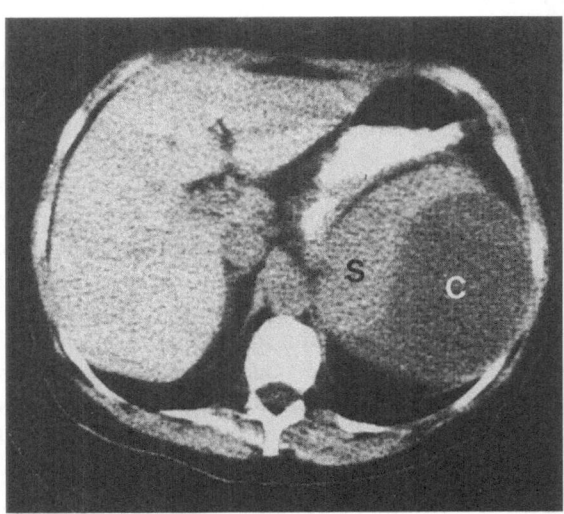

Figure 10.25(a)

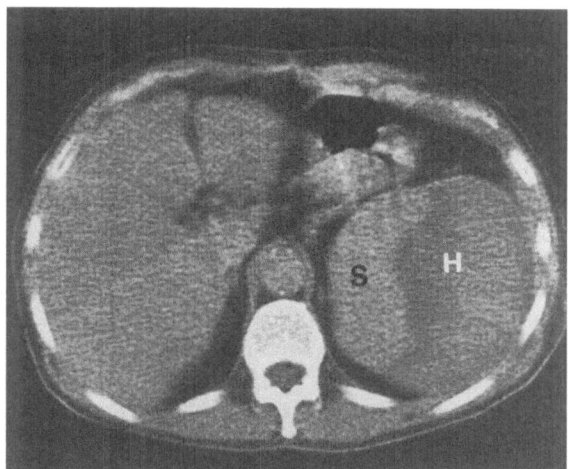

Figure 10.25(b)

Figure 10.25 Two lateral splenic masses. (a) Cyst (C) and spleen (S). The spleen and stomach are displaced medially by the mass which has a density close to that of water. (b) Subcapsular haematoma (H) which contains areas of varying density. Spleen (S)

A *haematoma* may have a similar appearance (figure 10.25b). Areas of high density are seen within the mass if the haematoma is relatively recent. Calcification in the spleen is easily shown with CT, although in most patients this has little clinical significance (figure 10.26). There has been much discussion in the literature regarding the ability of

CT to detect splenic involvement in malignant disease (*see* chapter 11). Unfortunately, CT is unable to identify lesions less than 1 cm in diameter. Diffuse involvement in such conditions as Hodgkin's disease cannot, therefore, be recognised. However, occasionally a large focal lesion is identified (figure 10.27) in a patient with Hodgkin's disease and this may have important influence on management.

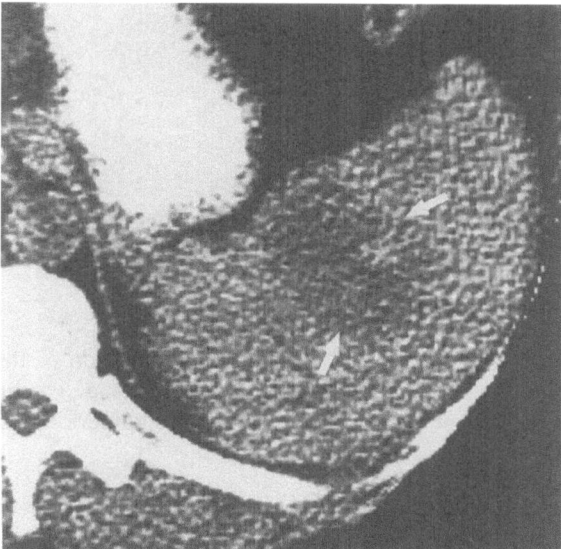

Figure 10.27 CT scan of a patient with Hodgkin's disease. Note large focal lesion (arrowed)

Uniform gross enlargement of the spleen may be seen in many conditions, but in general the CT examination is almost invariably carried out for another reason.

GASTROINTESTINAL TRACT

The application of CT to the investigation of the gastrointestinal tract is limited because the mucosal pattern cannot be seen and intraluminal masses are only occasionally identified. The technique is most useful for determining the extraluminal extent of malignant disease (Kressel *et al.*, 1978; Lee *et al.*, 1979). Occasionally, it may demonstrate a mass arising from the alimentary tract when this is not previously known (figure 10.28).

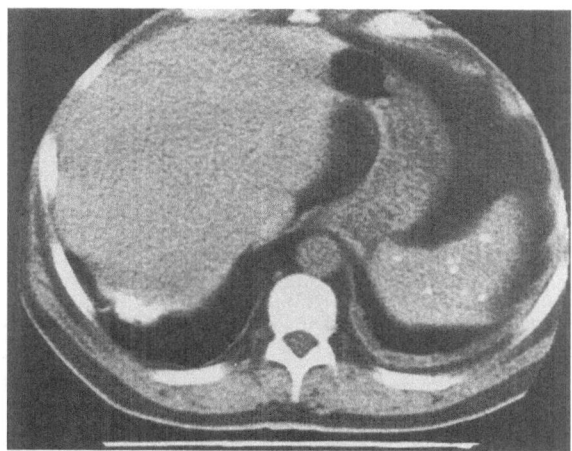

Figure 10.26 Calcification in the spleen

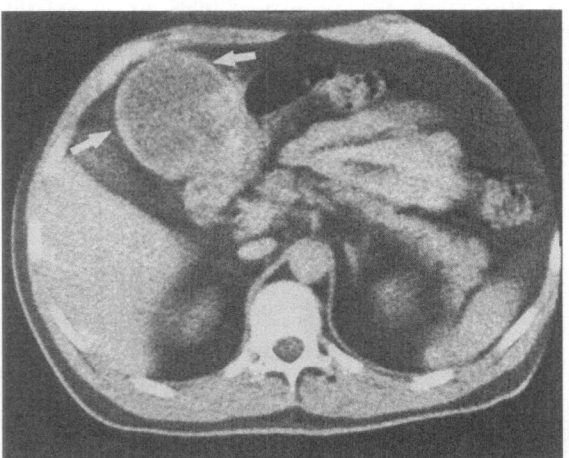

Figure 10.28 Leiomyoma arising from the lesser curvature of the stomach (arrowed). Barium examination showed only extrinsic compression

The application of CT to the examination of the oesophagus and rectum have been excluded from this discussion and are discussed in chapters 4 and 12.

ASPIRATION TECHNIQUES GUIDED BY COMPUTED TOMOGRAPHY

The technique of using CT for guiding various percutaneous procedures is now well established and several reports in the literature demonstrate that it is an accurate method of needling lesions in many different anatomical sites (Haaga *et al.*, 1977; Ferrucci and Wittenberg, 1978; Hardy *et al.*, 1980). It is beyond the scope of this text to describe the different techniques in detail. At the Royal Marsden Hospital, the procedure is based on that described by Haaga *et al.* (1977) and consists of three stages, as follows.

Selection of the Appropriate Scan

After a full series of diagnostic CT scans have been obtained, an appropriate slice demonstrating the mass to be aspirated is chosen. A CT scan is then repeated at the chosen level and the level of the slice is marked on the patient's skin.

Localisation of the Entry Point

The entry site on the skin is chosen according to the position of the mass and the structures in the proposed needle pathway. If necessary the patient is turned into the lateral oblique or prone position so that major vascular structures and other organs can be avoided. A metal marker is then placed on the skin in the longitudinal plane (figure 10.29) and the

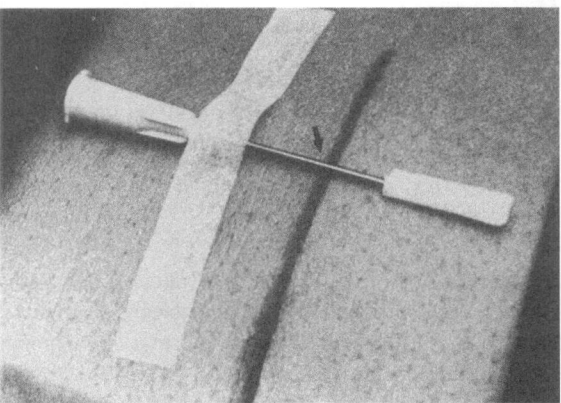

Figure 10.29 CT-guided aspiration procedure. The proposed entry site is marked on the patient's skin (arrowed)

scan repeated. The metal marker is clearly seen on the CT image (figure 10.30a). An injection of intravenous contrast medium is given before repeating the scan to demonstrate the vascular anatomy in the region of the mass and to avoid puncture of a highly vascular lesion, such as a haemangioma.

Aspiration

Percutaneous fine-needle aspiration is carried out under sterile conditions using local anaesthesia. An appropriate needle is selected which varies in length and gauge depending upon the site and size of the mass. Thus, a 22 French gauge spinal needle is used for aspiration of the pancreas. Other intra-

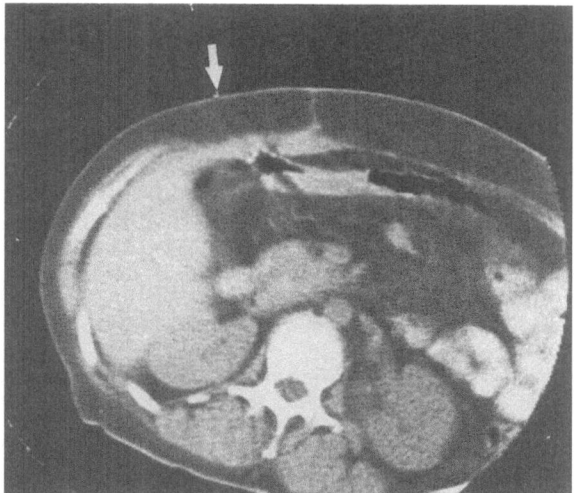

Figure 10.30(a)

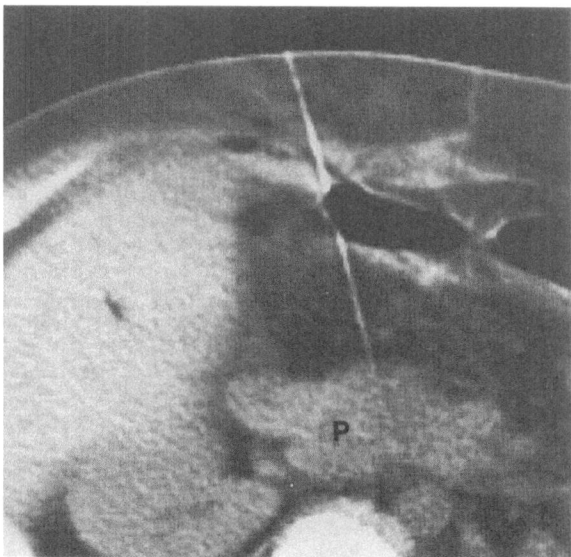

Figure 10.30(b)

Figure 10.30   Fine-needle aspiration of the pancreas. (a) The metal marker placed on the patient's skin is identified on the scan (arrowed). (b) A scan is taken just before aspiration to show the position of the needle in relation to the mass (P)

abdominal masses require a larger needle, e.g. an 18 gauge Menghini needle may be used for aspiration of retroperitoneal and liver lesions. The length of the needle chosen depends on the depth to which it is to be inserted, but it should not be excessively long because this may prevent the patient from entering the scanning gantry. The needle is directed to the predetermined depth during suspended respiration and the repeat scan obtained. If the needle is directly in line it is advanced into the mass and a further scan taken just before aspiration (figure 10.30b). A double-needle technique is sometimes used, whereby a fine needle (22 French gauge) is passed through a large needle (18 French gauge). This provides greater stability for directing the needle towards the lesion (Haaga *et al.*, 1977). Aspiration is obtained during suspended respiration.

Problems

In our experience, one of the main problems of using CT for guided aspiration techniques is that the needle is not always visualised on the repeat CT scan. This results from inaccuracy of couch movement and on the patient's inability to suspend respiration at the same degree of inspiration for each scan. Partial visualisation of the needle occasionally occurs if it has been directed obliquely so that it passes out of the CT section. Once this pitfall is appreciated, it can easily be recognised by measuring the portion of the needle seen on the CT image and comparing it with the actual length introduced into the patient. If this occurs, the needle should be redirected before attempting to aspirate the mass.

Apart from this technical difficulty, the main disadvantages of using CT for guiding percutaneous techniques are that it is a time-consuming and relatively cumbersome method. However, an excellent display of the anatomy in the region of a lesion is obtained, providing a degree of precision frequently unobtainable by other methods.

The Indications for Procedures Guided by Computed Tomography

(1) Intra-abdominal lesions not demonstrated by ultrasound or demonstrated better with CT. This may include lesions of the liver, the pancreas (figure 10.30) or the retroperitoneum (figure 10.31).

(2) Masses close to bone or close to the lateral pelvic side wall.

(3) Mediastinal lesions.

(4) Bone lesions (figure 10.32).

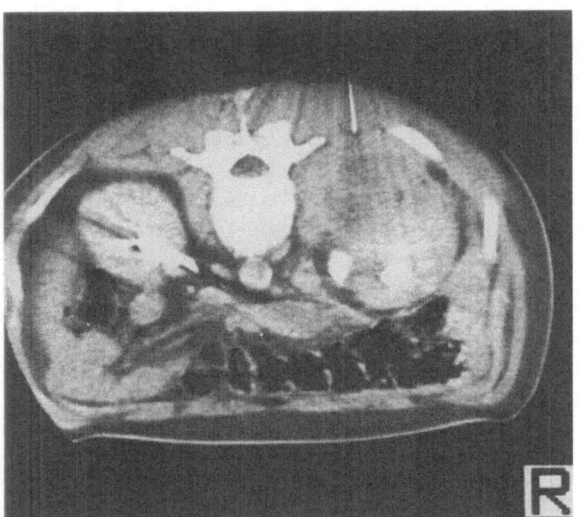

Figure 10.31 CT-guided aspiration of a large retroperitoneal abscess

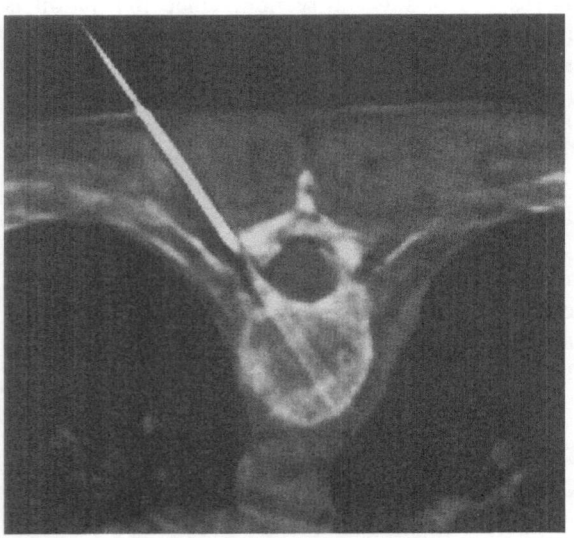

Figure 10.32 CT-guided bone biopsy of the ninth thoracic vertebra in a patient with Hodgkin's disease. The conventional film showed a generalised increase in density of the vertebral body following radiotherapy treatment for Stage I disease. The biopsy was normal

CT can be used to drain intra-abdominal abscesses as well as to obtain material for cytological and histological diagnosis.

REFERENCES

Amendola, M. A., Tisnado, J., Fields, W. R., Beachley, M. C., Vines, F. S., Cho, S.-R., Turner, M. A. and Konerding, K. F. (1979). Evaluation of retroperitoneal hemorrhage by computed tomography before and after translumbar aortography. *Radiology*, **133**, 401–404

Callen, P. W. (1979). Computed tomographic evaluation of abdominal and pelvic abscesses. *Radiology*, **131**, 171–175

Callen, P. W., Marks, W. M. and Filly, R. A. (1979). Computed tomography and ultrasonography in the evaluation of the retroperitoneum in patients with malignant ascites. *Journal of Computer Assisted Tomography*, **3** (5), 581–584

Daffner, R. H., Halber, M. D., Morgan, C. L., Trought, W. S., Thompson, W. M. and Rice, R. P. (1979). Computed tomography in the diagnosis of intra-abdominal abscesses. *Annals of Surgery*, **189** (1), 29–33

Dixon, A. K., Springall, R. G., Kelsey Fry, I. and Taylor, G. W. (1981). Computed tomography (CT) of abdominal aortic aneurysms: determination of longitudinal extent. *British Journal of Surgery*, **68** (1), 47–50

Ferrucci, J. T. and Wittenberg, J. (1978). CT biopsy of abdominal tumours: aids for lesion localisation. *Radiology*, **129**, 739–744

Gerzof, S. G., Robbins, A. H. and Birkett, D. H. (1978). Computed tomography in the diagnosis and management of abdominal abscesses. *Gastrointestinal Radiology*, **3**, 287–294

Gomes, M. N. (1978). CT scanning of the abdominal aorta. In *Abdominal Radiology: Abdomen CT*, eds. J. L. Lamarque and J. N. Bruel, Excerpta Medica, Amsterdam

Haaga, J. R., Reich, N. E., Havrilla, T. R. and Alfidi, R. J. (1977). Interventional CT scanning. *Radiologic Clinics of North America*, **XV** (3), 449–456

Hardy, D. C., Murphy, W. A. and Gilula, L. A. (1980). Computed tomography in planning percutaneous bone biopsy. *Radiology*, **134**, 447–450

Kressel, H. Y., Callen, P. W., Montagne, J.-P., Korobkin, M., Goldberg, H. I., Moss, A. A., Arger, P. H. and Margulis, A. R. (1978). Computed tomographic evaluation of disorders affecting the alimentary tract. *Radiology*, **129**, 451–455

Lee, K. R., Levine, E., Moffat, R. E., Bigongiari, L. R. and Hermreck, A. S. (1979). Computed tomographic staging of malignant gastric neoplasms. *Radiology*, **133**, 151–155

Marks, W. M., Korobkin, M., Callen, P. W. and Kaiser, J. A. (1978). CT diagnosis of tumor thrombosis of the renal vein and inferior vena cava. *American Journal of Roentgenology*, **131**, 843–846

Mendez, G., Jr., Isikoff, M. B. and Hill, M. C. (1980). Retroperitoneal processes involving the psoas demonstrated by computed tomography. *Journal of Computer Assisted Tomography*, **4** (1), 78–82

Meyers, M. A. (1976). In *Dynamic Radiology of the Abdomen: Normal and Pathology Anatomy*, Springer-Verlag, New York, Heidelberg and Berne

Ralls, P. W., Boswell, W., Henderson, R., Rogers, W., Boger, D. and Halls, J. (1980). CT of inflammatory disease of the psoas muscle. *American Journal of Roentgenology*, **134**, 767–770

Royal, S. A. and Callen, P. W. (1979). CT evaluation of anomalies of the inferior vena cava and left renal vein. *American Journal of Roentgenology*, **132**, 759–763

Sagel, S. S., Siegel, M. J., Stanley, R. J. and Jost, R. G. (1977). Detection of retroperitoneal haemorrhage by computed tomography. *American Journal of Roentgenology*, **129**, 403–407

Sterzer, S. K., Herr, H. W. and Mintz, I. (1979). Idiopathic retroperitoneal fibrosis misinterpreted as lymphoma by computed tomography. *Journal of Urology*, **122**, 405–406

Wolverson, M. K., Jagannadharao, B., Sundaram, M., Joyce, P. F., Riaz, M. A. and Shields, J. B. (1979). CT as a primary diagnostic method in evaluating intra-abdominal abscess. *American Journal of Roentgenology*, **133**, 1089–1095

11

Lymph Node Disease of the Abdomen and Pelvis

CT can demonstrate lymphadenopathy not only in those sites opacified at lymphography but also in those areas which are inaccessible, for example, the internal iliac and mesenteric nodes, and those in the porta hepatis and the retrocrural space. In this chapter, the CT findings in lymph node disease are described and the relationship of CT to lymphography in different tumour types is discussed.

TECHNIQUE OF EXAMINATION

If lymphadenopathy is suspected in the retroperitoneum, scans should be taken through the abdomen from the dome of the diaphragm to the aortic bifurcation. Intervals of 2 cm are generally regarded as acceptable because several nodes along the lymph node chains are usually involved if disease is present. However, if the primary disease is likely to involve the splenic hilar nodes or nodes in the mesentery and porta hepatis (e.g. lymphoma), it is preferable to scan the upper abdomen at intervals of 1.0 or 1.5 cm.

The investigation of pelvic lymphadenopathy is usually part of an examination to assess a primary pelvic tumour; in this situation, scans are taken at 1 cm intervals from the symphysis pubis to the middle of the fifth lumbar vertebra.

CT ANATOMY AND ABNORMAL APPEARANCES

The lymph nodes of the abdomen and pelvis consist of numerous small peripheral groups which are placed alongside the arterial tree and of central groups which are closely related to the aorta and receive the lymphatic drainage from the peripheral groups. Enlarged nodes can be detected in several major sites (figure 11.1). These include the para-aortic, retro-aortic and pre-aortic chains, the retrocrural space, the mesentery, porta hepatis, splenic and renal hila. The coeliac group of nodes form part of the pre-aortic chain, and peripancreatic nodes can also occasionally be identified. In the pelvis, enlarged nodes can be detected in the external iliac and internal iliac chains and occasionally in the obturator group of nodes.

In general, enlarged lymph nodes have a homogeneous density similar to other soft tissues, and the internal architecture of the node cannot be seen (figure 11.2). Thus, the only feature which distinguishes the normal from the abnormal node is enlargement. In most sites, nodes are considered to be enlarged if greater than 1.5 cm in diameter (Redman et al., 1977; Hodson et al., 1979). A notable exception is the retrocrural space, where normal structures, excluding the aorta, rarely exceed 6 mm in diameter (Callen et al., 1977) and soft-tissue structures larger than this are regarded as abnormal (figure 11.3).

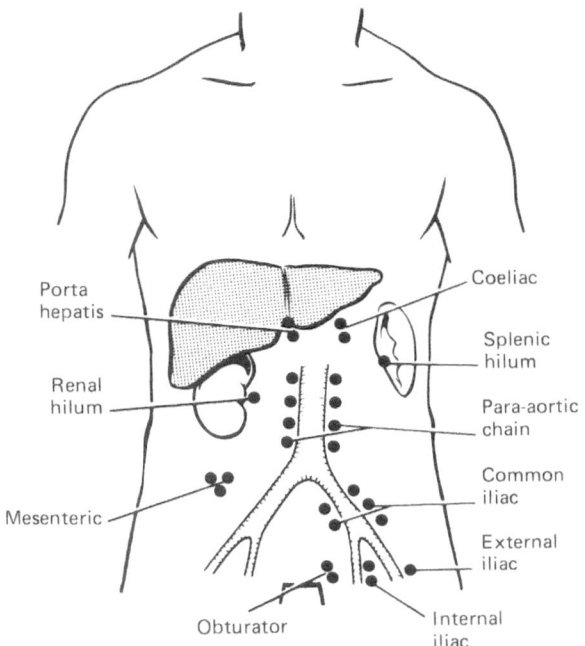

Figure 11.1 Diagram to show major sites where enlarged lymph nodes can be identified with CT

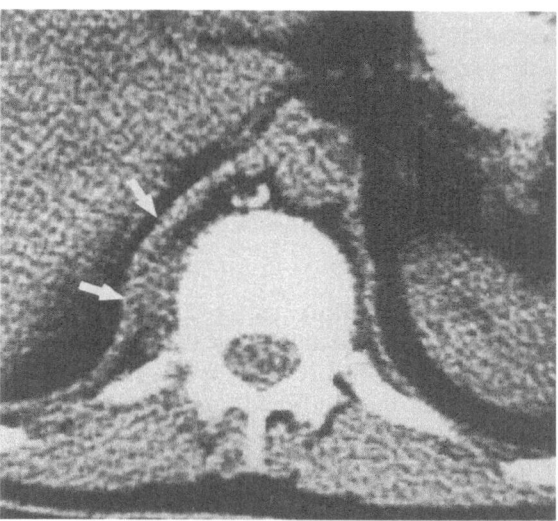

Figure 11.3 Enlarged retrocrural node on the right (arrowed). The right crus is elevated

The ability of CT to detect lymphadenopathy depends on the site of involvement and the degree of lymph node enlargement. By far the easiest areas to examine are the retroperitoneal and retrocrural

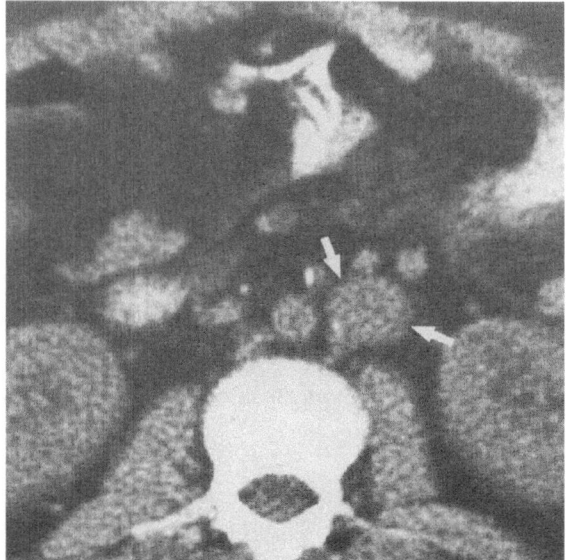

Figure 11.2 Enlarged lymph node (arrowed) adjacent to the aorta. The enlarged node has a similar density to other soft-tissue structures

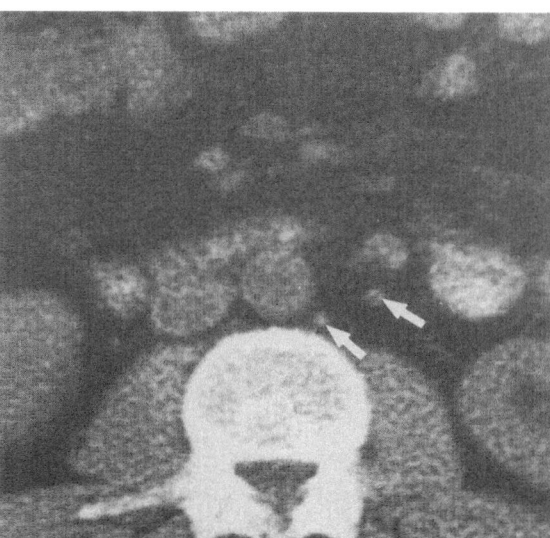

Figure 11.4 Small structures (arrowed) presumed to be normal nodes to the left of the aorta in a patient with abundant retroperitoneal fat

spaces, because here the lymph nodes are surrounded by fat. In obese patients, it is even possible to identify normal-sized lymph nodes in these areas (figure 11.4).

PARA-AORTIC AND RETROCRURAL NODES

Para-aortic Region

In the para-aortic region, enlarged nodes appear as discrete structures of soft-tissue density within the retroperitoneal fat (figure 11.5) or as a conglomerate mass in which the individual nodes cannot be distinguished (figure 11.6). A characteristic sign is obliteration of normal anatomical contours adjacent to the enlarged nodes. Thus, obliteration of the margin of the aorta and/or inferior vena cava is a very common observation, and, if there is gross disease, these vessels may be completely lost within the tumour mass (figure 11.7). Large nodes behind the aorta and inferior vena cava push these vessels forwards, the 'floating aorta' sign (figure 11.8). The anterior and lateral contours of the psoas muscles are also frequently obscured. Loss of these normal contours cannot, however, be regarded as pathognomonic of lymphadenopathy, as it may be seen in

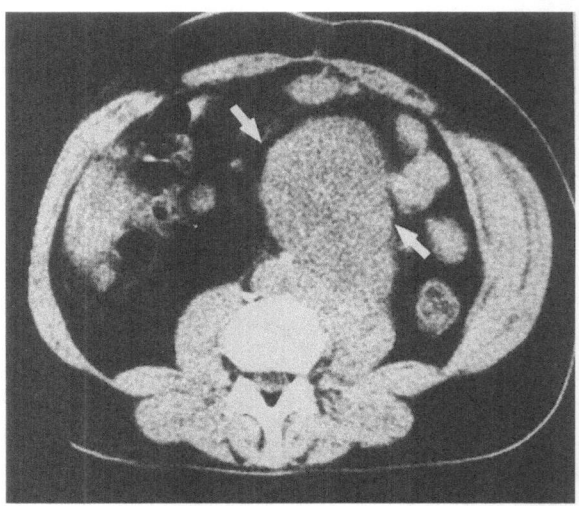

Figure 11.6   Conglomerate mass of enlarged nodes in the para-aortic region (arrowed)

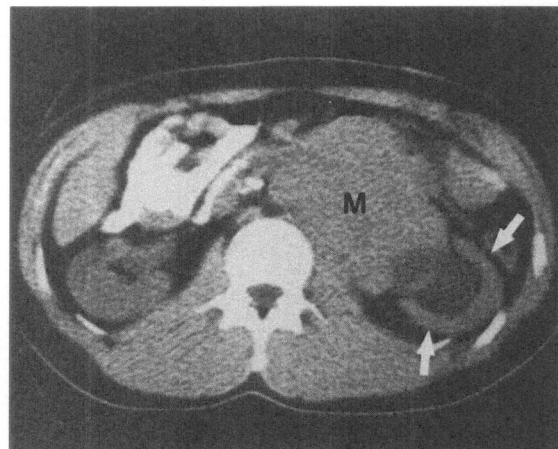

Figure 11.7   Enlarged para-aortic lymph nodes (M) in a patient with testicular teratoma. The mass has completely obscured the margin of the aorta so that it can no longer be identified. Note hydronephrosis of the left kidney (arrowed)

other conditions such as retroperitoneal haematoma, primary retroperitoneal tumours and primary retroperitoneal fibrosis (*see* chapter 9). Fibrosis can occur as a result of radiotherapy, and we have now seen several patients in whom the margins of the aorta and inferior vena cava are difficult to delineate

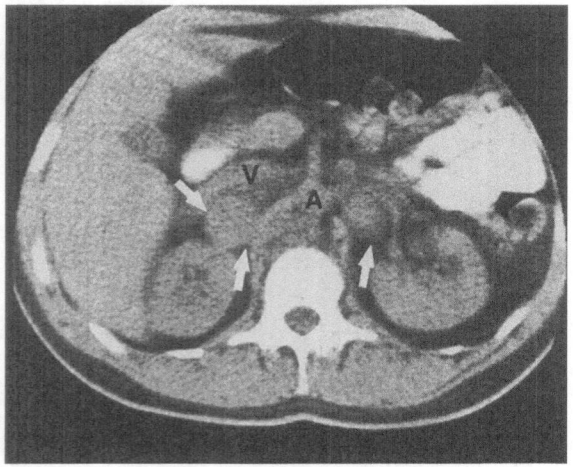

Figure 11.5   Discrete enlargement of lymph nodes in the para-aortic region (arrowed). Aorta (A), inferior vena cava (V)

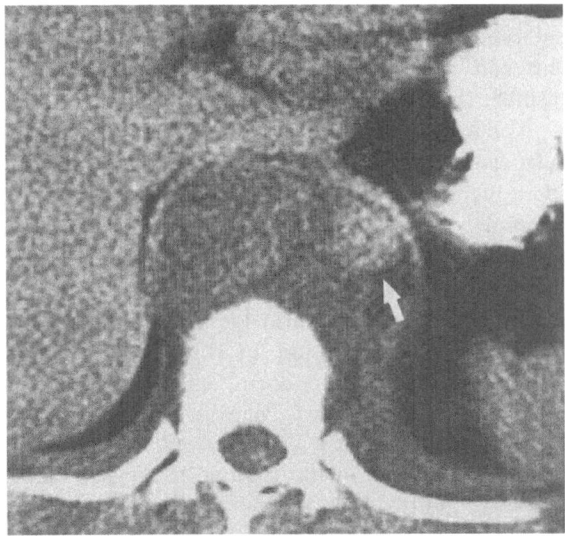

Figure 11.8(a)

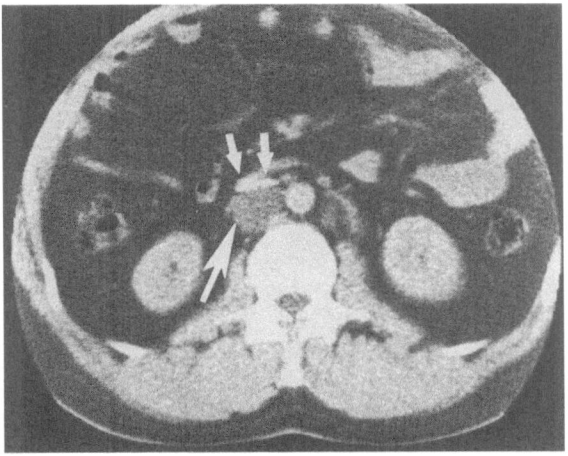

Figure 11.8(b)

Figure 11.8 Anterior displacement of the major vessels. (a) 'Floating aorta' sign. There is a mass of enlarged nodes in the retrocrural space which has pushed the aorta forwards (arrowed). (b) The inferior vena cava opacified with contrast medium (small arrows) has been pushed forwards by an enlarged node (large arrow)

following irradiation (figure 11.9). Continued clinical remission in two of these patients for a minimum period of two years indicates that the CT appearances are more likely to be due to fibrosis than any other pathology.

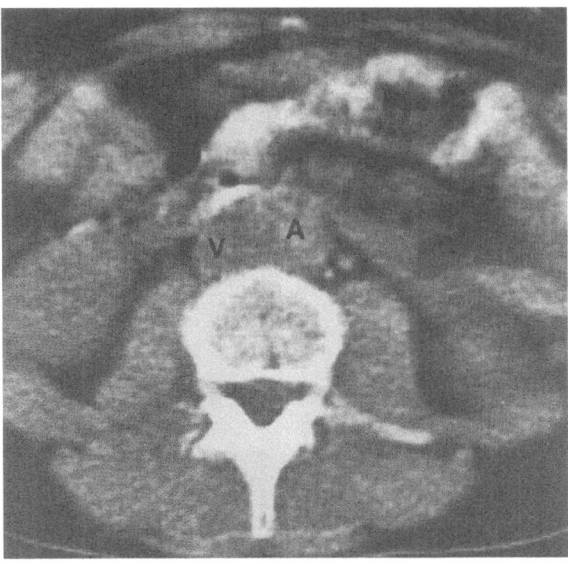

Figure 11.9 CT scan in a patient with a seminoma of the testis who had received radiotherapy to the para-aortic nodes. There is extra soft tissue between the aorta (A) and inferior vena cava (V) which has obscured the medial margins of these vessels. This appearance probably represents radiation fibrosis as the patient has remained well for over two years without any evidence of recurrent disease

The CT appearances of enlarged retroperitoneal lymph nodes does not permit reliable distinction between different types of disease, and, indeed, if the enlarged nodes are discrete, it is impossible to distinguish reactive hyperplasia from tumour. In patients with malignant testicular teratomas, the findings are, however, frequently characteristic. The lymphatic drainage of the testis is direct to the para-aortic lymph node chain and the metastases are, therefore, situated primarily in this region (*see* figure 11.6). The mass tends to be well circumscribed and many contain 'cystic' areas of low density (Husband *et al.*, 1980; *see also* chapter 17).

Retrocrural Space

The retrocrural space is one of the most rewarding areas for examination of lymphadenopathy by CT because it cannot be well demonstrated by any other

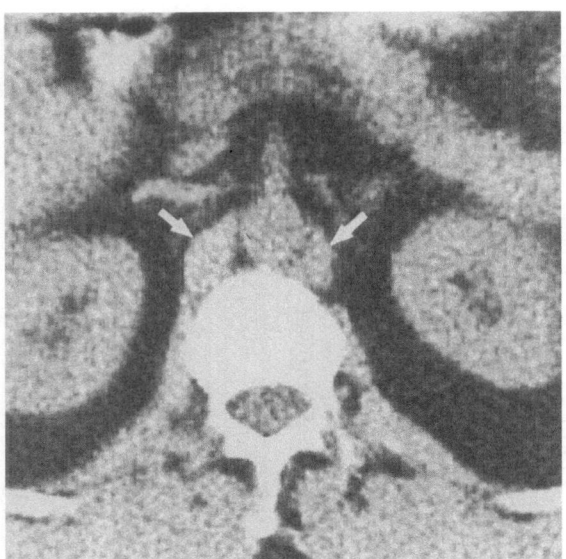

Figure 11.10(a)

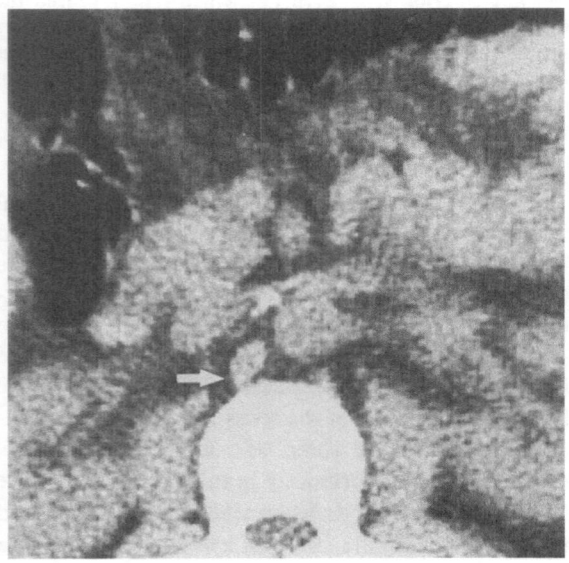

Figure 11.10(b)

Figure 11.10 Origin of crura. (a) The origins of the crura on both sides are bulky (arrowed). The margin of the aorta is obscured on the left. (b) The origin of the right crus (arrowed) is seen as a separate structure. It could be mistaken for an enlarged node unless its continuity with the remainder of the crus is recognised

technique. As already noted, minimal lymph node enlargement can be identified. If the nodes are much enlarged, they may fill the fat-containing space and displace the diaphragmatic crura (*see* figure 11.8a).

Although the para-aortic region and the retrocrural space are the easiest sites in which to identify large nodes, several difficulties occur. For example, the origins of the crura (from the anterolateral surfaces of the upper three lumbar vertebrae) are frequently seen in cross section as discrete rounded structures lying anteromedially to the psoas muscle (figure 11.10) and, if they are closely applied to the aorta, its margin may be obscured (figure 11.10a). These normal appearances may be mistaken for enlarged lymph nodes. Lymph node enlargement in the para-aortic region can be extremely difficult to diagnose with confidence in very thin patients (figure 11.11). Turning the patient

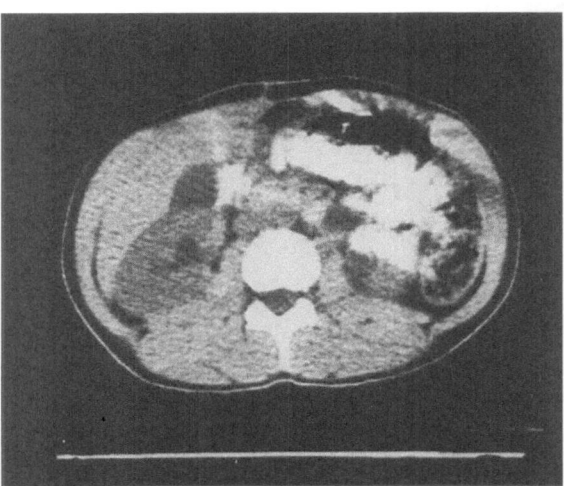

Figure 11.11 Thin patient. Evaluation of the retro-peritoneal space is difficult because the tissue planes are poorly defined and because bowel is closely applied to the great vessels

prone to displace loops of bowel and the use of a narrow window width to emphasise the fat planes will sometimes clarify the situation.

In general, minimal degrees of lymphadenopathy are easier to identify on the left side of the aorta than on the right, where the inferior vena cava, duodenum and head of the pancreas are so closely related to the

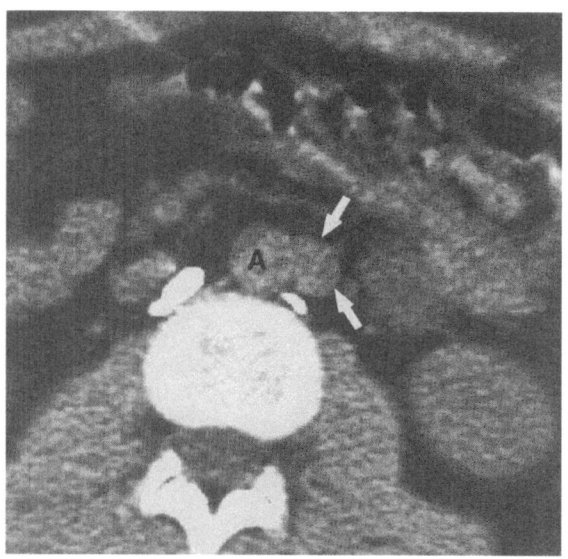

Figure 11.12(a)

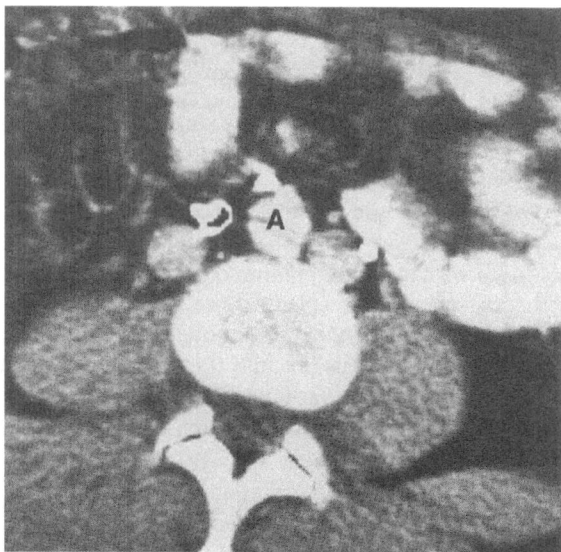

Figure 11.12(b)

Figure 11.12 Vessel imitating lymph node enlargement. (a) The pre-contrast scan shows a soft-tissue opacity (arrowed) adjacent to the left side of the aorta (A). (b) Post-contrast scan approximately 3 cm below (a). The structure has opacified and has the same shape and size as shown on the higher section

aorta that it can be difficult to differentiate these structures from enlarged nodes. Enlarged lymph nodes on the left must be distinguished from other normal structures such as the ureter, lumbar veins and arteries. Occasionally, a lumbar vessel is sufficiently large to be confused with an enlarged lymph node. However, the vessel is seen on several consecutive CT slices and, if doubt still exists, injection of iodinated intravenous contrast medium solves the problem (figure 11.12). A solitary enlarged node of similar dimensions to the aorta or vena cava, situated on the left side, may give an appearance that suggests that the patient has three major vessels, and this is a useful sign of lymphadenopathy (figure 11.13).

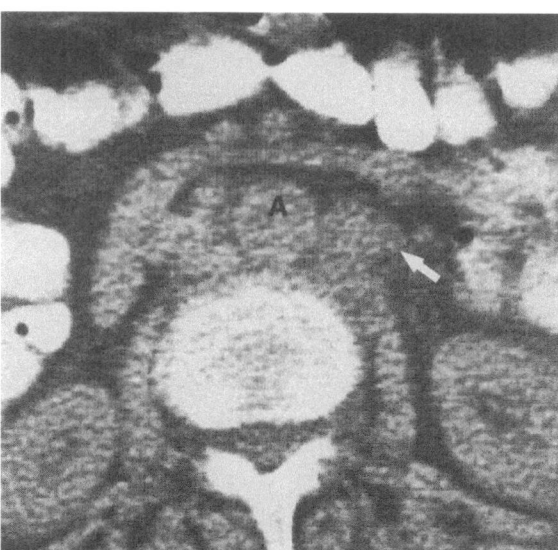

Figure 11.13 Enlarged lymph node (arrowed) adjacent to the aorta (A) looking like a third major vessel

NODES IN OTHER UPPER ABDOMINAL SITES

In sites such as the mesentery, porta hepatis and splenic hilar region, the degree of confidence in detecting lymphadenopathy is not as high as in the para-aortic region because there is often little surrounding fat and minimally enlarged nodes can be difficult to distinguish from other structures. Confidence increases with the size of the nodes involved. Inconstant shape and position of small bowel loops adds to the difficulty of diagnosis in those sites

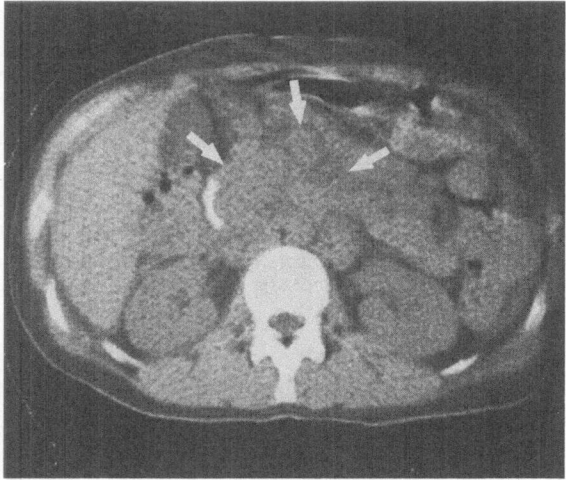

Figure 11.14(a)

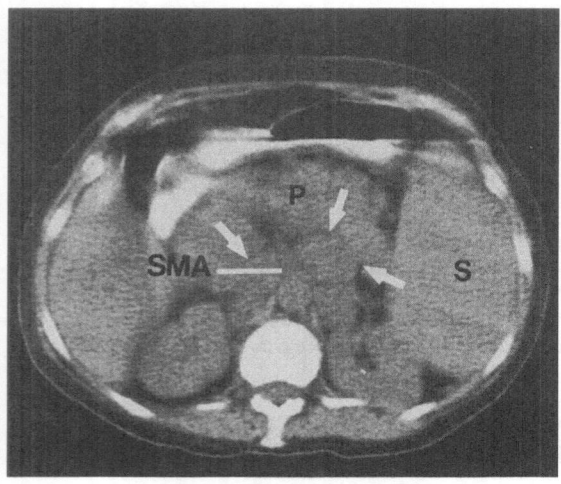

Figure 11.14(b)

Figure 11.14 Enlarged nodes (arrowed) in two patients with non-Hodgkin's lymphoma. (a) Mesenteric nodes with a lobulated outline. (b) Nodes are displacing the pancreas (P) anteriorly. Enlarged spleen (S)

where unopacified bowel may be closely related to lymph node chains.

Enlarged *mesenteric* and *coeliac* nodes are usually recognised as a mass or masses of soft-tissue density (figure 11.14). In the *porta hepatis*, nodes appear as discrete soft-tissue structures larger than the normal contents of the porta hepatis or as a conglomerate tumour mass (figure 11.15).

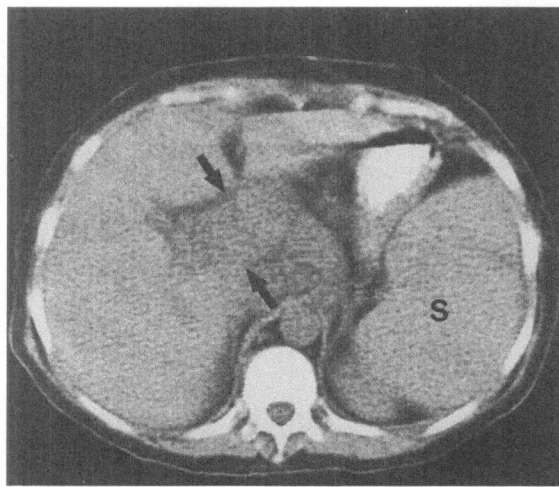

Figure 11.15 A conglomerate mass of enlarged nodes in the porta hepatis (arrowed) in non-Hodgkin's lymphoma. Enlarged spleen (S)

Splenic hilar nodes are closely related to the splenic artery and tail of the pancreas. They can be confused with loops of jejunum or, on rare occasions, with an accessory spleen (Lee *et al.*, 1978a). Enlargement of *peripancreatic* nodes can also cause a problem in diagnosis because they may be difficult to distinguish from an intrinsic pancreatic mass. Figure 11.16 shows an apparent mass in the head of the pancreas in a patient who presented with obstructive jaundice. A diagnosis of pancreatic carcinoma was made on the basis of the CT appearances, but at laparotomy the mass was found to be caused by enlarged peripancreatic nodes involved with lymphoma.

Renal hilar and *echelon* nodes are relatively easy to identify because they are situated in the perirenal fat at or below the renal hilum. Enlarged nodes at this site may cause hydronephrosis (figure 11.17). In

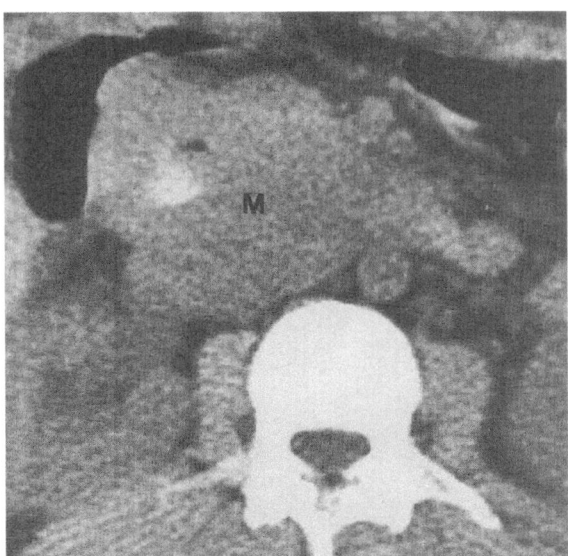

Figure 11.16 Enlarged peripancreatic nodes in non-Hodgkin's lymphoma. The mass (M) could not be distinguished from a pancreatic carcinoma on the basis of the CT scan appearances alone

patients with testicular tumours, such node enlargement may be the only site of abdominal disease (Macdonald, 1981).

Pelvic Nodes

The diagnosis of pelvic lymphadenopathy, as in other sites, depends on the size of the abnormal nodes. Diagnosis is more difficult than with para-aortic nodes because the external and internal iliac nodes are so closely applied to the vascular bundles and the pelvic muscles that they may be difficult to separate from them. Enlargement of external iliac nodes is seen as a soft-tissue bulge on one or both lateral pelvic walls adjacent to the iliac bones (figure

Figure 11.17 A patient with a testicular teratoma. The lymphogram was normal. (a) Intravenous urogram showing right hydronephrosis. This was considered to be due to congenital pelvi-ureteric junction obstruction. (b) The CT scan showed an enlarged mass of involved lymph nodes (arrowed) just below the hilum of the right kidney. The mass was subsequently excised

11.18). Enlarged internal iliac and obturator nodes are seen more posteriorly, adjacent to the obturator internus muscle (figure 11.19).

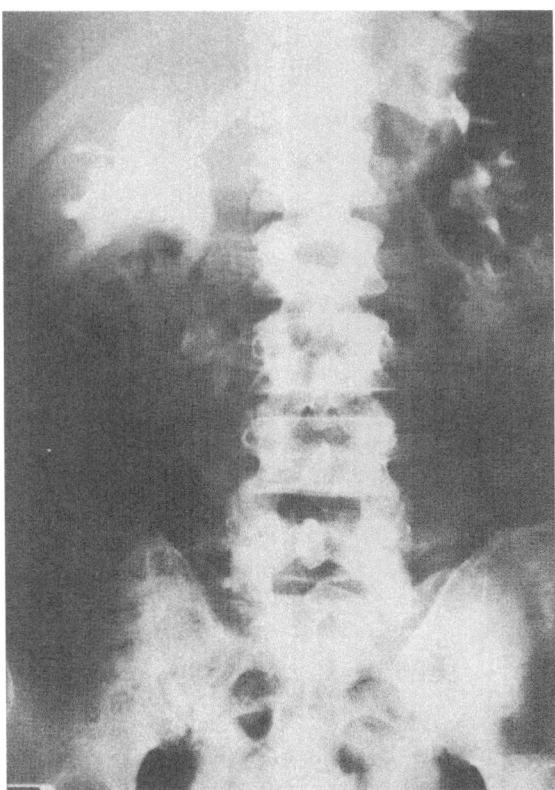

Figure 11.17(a)

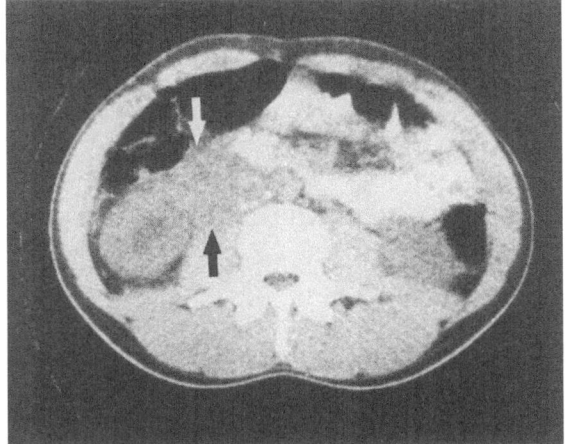

Figure 11.17(b)

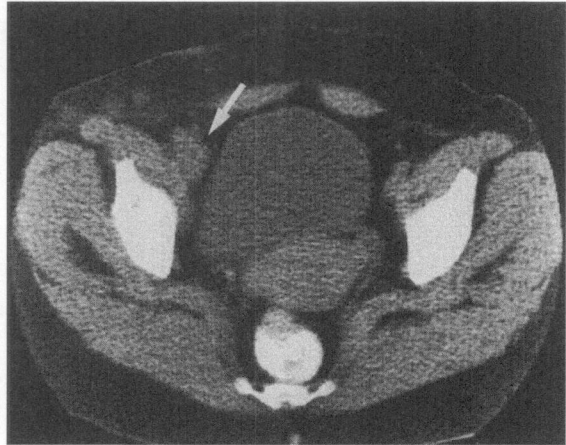

Figure 11.18(a)

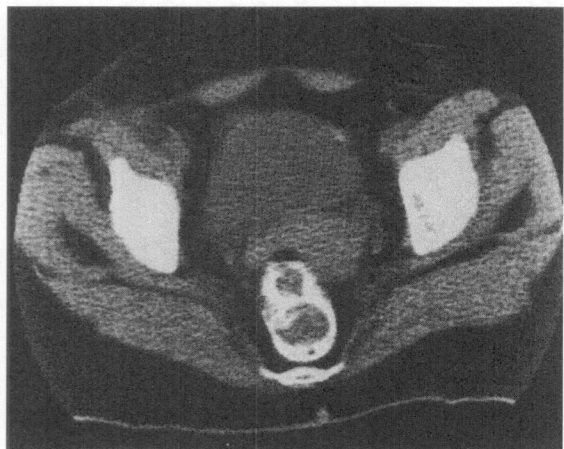

Figure 11.18(b)

Figure 11.18   Enlarged external iliac nodes on the right (arrowed) (a) before treatment (b) after treatment

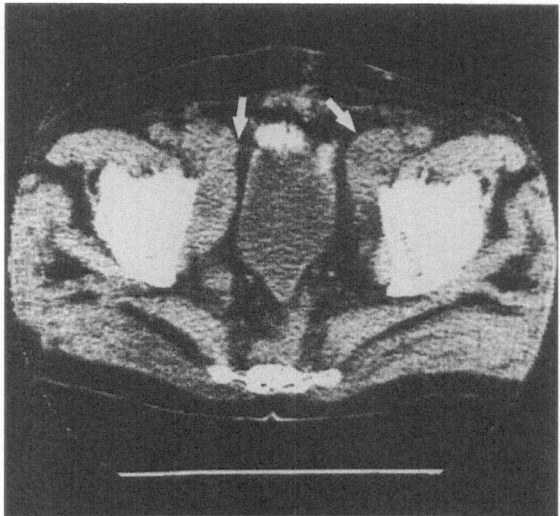

Figure 11.19   Bilateral enlarged external iliac nodes (arrowed). There is also enlargement of the internal iliac nodes on the right

investigations. In patients with metastatic carcinoma, radical lymphadenectomy is rarely performed and, as yet, there are few reports correlating CT with surgical findings in those patients undergoing exploratory laparotomy. The advent of percutaneous lymph node biopsy opens the way to further correlative studies.

Lymphoma

In patients with lymphoma, several studies have been reported correlating CT with both surgery and lymphography. All show that both techniques are highly accurate for demonstrating para-aortic node enlargement (Redman *et al.*, 1977; Breiman *et al.*, 1978; Lee *et al.*, 1978a; Best *et al.*, 1978). This is so even in patients undergoing staging laparotomy for Hodgkin's disease, in the majority of whom the nodes are either normal or only minimally enlarged. In a study at the BUPA Medical Centre and St Bartholomew's Hospital, abnormal nodes were found at surgery in the para-aortic region in four out of 39 patients with Hodgkin's disease who underwent laparotomy (Earl *et al.*, 1980). CT correctly identified the patients with nodal involvement. The overall accuracy was 87% compared with

ACCURACY OF COMPUTED TOMOGRAPHY

Lymph Node Disease

The accuracy of CT in the detection of lymph node disease can only be properly assessed by histological confirmation. This is relatively easy in the abdomen of patients with lymphoma because staging laparotomy is performed as part of the initial

79% with lymphography. The higher accuracy of CT was due to the number of false positive examinations with lymphography (five patients) compared with CT (two patients). The findings were equivocal in three out of the 39 patients with each technique, in all of whom the nodes were normal at surgery. Both this study and the study by Best *et al.* (1978) show that CT is an unreliable method for showing enlargement of nodes outside the retroperitoneum in Hodgkin's disease. Thus, in the study by Earl *et al.* (1980), seven patients had coeliac axis node involvement at laparotomy but CT was abnormal in only two of these. Splenic hilar nodes were involved in three patients but in only one were the enlarged nodes detected with CT. The size of the involved nodes is clearly important because in four out of the five patients with coeliac node involvement and in both of the patients with splenic hilar involvement in whom CT did not detect the abnormalities, the nodes at laparotomy measured less than 1.5 cm in diameter. In this study, there were two instances of enlarged nodes demonstrated with CT which did not contain Hodgkin's disease. In one patient, coeliac node involvement was shown on CT (1.5 cm diameter), but, at histological examination, the nodes were found to contain sarcoid-type granulomata. In another patient, enlarged splenic hilar nodes were shown, which proved to be due to lymphoid hyperplasia. This emphasises the general point that, while CT can demonstrate enlarged nodes, it gives no indication of the internal architecture of the node.

Nodal Metastases

Nodal metastases from primary cancers frequently cause little, if any, enlargement of the nodes and it is, therefore, not surprising that CT is less accurate than in the diagnosis of lymphomatous involvement, particularly in the pelvis, where the anatomy is not so clearly defined. Lee *et al.* (1978b) have correlated CT findings with surgery in 26 patients with pelvic cancer, 15 of whom had nodal involvement. False negative examinations occurred in six patients, emphasising the inability of CT to detect metastases in normal-sized nodes. There were no false positive examinations. Lymphography was compared with CT in 14 patients in whom surgical confirmation

was available, and as expected there was a greater number of false negative examinations with CT than with lymphography. Experience at the Royal Marsden Hospital supports the view that CT is inferior to lymphography for detecting nodal metastases from pelvic cancers. In a series of 95 patients, CT failed to identify metastases in 14 out of 26 patients with positive lymphograms. The accuracy of lymphography was assessed by histology or by follow up for a minimum period of one year. Rather alarmingly, there were also 10 false positive examinations with CT, the causes of which are outlined in table 11.1

Table 11.1 Positive CT compared with negative lymphogram in pelvic cancer (11 patients)

True positive = 1	
Unopacified node – surgically confirmed	
False positives = 10	
Vessels	3
Reactive hyperplasia	2
Inflammatory mass	1
Bowel, etc.	4

Testicular Tumours

Testicular tumour deposits differ from those of primary pelvic tumours because the nodal metastases tend to be large, breaking out beyond the confines of the normal node, and because these tumours predominantly involve the upper para-aortic chain. For these reasons, CT is well suited to examination of this type of tumour. Surgical confirmation of abnormalities is uncommon because, in the United Kingdom, lymphadenectomy is usually only undertaken in selected patients after chemotherapy and irradiation (Hendry *et al.*, 1980). CT findings can, however, be compared with the results of lymphography, which is known to be a highly accurate technique for demonstrating metastases from testicular teratoma (Wilkinson and Macdonald, 1975; Wallace, 1969). At the Royal Marsden Hospital, CT findings have been compared with those of lymphography in 88 patients (table 11.2). Overall, there was good agreement between

Table 11.2   Comparison of CT with lymphography in 88 patients with testicular teratomas examined before treatment

Lymphogram		CT findings	
	No. of patients	Negative	Positive
Negative	32	28	4*
Positive	50	2	48*
Equivocal	6	5	1*
Total	88	35	53

*Additional information obtained with CT.

CT and lymphography, but CT missed lymph node metastases in one patient with a single abnormal node shown at lymphography (figure 11.20). CT detected retrocrural lymph node involvement in three patients in whom the lymphogram was normal and in a further patient an abnormal renal hilar node was identified (*see* figure 11.17b). When both techniques were positive, CT demonstrated the full extent of disease more precisely than the lymphogram (figure 11.21). This subject is discussed in depth elsewhere (Husband, 1981; Macdonald, 1981).

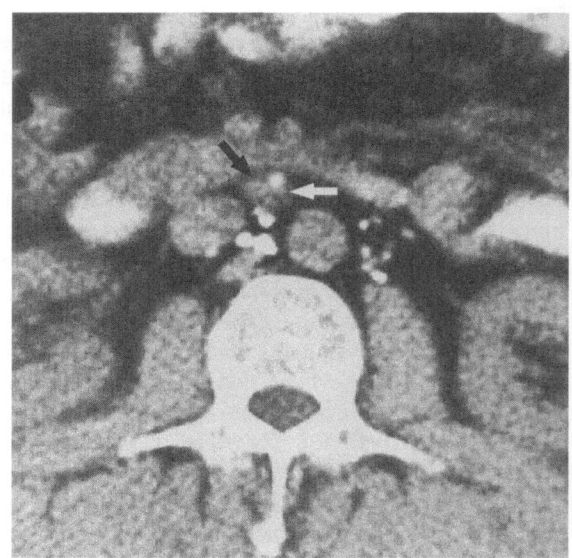

Figure 11.20(b)

Figure 11.20   Metastasis in a normal-sized node in a patient with testicular teratoma. (a) Lymphogram (oblique view) showing filling defect (arrowed). (b) CT scan of the same patient. The abnormal node was identified in retrospect (arrowed), but was missed at the time of reporting the examination

USE OF COMPUTED TOMOGRAPHY IN LYMPH NODE DISEASE

Both lymphography and CT have advantages and disadvantages for the diagnosis of lymph node disease, and the technique used will depend not only on the availability of equipment but also on the experience of the observer, on the tumour type and on the clinical problem. Lymphography has the advantage that experience in the technique and reporting of lymphograms is in general readily available. The clinician accepts the positive or negative lymphogram more easily than CT at the present time, and follow-up examinations are carried out with little inconvenience to the patient. One of the major advantages of lymphography is the ability to show the internal architecture of the opacified nodes. Thus, distinction between tumour deposits and reactive hyperplasia can be made in the

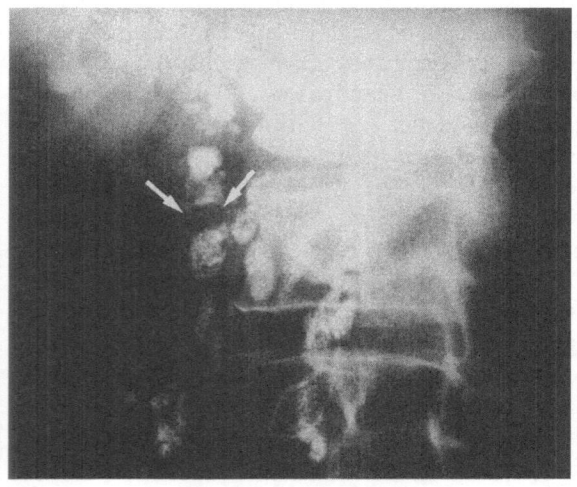

Figure 11.20(a)

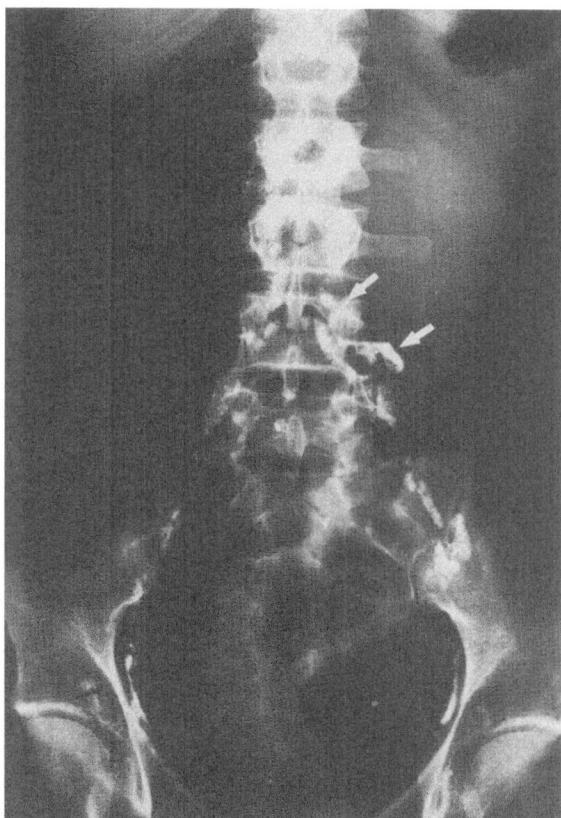

Figure 11.21(a)

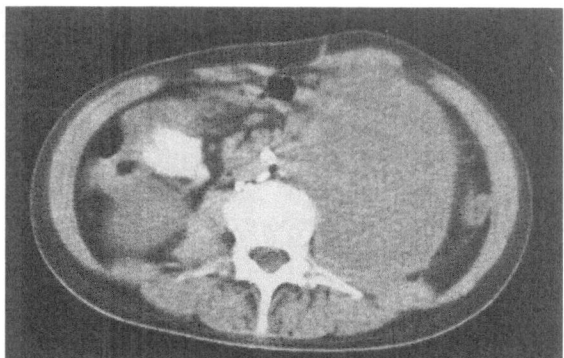

Figure 11.21(b)

Figure 11.21 **Abdominal mass from testicular teratoma. (a) Displacement of normal opacified lymph nodes (arrowed) by lymph node mass which has not taken up the contrast medium. (b) CT scan defines the full extent of the mass**

majority of cases, but with CT such distinction is impossible if nodal enlargement is discrete (figure 11.22).

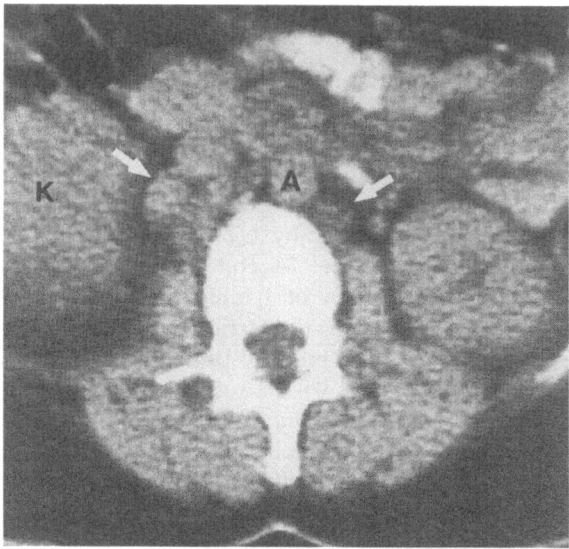

Figure 11.22 **Discrete enlargement of para-aortic lymph nodes (arrowed) due to inflammatory changes in a patient with xanthogranulomatous pyelonephritis. The appearances are indistinguishable from enlargement due to tumour. Aorta (A). Note enlarged right kidney (K)**

The main drawbacks of lymphography are that it is an unpleasant procedure and that, in many centres, the patient is admitted overnight for the examination. This makes lymphography as expensive as CT scanning. In addition, lymphography is best avoided in patients with respiratory problems or in those who are allergic to iodine-based contrast medium.

CT scanning causes little patient discomfort and can demonstrate abnormal nodes in areas which are inaccessible to lymphography. Extranodal sites of disease, such as the liver and bone, can be assessed at the same examination. Follow-up examinations cannot be carried out as frequently and as simply with CT as with a plain abdominal radiograph, but, if accurate delineation of tumour regression is required, particularly if the nodal mass is not outlined with contrast medium, CT is the best method for follow-up purposes.

There is still considerable controversy regarding the relative roles of CT and lymphography. The following summary suggests a possible approach to the way in which CT and lymphography can be used to best advantage in different tumour types.

Primary Pelvic Cancers (e.g. Carcinomas of the Bladder, Cervix and Ovary)

Since minimal degrees of pelvic lymphadenopathy are difficult to identify by CT, it seems clear that lymphography will not be completely replaced by CT for the detection of lymph node metastases. Most scans are, however, carried out for determining the extent of the primary tumour and in many cases involved nodes will be sufficiently enlarged to be shown at the same time. If no enlarged nodes are shown on the scan, lymphography is indicated. In our opinion, lymphography remains the method of choice for investigations of primary pelvic tumours.

Testicular Tumours

CT is at least as accurate as lymphography in detecting nodal involvement in this type of tumour. In addition, it provides unique information regarding the extent and volume of metastatic tumour. This is important because the volume of metastases influences prognosis and hence patient management (Peckham *et al.*, 1979). At the same time, CT will demonstrate the liver, which is a relatively common site for metastases in patients with advanced disease. CT would thus appear to be the preferred technique for the initial examination in this tumour. If CT is negative, lymphography would be indicated to exclude metastases in normal or only minimally enlarged nodes.

Lymphomas

Both CT and lymphography are in general equally effective in detecting the presence of para-aortic node enlargement. A CT scan can, however, define the extent of the involvement more precisely by identifying unopacified abnormal nodes, especially in areas inaccessible to lymphography. Even so, CT scanning with present techniques cannot replace staging laparotomy in patients with Hodgkin's disease and non-Hodgkin's lymphoma because of its inability to exclude splenic involvement (*see* chapter 10) (Redman *et al.*, 1977; Earl *et al.*, 1980).

The main advantages of lymphography are its ability to detect finer changes in size of the nodes during the course of treatment (Haefliger *et al.*, 1979) and the simplicity of obtaining follow-up examinations. It also has the advantage that discrete enlargement of nodes due to reactive hyperplasia can be differentiated from tumour deposits.

There are, of course, situations when CT scanning is clearly indicated and can provide unique information which is helpful to management. For example, in patients with primary gut lymphomas, lymphography does not demonstrate the primary tumour and CT can be used to define the full extent of disease at presentation and to monitor therapeutic response. CT is also indicated in patients with gross obstruction to the lymphatic system which prevents contrast entering the nodes, or when there is poor filling of the nodes following radiotherapy treatment when recurrence is suspected. It also provides an alternative procedure in patients who are unfit for lymphography and is an effective method of demonstrating bony disease in the vertebrae or pelvis.

Lymphography and CT should be regarded as complementary procedures, the method of choice depending on the particular clinical problem as well as on the availability of equipment and relative expertise in the two procedures.

REFERENCES

Best, J. J. K., Blackledge, G., Forbes, W. St C., Todd, I. D. H., Eddleston, B., Crowther, D. and Isherwood, I. (1978). Computed tomography of the abdomen in the staging and clinical management of lymphoma. *British Medical Journal*, 2, 1675

Breiman, R. S., Castellino, R. A., Harell, G. S., Marshall, W. H., Glatstein, E. and Kaplan, H. S. (1978).

CT–pathologic correlations in Hodgkin's disease and non-Hodgkin's lymphoma. *Radiology*, **126**, 159–166

Callen, P. W., Korobkin, M. and Isherwood, I. (1977). Computed tomographic evaluation of the retrocrural pre-vertebral space. *American Journal of Roentgenology*, **129**, 907–910

Earl, H. M., Sutcliffe, S. B. J., Kelsey Fry, I., Tucker, A. K., Young, J., Husband, J. E., Wrigley, P. F. M. and Malpas, J. S. (1980). Computerised tomographic (CT) abdominal scanning in Hodgkin's disease. *Clinical Radiology*, **31**, 149–153

Haefliger, J. M., Peckham, M. J. and Steel, G. G. (1979). Changes in lymph node size following systemic irradiation for malignant teratoma. *Clinical Radiology*, **30**, 5–10

Hendry, W. F., Barrett, A., McElwain, T. J., Wallace, D. M. and Peckham, M. J. (1980). The role of surgery in the combined management of metastases from malignant teratomas of the testis. *British Journal of Urology*, **52**, 38–44

Hodson, N. J., Husband, J. E. and Macdonald, J. S. (1979). The role of computed tomography in the staging of bladder cancer. *Clinical Radiology*, **30**, 389–396

Husband, J. E. (1981). The role of computed tomography in testicular teratomas. In *The Management of Testicular Tumours*, ed. M. J. Peckham, London, Edward Arnold

Husband, J. E., Macdonald, J. S. and Peckham, M. J. (1980). The role of abdominal computed tomography in the management of abdominal metastases from teratoma of the testis. A review of 85 patients. *Computerised Tomography*, **4**, 1–16

Lee, J. K. T., Stanley, R. J., Sagel, S. S. and Levitt, R. R. (1978a). Accuracy of computed tomography in detecting intra-abdominal and pelvic adenopathy in lymphoma. *American Journal of Roentgenology*, **131**, 311–315

Lee, J. K. T., Stanley, R. J., Sagel, S. S. and McClennan, B. L. (1978b). Accuracy of CT in detecting intra-abdominal and pelvic lymph node metastases from pelvic cancers. *American Journal of Roentgenology*, **131**, 675–679

Macdonald, J. S. (1981). Lymphography in testicular tumours. In *The Management of Testicular Tumours*, ed. M. J. Peckham, London, Edward Arnold

Peckham, M. J., McElwain, T. J., Hendry, W. F., Juttner, C. and Barrett, A. (1979). The combined treatment of malignant testicular teratoma: a preliminary report. *Lancet*, **ii**, 267–270

Redman, H. C., Glatstein, E., Castellino, R. A. and Federal, W. A. (1977). Computed tomography as an adjunct in staging of Hodgkin's disease and non-Hodgkin's lymphoma. *Radiology*, **124**, 381–385

Wallace, E. M. K. (1969). Lymphography in the management of testicular tumours. *Clinical Radiology*, **20**, 453–458

Wilkinson, D. J. and Macdonald, J. S. (1975). A review of the role of lymphography in the management of testicular tumours. *Clinical Radiology*, **26**, 89–98

12

The Pelvis

Even with a detailed knowledge of anatomy, the pelvis is one of the most difficult regions to analyse with CT. Several factors contribute to the problems of interpretation. First, there is relatively little intervening fat between adjacent organs and structures. Secondly, small bowel loops have an inconstant shape and position and may be interpreted as representing a pelvic mass. Thirdly, many small structures pass through the pelvic adipose tissue (vessels and nerves) and these may cause confusion when attempting to identify minimal pelvic abnormalities such as parametrial extension of a cervical cancer or extravesical extension of a bladder tumour. In addition, and perhaps most importantly, in the female the long axes of the vagina, cervix and uterus lie in a longitudinal/oblique plane, so that the cross sectional display with CT is not the ideal format for demonstrating these organs.

TECHNIQUE OF EXAMINATION

The first requirement for a good-quality scan of the pelvis is a full bladder, because it displaces the small bowel out of the pelvis into the abdomen (figure 12.1). Confusion between soft-tissue masses in the pelvis and unopacified bowel is thus avoided and, in addition, there are fewer streak artefacts from gas in the moving bowel.

Dilute oral and rectal contrast medium are given

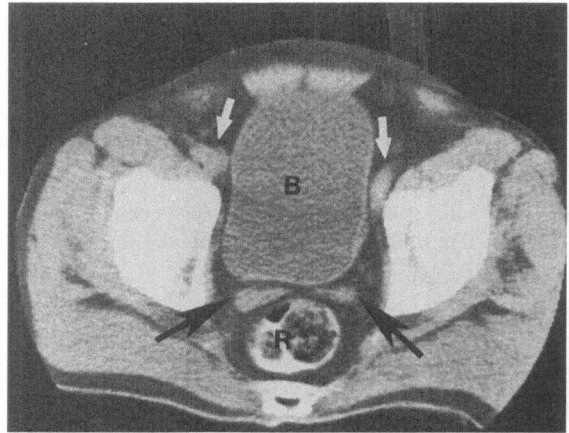

Figure 12.1   Normal scan in a male patient. Bladder (B), seminal vesicles (large arrows), rectum (R), iliac vessels (small arrows)

before the scan in order to delineate any small bowel loops remaining in the pelvis and as much of the colon as possible (figure 12.1). Sufficient time must be allowed for the oral contrast medium to reach the distal ileum before the examination is begun. Since transit time varies greatly from patient to patient, it is useful to check that contrast medium has reached the distal ileum and caecum by taking a plain abdominal radiograph or scanogram before the scan.

Insertion of a tampon in the vagina helps to identify the vaginal vault and above this the cervix and corpus uteri (figure 12.2).

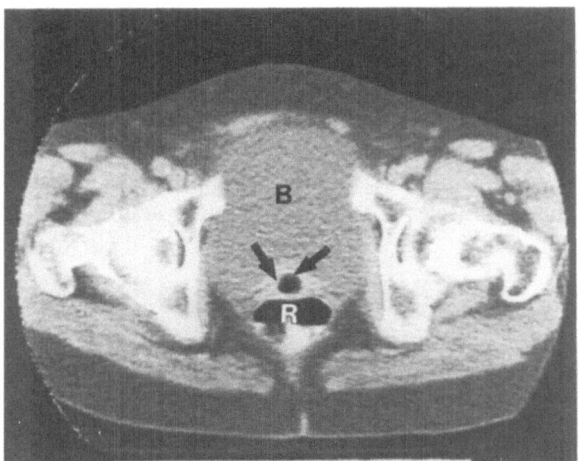

Figure 12.2 Normal scan in a female patient. Tampon in the vagina (arrowed) seen as a circular area of low density due to air trapped within its fibres. Bladder (B), rectum (R)

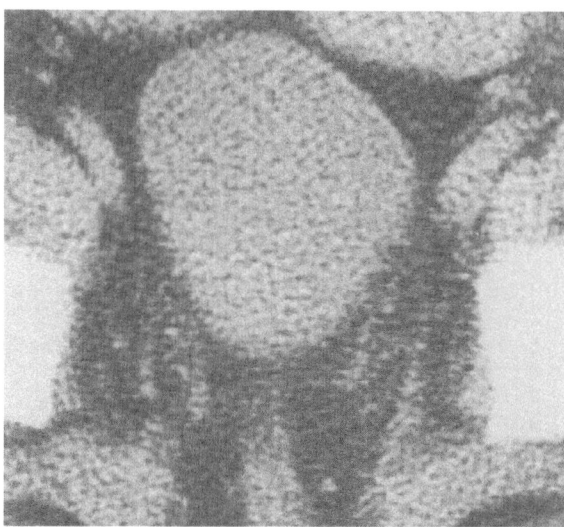

Figure 12.3(a)

In most patients having pelvic scans, the bladder is easily identified by the low-density urine within it, but sometimes opacification with intravenous contrast medium, e.g. 30 ml meglumine iothalamate is required especially in patients with small-capacity bladders or those who are incontinent. Intravenous contrast medium also demonstrates the intravesical portion of a bladder tumour (figure 12.3); occasionally, it will help to distinguish the bladder from a cystic mass in the pelvis. It is best to use a relatively low dose of contrast medium, e.g. 30 ml meglumine iothalamate (Conray 280), because larger doses produce such dense opacification that intravesical tumours may be obscured.

Intravenous contrast medium also opacifies the ureters to show their course (figure 12.4), their relationship to a pelvic mass and the presence of any dilatation. Larger doses of contrast medium (60 ml Conray 420 sodium iothalamate given as a bolus injection) may be useful for distinguishing normal vessels from suspected enlarged lymph nodes or other pelvic lesions. Vascular enhancement may also be of value before surgery in order to delineate the precise relationship of a mass to the major vessels or whether they are directly involved.

Seidelmann *et al.* (1978) have used negative contrast medium (carbon dioxide) introduced by

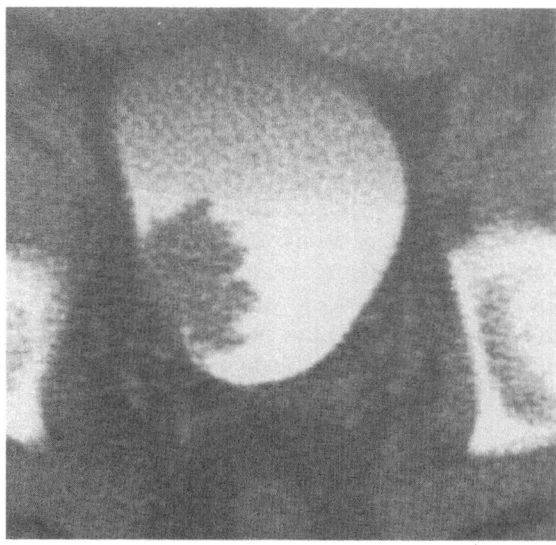

Figure 12.3(b)

Figure 12.3 Carcinoma of the bladder. (a) The intravesical tumour is not identified because the density of the tumour is similar to that of the surrounding urine. (b) The tumour arising from the right bladder wall is clearly seen after injection of intravenous contrast medium. (Reproduced by kind permission of *Radiology*)

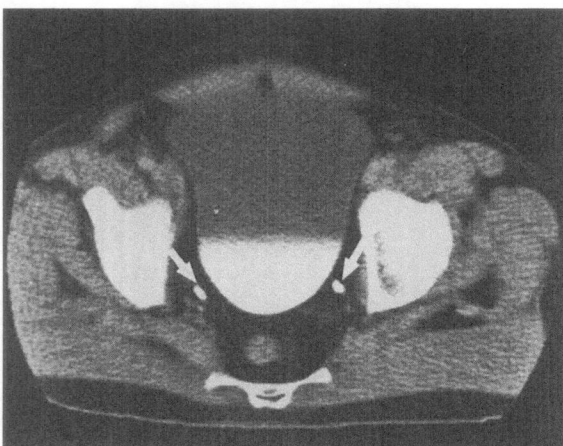

Figure 12.4   Normal scan in a male patient. There is layering of contrast medium in the posterior aspect of the bladder in the supine position. The opacified ureters are clearly seen in the perivesical fat (arrows)

catheterisation to demonstrate bladder tumours. They consider that this is the best method for demonstrating both the intraluminal growth and the bladder wall. In our experience, this relatively invasive procedure is not necessary.

The initial series of pelvic scans is carried out in the supine position and is taken from the lower border of the symphysis pubis to the middle of the fifth lumbar vertebra at 1 or 1.5 cm intervals. When the initial series of scans has been studied, further scans can be obtained in the supine position after injection of intravenous contrast medium or in the prone or lateral decubitus positions. The latter positions are particularly helpful in demonstrating tumours of the bladder base or dome and for distinguishing mobile loops of bowel from a suspected mass.

CT ANATOMY

Although the pelvis contains many different organs, their constant relationship to each other helps CT interpretation. The symmetrical arrangement of muscles, vessels and lymph nodes makes comparison with the opposite side a useful guide to correct interpretation.

Scans through the symphysis pubis demonstrate the perineal muscles surrounding the urethra, vagina and rectum in the female (figure 12.5a) and the prostate and rectum in the male (figure 12.5b). The other important structures at this level are the obturator internus and gluteus maximus muscles. These muscles form the lateral and posterior

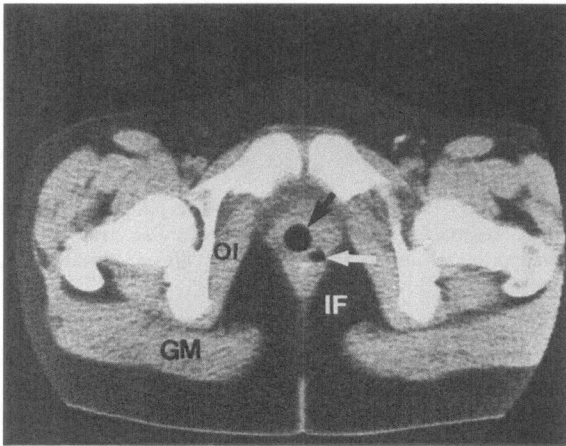

Figure 12.5(a)

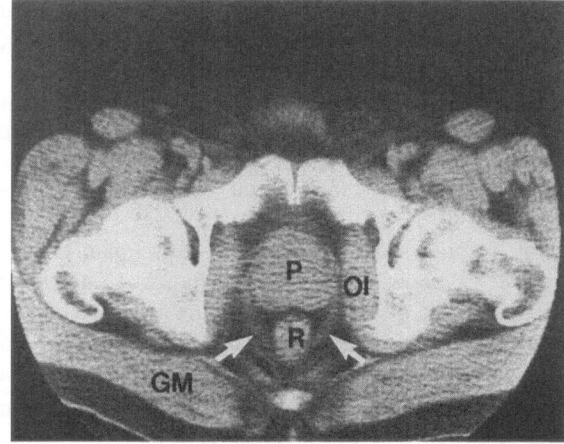

Figure 12.5(b)

Figure 12.5   Normal scans through the symphysis pubis. (a) Female patient. Tampon in the vagina (black arrow), air in the rectum (white arrow). Ischiorectal fossa (IF). (b) Male patient. Prostate (P), rectum (R), levator ani (small arrows), obturator internus muscle (OI), gluteus maximus muscle (GM)

boundaries of the ischiorectal fossae. Occasionally, inferior rectal and pudendal vessels can be identified in the ischiorectal fossa (van Engelshoven and Kreel, 1979).

Higher scans passing just above the symphysis demonstrate the base of the bladder and rectum. In the female, the vagina lies behind the bladder (figure 12.6a). In the male, the upper portion of the prostate may be seen at this level (figure 12.6b) and just

above it the seminal vesicles can be identified lying immediately behind the bladder (*see* figure 12.1). Fat in this region forms a well defined angle between the posterior bladder wall and the anterior surface of each seminal vesicle, and loss of this angle is a useful sign of extravesical spread in bladder cancer. In addition to these major structures, the ureters and numerous small vessels and nerves pass through the extraperitoneal adipose tissue; phleboliths are commonly visible in the pelvic veins. At the same level, the side walls of the pelvis consist of the internal obturator muscles on either side and the coccygeus muscles. Since the peritoneal cavity extends into the pelvis on both sides and in front of the bladder, small bowel loops are frequently seen lying adjacent to the bladder wall, particularly if it is not filled to capacity.

When the bladder is filled, it appears as a square-shaped structure in cross section (*see* figure 12.1). The density of urine usually approximates to that of water, so that the bladder wall can be delineated between it and the surrounding fat. When the bladder is full, the wall is no more than 3 to 4 mm thick in the majority of patients.

Scans through the dome of the bladder may contain only bladder wall which will then appear as a rounded soft-tissue shadow. This may be interpreted as a mass unless contiguous scans are taken down into the pelvis to show its continuity with the rest of the bladder (figure 12.7). Similarly,

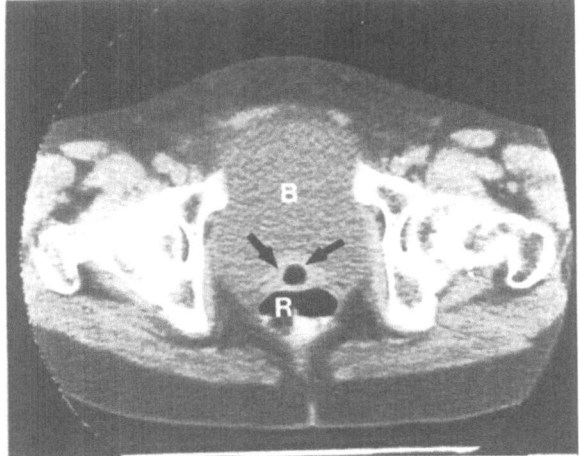

Figure 12.6(a)

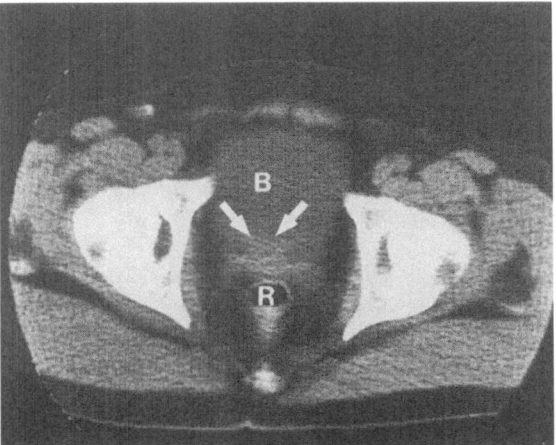

Figure 12.6(b)

Figure 12.6 Normal scans of the pelvis. (a) Female patient. Bladder (B), vagina (arrowed), rectum (R). (b) Male patient. Bladder (B), upper portion of prostate (arrowed), rectum (R)

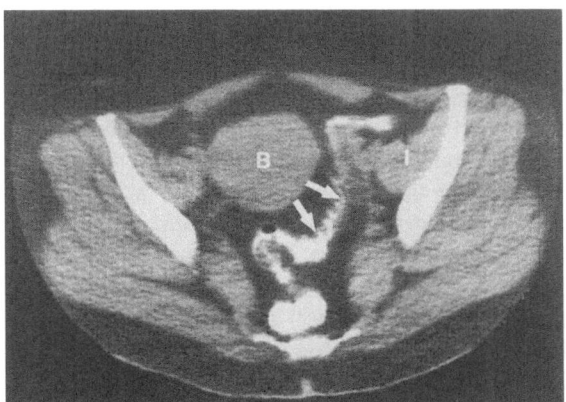

Figure 12.7 CT scan through the dome of the bladder which appears as a mass of soft-tissue density (B). Sigmoid colon (arrowed), iliopsoas (I)

when the bladder is empty, it appears as a central soft-tissue structure. In this situation, the use of intravenous contrast medium or the injection of a diuretic is usually needed to clarify the anatomy.

The vaginal vault appears as a soft-tissue structure with its long axis in the transverse plane. The cavity is outlined by air in the tampon (*see* figures 12.2 and 12.6a). Immediately above this, the cervix is identified as a smooth, soft-tissue, rounded structure approximately 3 cm in diameter (figure 12.8). Occasionally it is seen lying laterally or

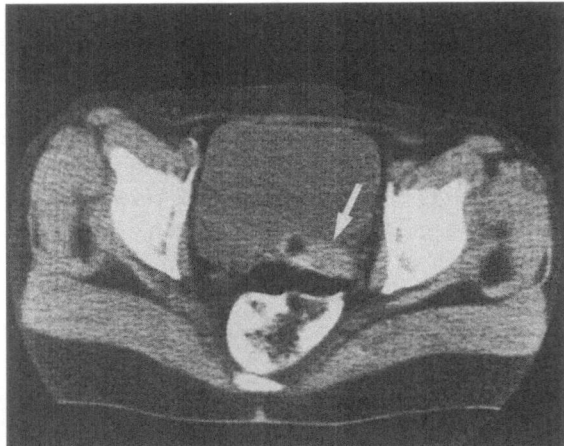

Figure 12.9   Normal female pelvis showing the cervix (arrowed) to the left of the vaginal tampon

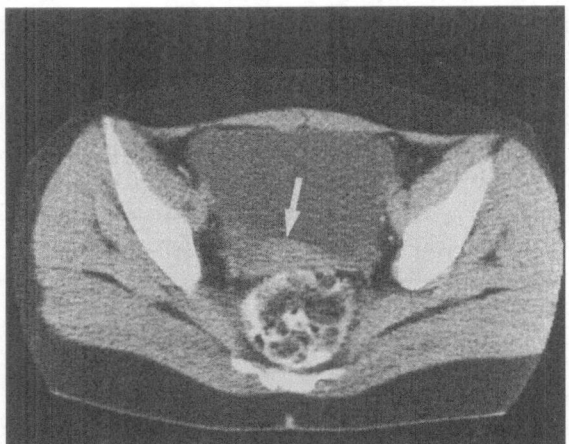

Figure 12.8   Normal female pelvis at the level of the cervix (arrowed)

posteriorly to the tampon. This is presumably because the tampon has been placed in one of the vaginal fornices rather than centrally (figure 12.9). The cervix cannot be reliably distinguished from the lower part of the body of the uterus, but scans 1 to 1.5 cm above the cervix show the characteristic shape of the uterus. The posterior surface is smooth, convex and extends laterally on either side into the broad ligaments (figure 12.10). There is usually sufficient intrapelvic fat to delineate this posterior uterine surface clearly. The anterior margin of the body of the uterus is less clearly defined, the appearance varying with its position and the degree of bladder filling. The more vertical the uterus lies, the smaller it will appear on a single section, the more sharply defined will be its margins and the

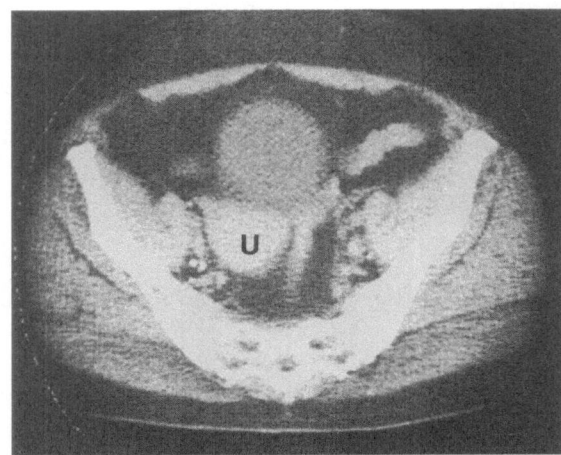

Figure 12.10   Normal female pelvis showing the uterus (U). Note the smooth convex posterior border

more oval will be its shape (figure 12.11). When anteverted it is viewed in longitudinal plane and will appear relatively larger and its outer and lateral margins will be less well defined (figure 12.12). When part of the bladder and uterus are included in the same section, partial volume averaging can produce a confusing appearance suggesting an abnormal mass. The density of the uterus is similar to that of other soft tissues; the intra-uterine cavity cannot be seen.

The ovaries are situated on the side walls of the

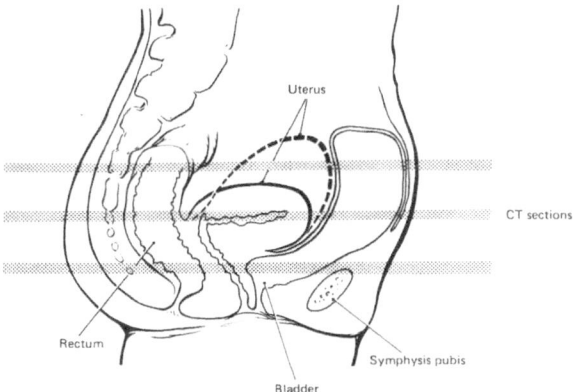

Figure 12.11(a)

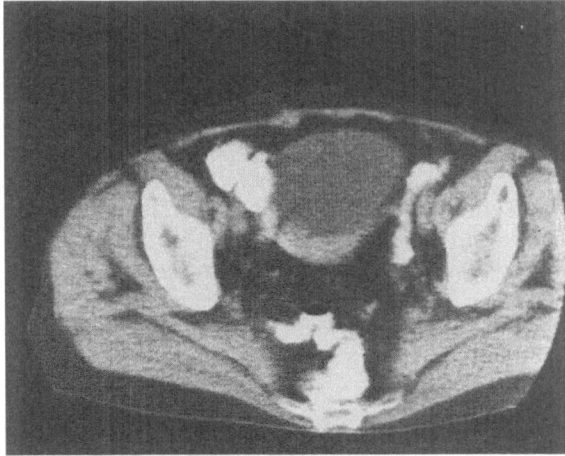

Figure 12.11(b)

Figure 12.11 (a) Diagram to show the position of the normal and the anteverted uterus in relation to CT sections: – – – – normal; ——— anteverted. (b) Normal female pelvis showing uterus in a vertical position

bony pelvis closely related to the obturator vessels but are rarely identified as separate structures. This is presumably because there is little surrounding fat and because they are confused with other normal structures in this region.

Scans at higher levels through the pelvis show the sigmoid colon curving towards the left and an increasing number of small bowel loops which are situated in front and beside the bladder vault (*see* figure 12.7). The most important muscles to be identified in this region are the symmetrically paired

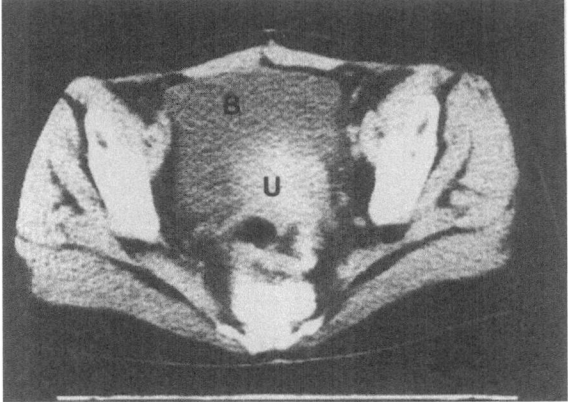

Figure 12.12 Normal female pelvis showing an anteverted uterus (U) indenting the posterior aspect of the bladder (B)

iliacus and psoas muscles. The iliacus forms a triangular sheet which arises from the cavity of the iliac fossa. Its fibres converge into the lateral side of the tendon of the psoas muscle. The junction of the psoas and iliacus muscles produces a characteristic comma shape on the axial scan (*see* figure 12.7). The pyriformis muscle is seen lying between the sacrum from which it arises and the posterior margin of the iliac bone. It lies anteromedially to the gluteus maximus muscle and leaves the pelvis through the greater sciatic foramen.

The external and internal iliac arteries and veins and their accompanying lymph nodes lie close to the pelvic side wall (*see* figure 12.1). Although the external iliac vessels can usually be seen as individual structures, the internal iliac vessels and lymph nodes are more difficult to identify.

BLADDER

CT scans of the bladder are virtually all undertaken to assess patients known to have bladder cancer. A bladder tumour appears on CT as a mass of soft-tissue density projecting into the bladder lumen. It is either pedunculated or sessile and is continuous with the bladder wall (figure 12.13, and *see* figure 12.3b). Occasionally, with large tumours, calcification may be seen encrusted on the surface of the tumour (figure 12.14). Tumours as small as 1 to 2 cm in diameter can usually be identified, but even large

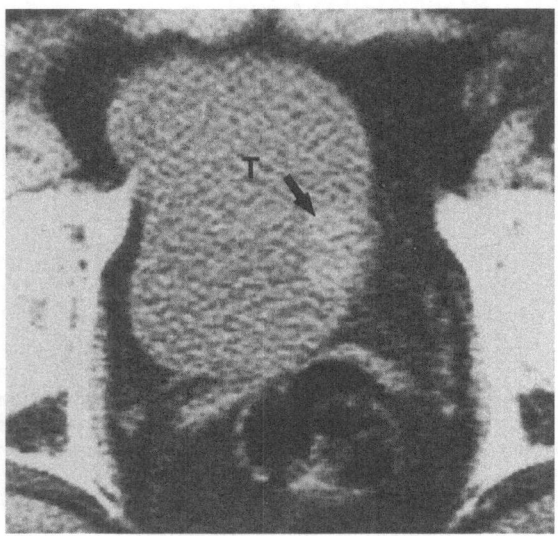

Figure 12.13   Carcinoma of the bladder. The tumour (T) arises from the left bladder wall and is continuous with it. Note minimal tumour extension into the perivesical fat. (Reproduced by kind permission of *Radiology*)

growths may be missed, especially if situated at the dome or bladder base.

Bladder tumours infiltrate into the deep layers of the bladder wall, into the extravesical tissues and into adjacent organs, and one of the main advantages of CT is the ability to detect such tumour invasion. Superficial tumours which involve the mucosa and submucosa cannot be distinguished from each other with CT, but it may be possible to identify involvement of the deep muscles by thickening of the bladder wall in the region of the intravesical tumour (Hodson *et al.*, 1979). Minimal extravesical tumour spread through the bladder wall is recognised as loss of definition of the extravesical fat margin in the region of the tumour (*see* figure 12.13). Advanced tumour spread is easily recognised as a definite mass extending beyond the bladder wall into the surrounding fat (figure 12.15a) or even as far as the lateral pelvic or anterior abdominal wall (figure 12.15b).

Spread of tumour into adjacent organs such as the rectum, vagina, uterus and prostate may be more difficult to identify because there is little fat between the organs and the tumour may lie adjacent to a structure without necessarily invading it. Involvement of the seminal vesicles is an exception to this

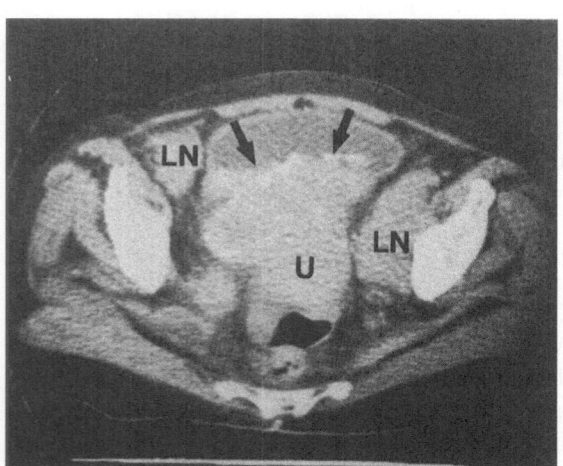

Figure 12.14   Carcinoma of the bladder. Note calcification on the surface of the tumour (arrowed). The tumour has spread posteriorly and involves the uterus (U). There are bilateral enlarged external iliac lymph nodes (LN). (Reproduced by kind permission of *Radiology*)

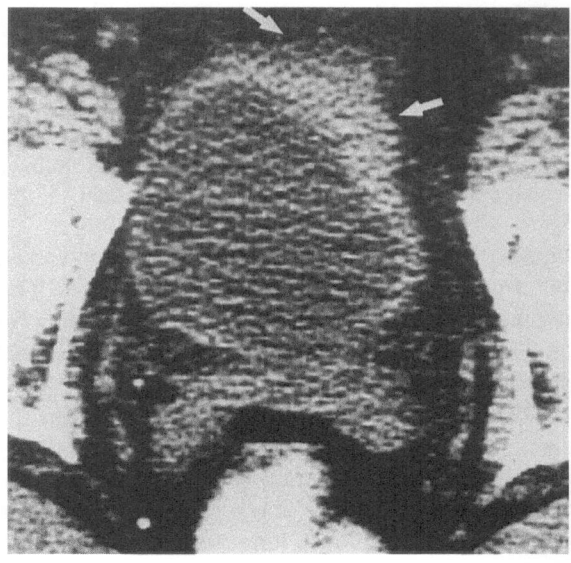

Figure 12.15(a)

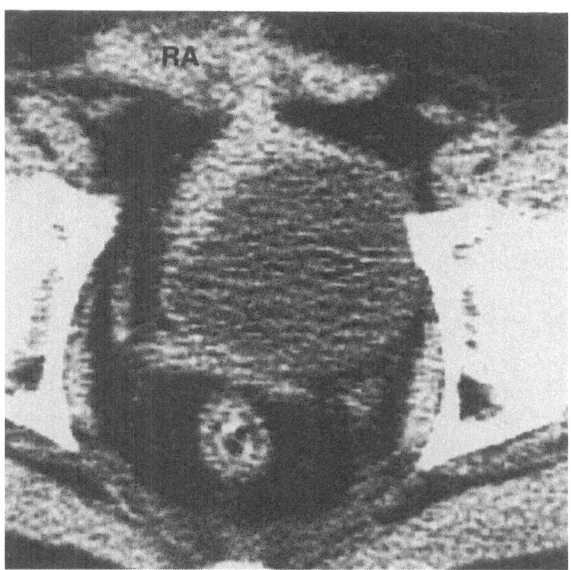

Figure 12.15(b)

Figure 12.15 Carcinoma of the bladder. (a) The tumour
on the left anterior lateral wall extends into the perivesical
fat (arrowed). (b) The tumour on the right anterior lateral
wall has extended as far as the anterior abdominal wall
involving the rectus abdominis muscle (RA)

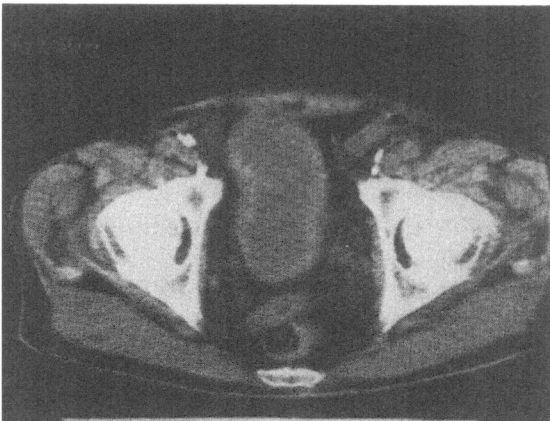

Figure 12.17(a)

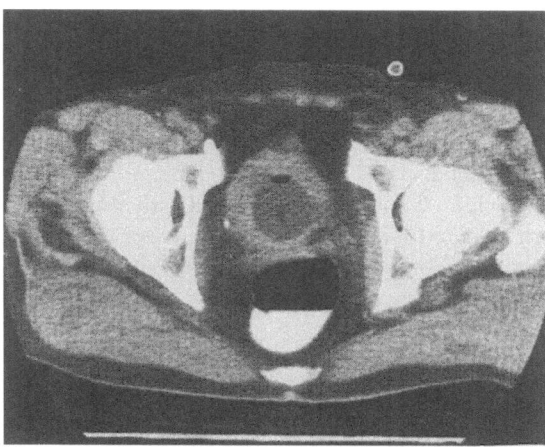

Figure 12.17(b)

Figure 12.17 Two patients with carcinoma of the
bladder. (a) Generalised thickening of the bladder wall
after radiotherapy. (b) A similar appearance in a patient
who had received no treatment. The whole of the bladder
wall was grossly infiltrated by tumour at cystoscopy.
Note catheter in the bladder lumen

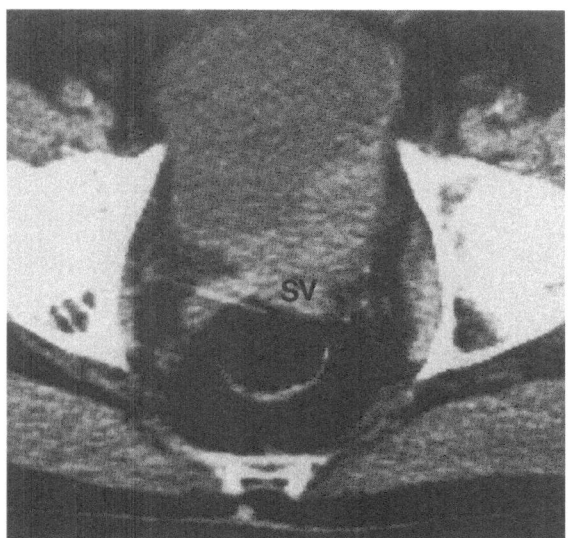

Figure 12.16 Carcinoma of the bladder. The tumour
has spread posteriorly and involves the left seminal vesicle
(SV). Note loss of the seminal vesicle angle on the left.
(Reproduced by kind permission of *Radiology*)

rule because the well defined fat angle between the
posterior bladder wall and the seminal vesicles in the
supine position is obliterated (figure 12.16). In
advanced disease, invasion of adjacent organs such
as the uterus is obvious (*see* figure 12.14).

There are several difficulties associated with
interpretation of pelvic scans in patients with bladder
cancer. For instance, loops of bowel which have
remained unopacified by contrast medium may be

misinterpreted as tumour extension if closely related to the bladder wall. A tumour at the bladder base may be difficult to distinguish from an enlarged prostate gland. Following endoscopic resection, oedema and inflammation of the bladder wall may be confused with deep muscle involvement. In addition, blood clot may be misinterpreted as tumour.

Radiotherapy treatment may cause difficulty in interpretation because it results in generalised thickening of the bladder wall, and, unless an intraluminal mass is present, it is impossible to distinguish thickening due to irradiation from that due to tumour (figure 12.17). In addition, the bladder may be so small after radiotherapy that any intraluminal tumour may be difficult to visualise (Husband and Hodson, 1980).

RECTUM

For practical purposes, mass lesions of the rectum investigated by CT are malignant tumours. Although CT may occasionally demonstrate an intraluminal mass, its major value lies in the detection of the extent of extraluminal tumour, either as part of preoperative assessment or for the diagnosis of local tumour recurrence.

Primary Rectal Tumours

CT can show the extent of local spread outside the rectal wall, particularly when there is plenty of fat in the ischiorectal fossa (figure 12.18) (van Voorthuisen, 1980).

Recurrent Rectal Tumours

The diagnosis of recurrent rectal tumours is difficult by clinical examination and conventional radiological techniques, particularly in male patients who have undergone abdominoperineal (AP) resection. CT provides a unique diagnostic tool for investigating the presence and extent of tumour recurrence.

The abnormal anatomy following abdominoperineal resection presents some problems in interpretation. Small bowel frequently extends into the sacral hollow (figure 12.19a). Unless opacified with contrast medium, this small bowel may be mistaken for recurrent tumour (figure 12.19b). In female patients, the uterus also lies in the sacral hollow and

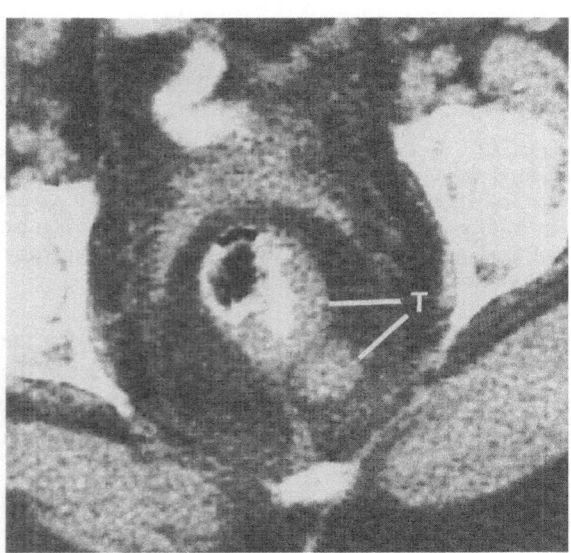

Figure 12.18 Carcinoma of the rectum showing the tumour (T) spreading into the perirectal fat

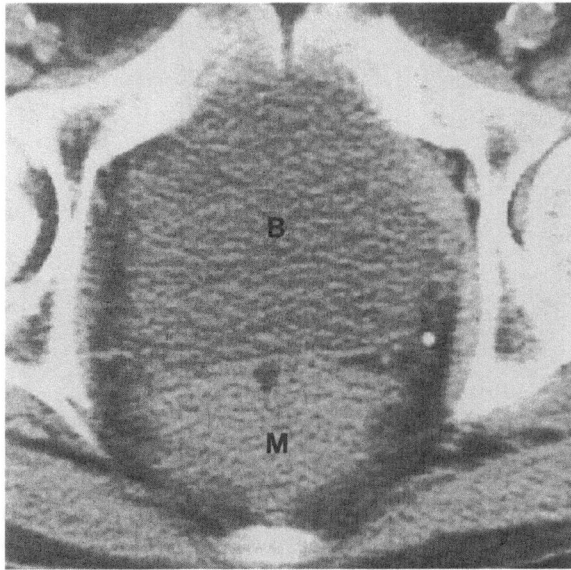

Figure 12.19(a)

must not be confused with recurrent tumour (figure 12.20). In addition, normal postoperative granulation tissue may present as a soft-tissue mass. It tends to lie centrally, has ill defined margins, does not invade neighbouring muscle and is frequently related to surgical clips (figure 12.21). Even so, it may sometimes be impossible to distinguish such a mass

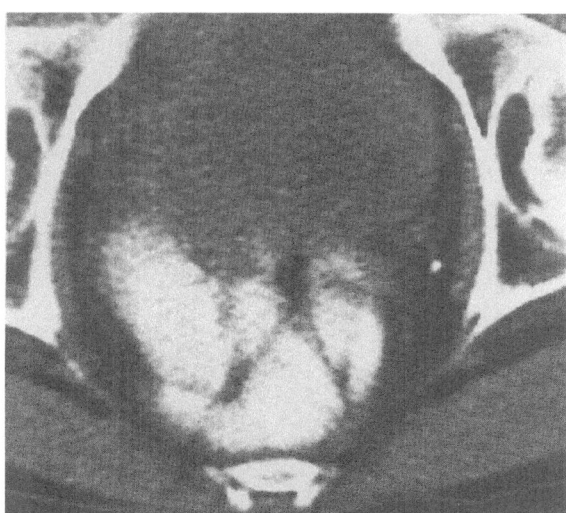

Figure 12.19(b)

Figure 12.19 Male patient with suspected recurrence of rectal carcinoma after abdominoperineal resection. (a) There is a soft-tissue mass (M) lying behind the bladder (B). (b) The scan was repeated following further oral Gastrografin. The soft-tissue mass seen in scan (a) has been opacified and represents loops of small bowel. (Reproduced by kind permission of *Radiology*)

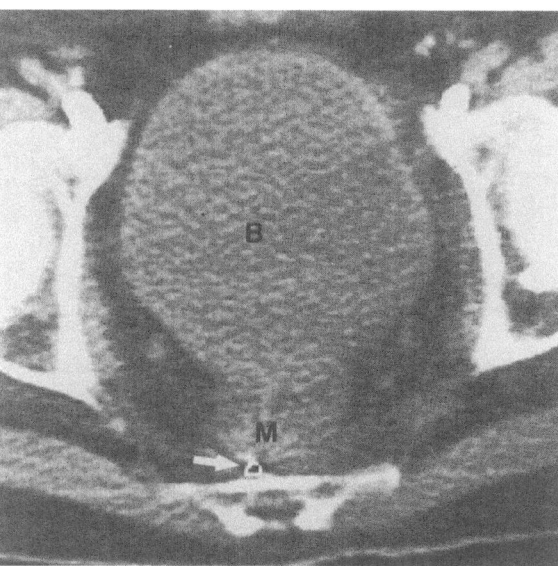

Figure 12.21 Another male patient with suspected recurrence of rectal carcinoma following abdominoperineal resection. The soft-tissue mass (M) behind the bladder (B) represents postoperative granulation tissue. The patient has been followed up for over one year with no evidence of recurrent tumour. Note surgical clip (arrowed). (Reproduced by kind permission of *Radiology*)

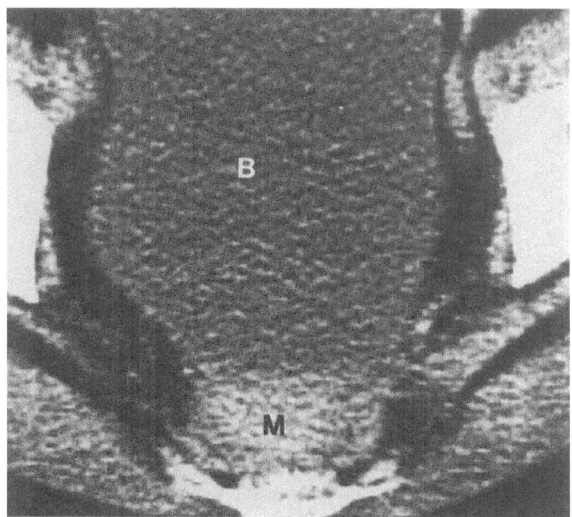

Figure 12.20 Female patient with suspected recurrence of rectal carcinoma after abdominoperineal resection. There is a soft-tissue mass (M) behind the bladder (B). At subsequent laparotomy, this was shown to be the normal uterus

of granulation tissue from a mass of recurrent tumour; percutaneous fine-needle aspiration may then be required.

Recurrent tumours from carcinoma of the rectum often lie more on one side of the pelvis than on the other and have a sharply defined, although irregular, shape (figure 12.22). The density of the mass is similar to that of soft tissue in the majority of patients but occasionally low-density areas, presumably due to necrosis, are seen. Invasion of structures, such as muscle, adjacent organs or the

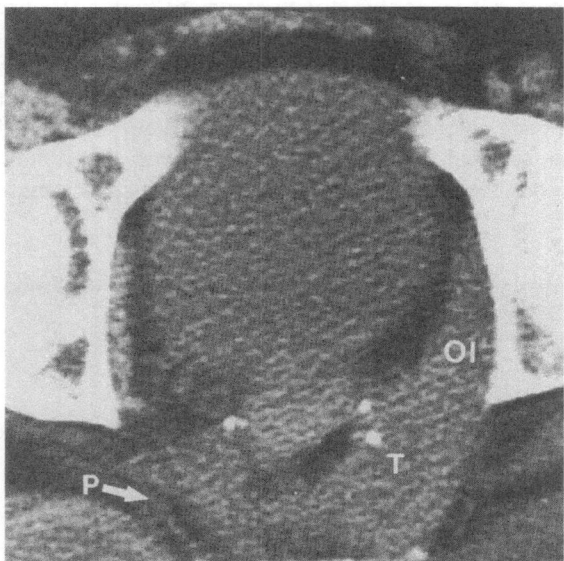

Figure 12.22(a)

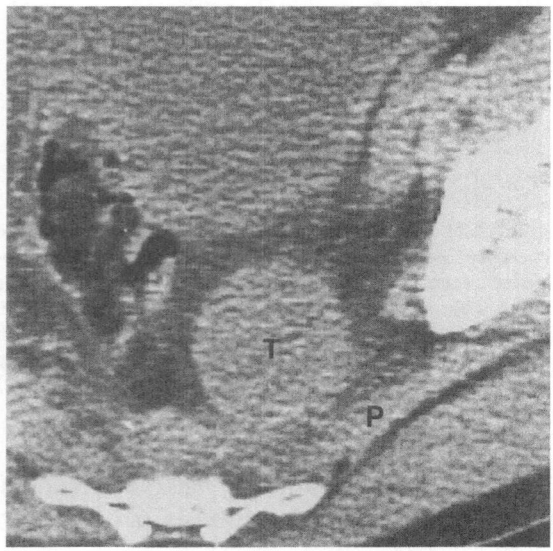

Figure 12.22(b)

Figure 12.22 Two patients with recurrent rectal carcinoma after abdominoperineal resection. (a) The tumour (T) lies on the left side of the pelvis. It involves the obturator internus muscle (OI) and the pyriformis muscle (P) which cannot be identified as a separate structure. Note normal pyriformis muscle on the right. (b) The tumour (T) has a well defined margin. The left pyriformis muscle (P) does not appear to be involved

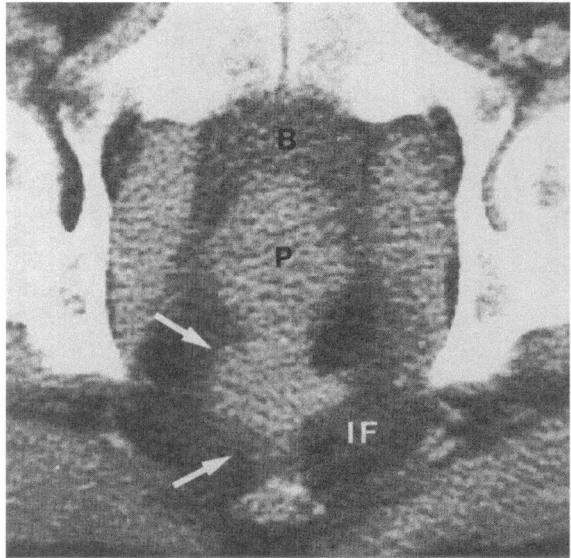

Figure 12.23 Recurrent carcinoma of the rectum (arrowed) in a male patient involving the ischiorectal fossa (IF). Prostate (P), bladder (B)

ischiorectal fossa, is common (figure 12.23) (Husband *et al.*, 1980). Advanced tumours may invade and almost completely destroy the sacrum (figure 12.24).

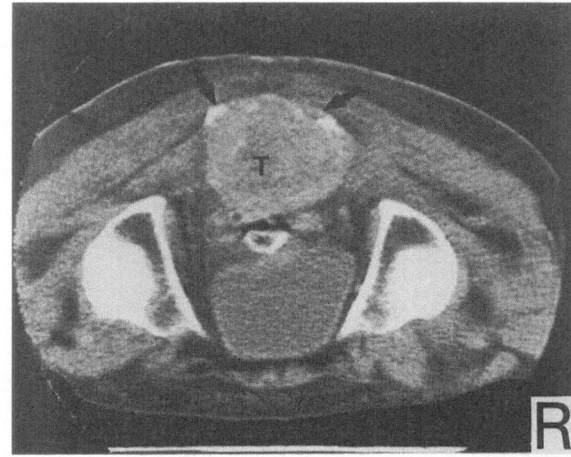

Figure 12.24 Recurrent carcinoma of the rectum in a male patient. Tumour (T) has almost completely destroyed the sacrum (arrowed). The patient was scanned prone because of severe pain

FEMALE GENITAL TRACT

The cervix and body of the uterus present particular problems with CT because they appear as solid organs of soft-tissue density, and tumours within them which have a similar density cannot be distinguished from the surrounding normal tissues. Furthermore, since there is no fat plane between the cervix and uterus, it is difficult to delineate the precise boundaries of these structures.

The Cervix

The normal cervix rarely exceeds 2–3 cm in diameter and tumours are only seen if larger than this (figure 12.25) or if they extend beyond its confines (figure 12.26) or into adjacent structures. The

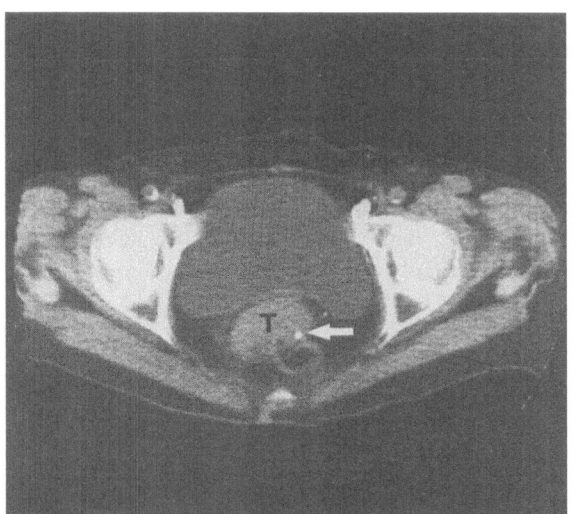

Figure 12.25　Carcinoma of the cervix (T). Note high-density radium implant within the tumour (arrowed)

enlargement of the cervix is generally uniform, but, even with tumours known to be contained within the organ, the edge of the mass is frequently ill defined (figure 12.27). For this reason, it is difficult to identify early tumour spread into the parametria. Another major difficulty with CT is attempting to define upper and lower limits of the tumour spread either into the lower portion of the corpus or into the upper vagina.

The Body of the Uterus

Tumours are the commonest abnormality of the body of the uterus seen with CT, although rare conditions such as haematocolpos have been identified. Both benign tumours (myomyomata) and malignant tumours (adenocarcinoma) can be seen with CT if the organ is enlarged. A benign myoma often produces a lobulated outline to the uterus. It has

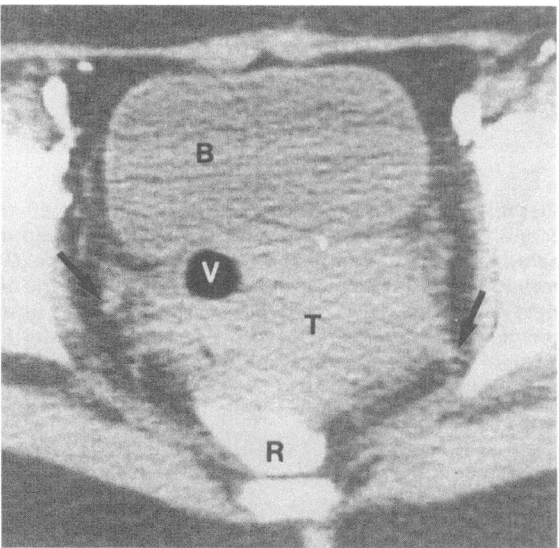

Figure 12.26(a)

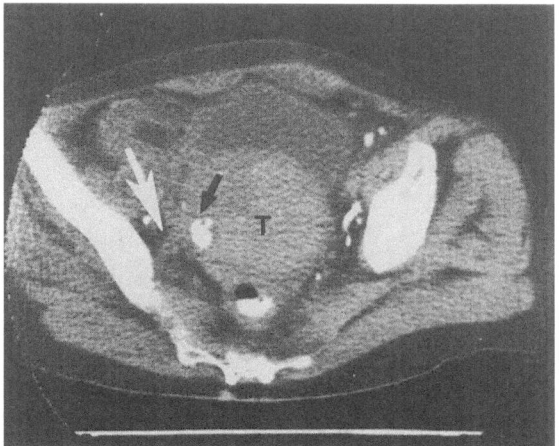

Figure 12.26(b)

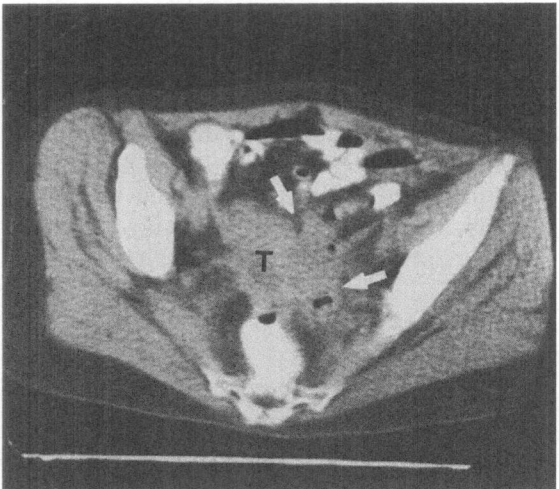

Figure 12.26(c)

Figure 12.26   Three patients with carcinoma of the cervix. (a) The tumour (T) has spread bilaterally into the parametral tissues (arrowed). Bladder (B), vagina (V), rectum (R). (b) The large tumour (T) has spread to the right pelvic wall (large arrow). Note contrast in the bowel surrounded by tumour (small arrow). (c) The tumour (T) involves the sigmoid colon and loops of the small bowel (arrowed)

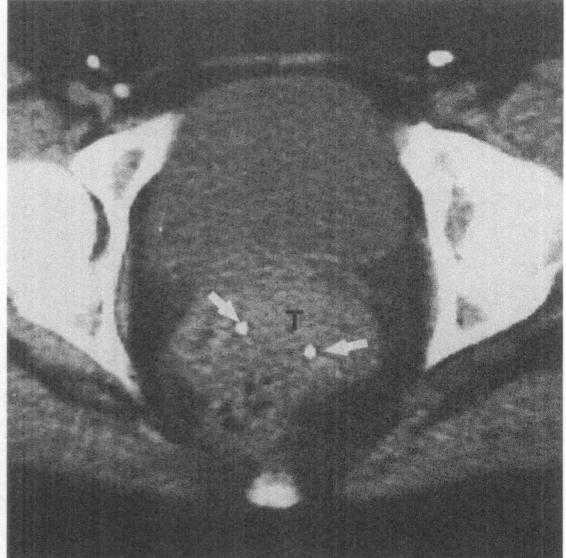

Figure 12.27   Carcinoma of the cervix. The tumour (T) has an ill-defined edge. Hysterectomy was performed and there was no evidence of parametral tumour spread. Note radium implants in the tumour

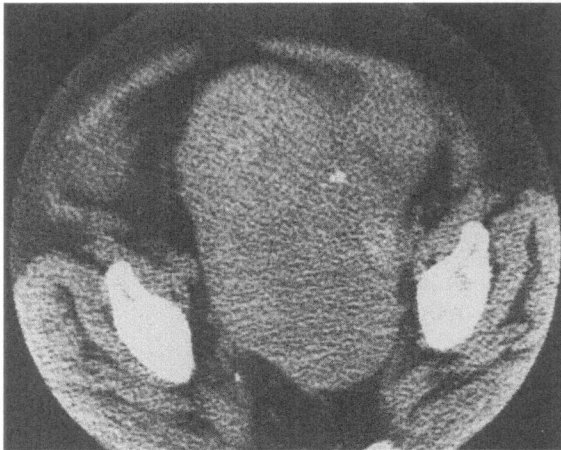

Figure 12.28   Huge fibroid uterus. The mass has a lobulated outline and contains calcification

uniform soft-tissue density unless it contains areas of degeneration (low density) or calcification (high density) (figure 12.28). Malignant tumours also have a soft-tissue density and therefore cannot be reliably distinguished from a benign tumour unless they have spread beyond the primary organ. Tumour spread beyond the uterus appears as a soft-tissue mass with an irregular edge extending into the surrounding adipose tissue and adjacent structures.

The Ovaries

Although the normal ovaries are rarely seen with CT, ovarian masses can be recognised. *Cysts* have a

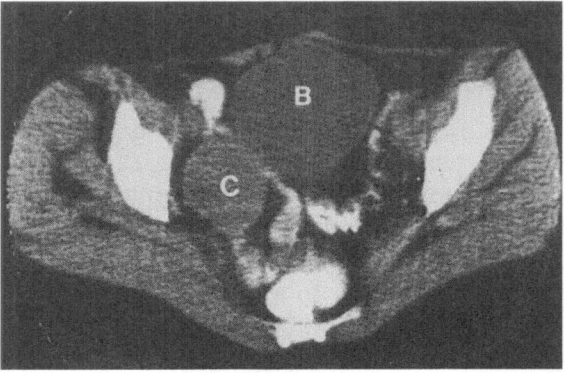

Figure 12.29(a)

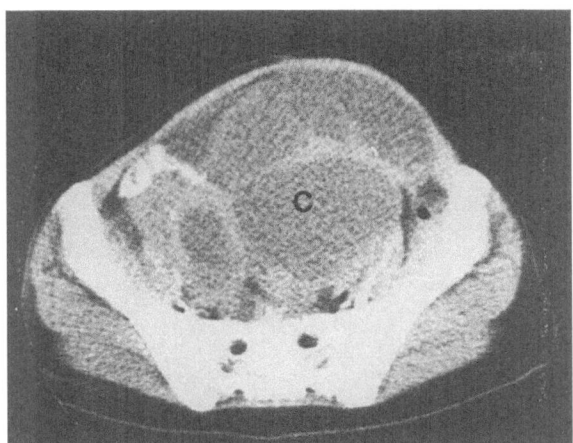

Figure 12.29(b)

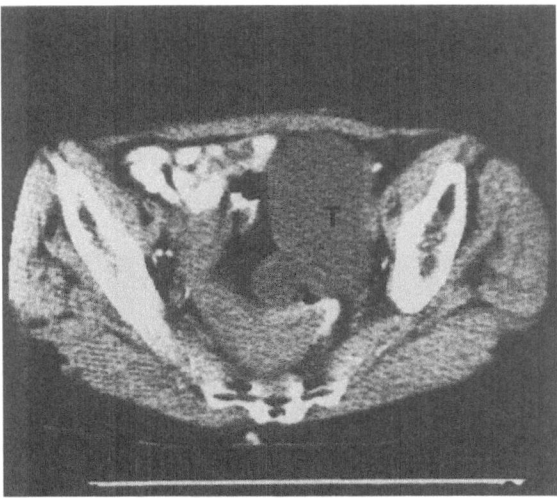

Figure 12.29(c)

Figure 12.29 Three patients with ovarian cysts. (a) Benign unilocular ovarian cyst (C). Bladder (B). (b) Benign multilocular ovarian cyst (C). (c) Carcinoma of the ovary. The tumour (T) is cystic and has a similar appearance to the benign ovarian cyst

low density and may be unilocular or multilocular (figure 12.29a and b). The wall of the cyst can frequently be identified, having a density similar to that of soft tissue, but differentiation between a benign and a malignant cyst is not possible (figure 12.29c). Dermoid cysts may show a characteristic appearance because the components of the tumour

(fat, calcium, soft tissue) can be distinguished from each other. But, with this exception, it seems unlikely that benign cysts can be distinguished from those that are malignant.

Solid ovarian *tumours* appear as soft-tissue masses, whether benign or malignant (figure 12.30). Depending on size, the mass may displace adjacent organs, such as the bladder, cervix and uterus, and may even extend into the abdomen.

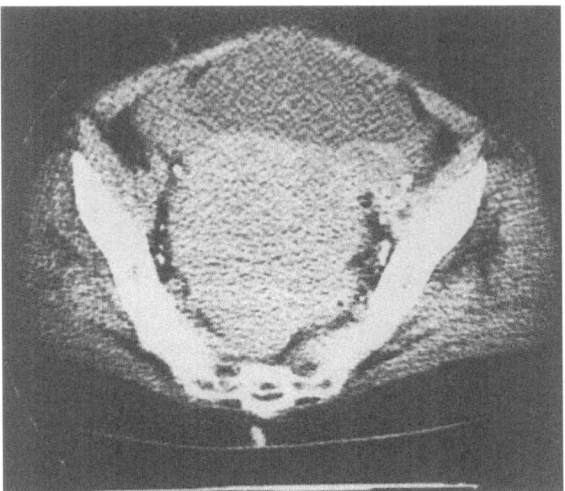

Figure 12.30 Carcinoma of the ovary

PROSTATE

Calcification is commonly seen in the prostate and, as with calcification elsewhere, is more readily shown on CT than with conventional radiography. *Benign prostatic hypertrophy* appears as uniform enlargement of the gland in the lower cuts and may be seen above the symphysis pubis indenting the base of the bladder (figure 12.31).

Carcinoma of the prostate presents the same diagnostic problems as other solid organs in the pelvis; that is, tumours can only be demonstrated if they cause enlargement of the gland or extend through the prostatic capsule. Enlargement of the prostate due to cancer is usually uniform in density and cannot be distinguished from benign prostatic

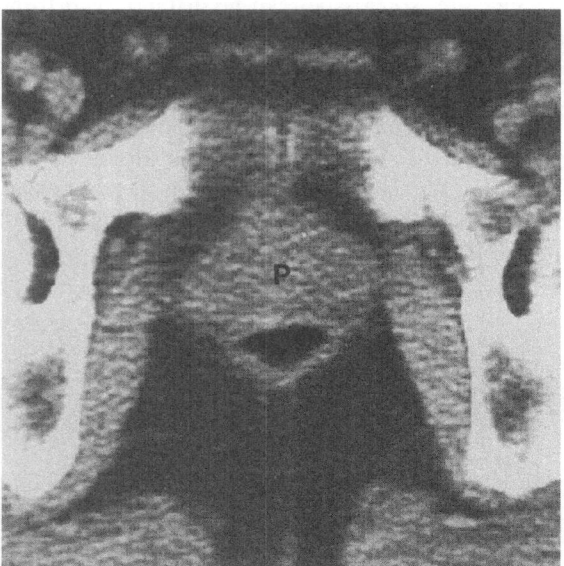

Figure 12.31(a)

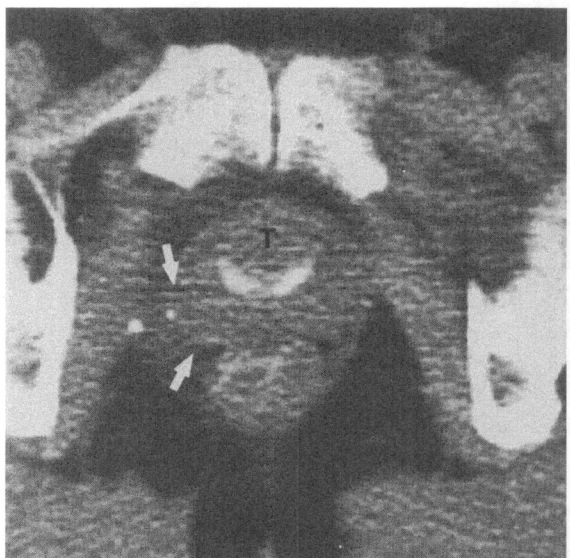

Figure 12.32   Carcinoma of the prostate. The tumour (T) extends into the ischiorectal fossa on the right (arrowed). Note calcification in the prostate

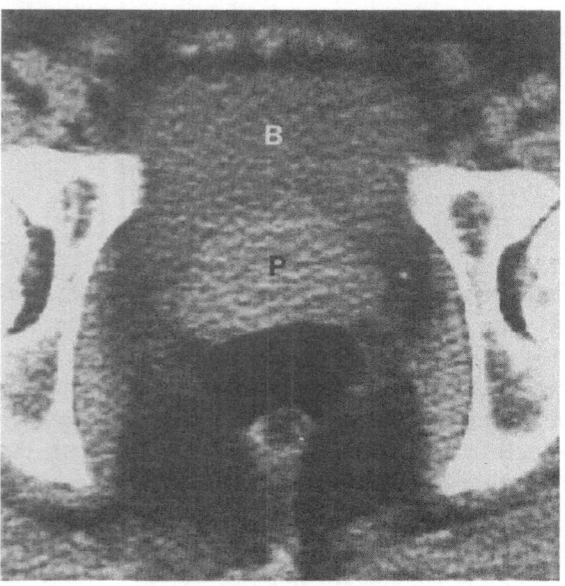

Figure 12.31(b)

Figure 12.31   (a) and (b) Benign prostatic hypertrophy (P) seen on two consecutive slices. The mass indents the base of the bladder (B)

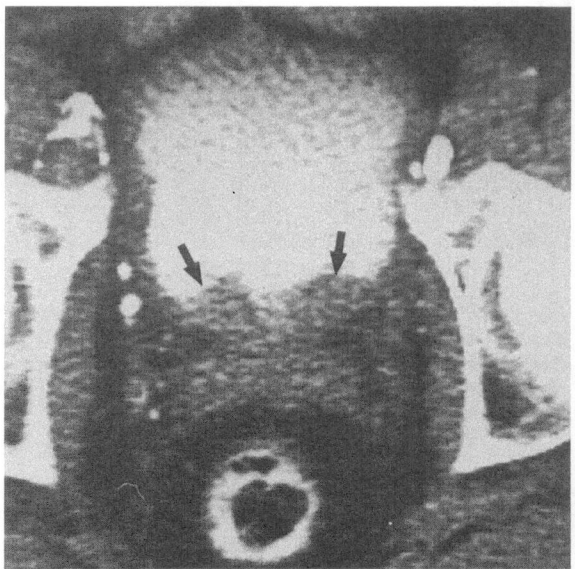

Figure 12.33   Carcinoma of the prostate. The enlarged gland extends into the bladder base (arrowed), but it is impossible to determine whether the bladder mucosa is involved by tumour or not

hypertrophy (figure 12.31) (Price and Davidson, 1979) unless the tumour is advanced and has spread through the prostatic capsule into adjacent structures and organs (figure 12.32).

Early spread of prostatic cancer beyond the capsule is difficult to see, especially if there is little fat between the lateral margins of the prostate and the levator ani muscles. Furthermore, a tumour contained within the gland may displace the fat plane without necessarily invading it. Extension of tumour into the bladder base beyond the primary organ is usually impossible to assess unless gross tumour invasion is present (figure 12.33).

MISCELLANEOUS PELVIC CONDITIONS

Pelvic Lipomatosis

This is elegantly demonstrated with CT because the attenuation value of fat is so low compared to other tissues (figure 12.34).

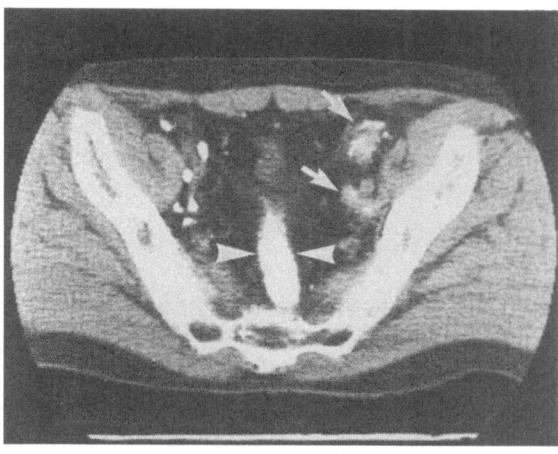

Figure 12.34(b)

Figure 12.34   Pelvic lipomatosis in a patient with Stage IV Hodgkin's disease. (a) The intravenous urogram shows medial deviation of the ureters. At lymphography, the lymph nodes on the right side of the pelvis appear normal, but there has been poor opacification on the left. A large pelvic mass was suspected. (b) The CT scan demonstrated pelvic lipomatosis and only minimal enlargement of lymph nodes on the left side of the pelvis (arrowed). Note the abundant pelvic fat and the centrally placed sigmoid colon (arrowheads)

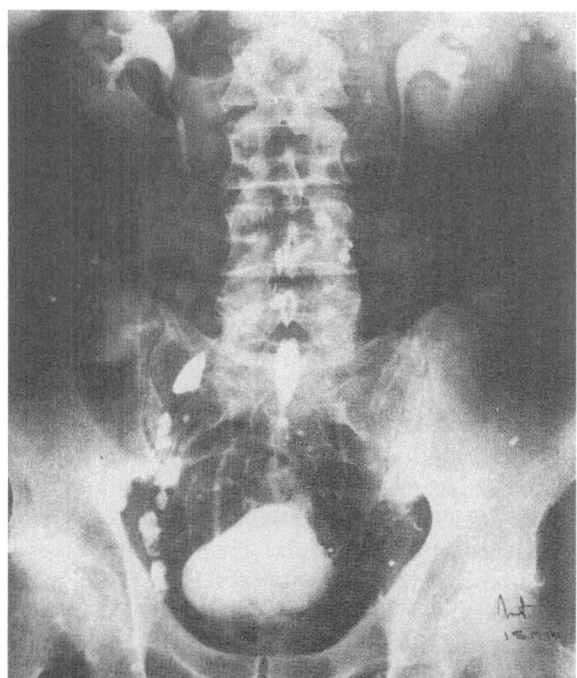

Figure 12.34(a)

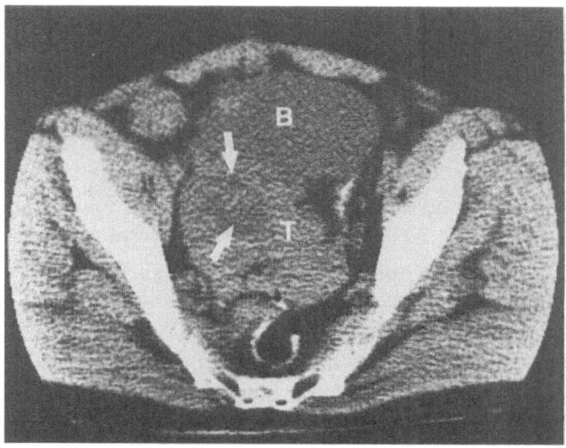

Figure 12.35   Soft-tissue fibrosarcoma of the pelvis. The tumour (T) contains a central area of low density (arrowed). Differentiation between a benign and malignant tumour is not possible. Bladder (B)

Miscellaneous Tumours

There are several different tumour types which have not been discussed, but, in general, CT is not able to distinguish one tumour type from another unless the components of the tumour (for example, fat or calcium) indicate its nature (figure 12.35).

USE OF COMPUTED TOMOGRAPHY

The majority of CT examinations of the pelvis are carried out to identify a suspected pelvic mass or to define the extent and spread of known pelvic disease.

One of the most effective uses of CT in the pelvis is in the assessment of *bladder cancer*, because conventional methods of staging are known to be inaccurate (Whitmore *et al.*, 1977). These conventional methods include intravenous urography, cystoscopy with biopsy and bimanual examination under general anaesthesia. More sophisticated techniques such as arteriography (Lang *et al.*, 1966) and intravesical and perivesical gas insufflation (Gosalbez and Gil-Vernet, 1962) have not found widespread acceptance on account of their invasive nature. Ultrasound, although a non-invasive technique, is only of value in those centres where sufficient expertise is available to provide accurate results (Morley, 1978). The majority of errors using these techniques occur in attempting to define the extent of deep muscle invasion and extravesical tumour spread.

CT is relatively non-invasive, and, from studies correlating CT findings with pathological staging, appears to be a highly accurate method (Seidelmann *et al.*, 1977; Kellett *et al.*, 1980; Husband and Hodson, 1981). Comparison of CT staging with clinical staging has therefore not surprisingly shown that CT is superior (Husband and Hodson, 1981). With reference to the International Union Against Cancer (UICC) classification of bladder tumours (UICC, 1978), this study showed that CT provided additional information over clinical staging in 57% of the patients. This study and other similar studies (Seidelmann *et al.*, 1977; Kellett *et al.*, 1980) have indicated that the main advantage of CT is in the

distinction between intravesical disease and early extravesical disease.

Patients with bladder cancer who have been treated with radiotherapy present special problems. Clinical evaluation is difficult due to irradiation fibrosis, resulting in overestimation of the extent of disease. Kellett *et al.* (1980) suggest that CT may be particularly helpful in distinguishing a clinical frozen pelvis due to radiation fibrosis from one due to tumour recurrence.

The role of CT in the detection of lymph node involvement is discussed in chapter 11.

In patients with *rectal cancer*, the major role of CT is in the detection of local recurrence following surgery (especially after abdominoperineal resection).

The value of CT as an investigation in the preoperative assessment of rectal cancer is still unclear. Local lymph node involvement is frequently microscopic and cannot be detected. The ability of CT to detect extensive spread outside the rectum may prove to be of value in deciding on the use of radiotherapy prior to surgery in selected patients (Dixon *et al.*, 1981).

The primary role of CT in *female pelvic disease* is likely to be in staging of malignant tumours and in the detection of recurrence, although a diagnosis of a suspected pelvic mass, not necessarily malignant, is also an indication for its use. The dose of x-radiation received by the pelvic organs must be considered, and in young females the examination is only justified if the same information cannot be obtained by other methods, such as ultrasound and conventional radiology. The precise relationship of CT to these other techniques in diagnosis and staging still awaits full evaluation. At the present time, it is, therefore, only possible to discuss the potential value of CT and definite conclusions cannot be drawn.

CT has no place in the primary diagnosis of *carcinoma of the cervix and uterus* but may be a useful adjunct to other methods currently used in the staging of these tumours. From studies already undertaken at the Royal Marsden Hospital, it is clear, however, that CT is less accurate for evaluation of the cervix than for evaluation of the bladder. Additional information over clinical methods of investigation were only obtained in 28% of a total of

34 patients with cervical cancer. As with cancer of the bladder, CT is of particular value following radiotherapy, helping to distinguish between a frozen pelvis due to radiation fibrosis and one due to recurrent tumour (figure 12.36). In this group of 19 patients, CT provided useful additional information in 70% of such cases.

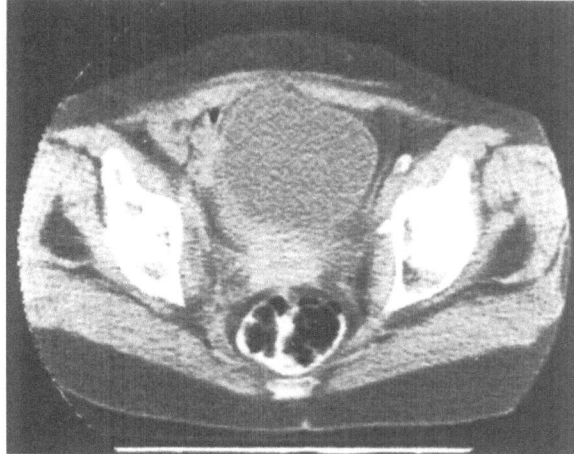

Figure 12.36(a)

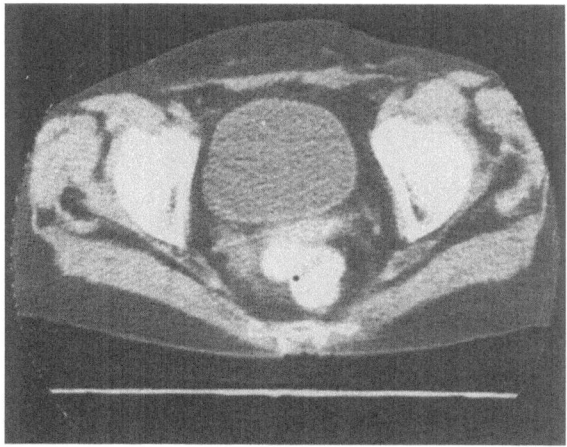

Figure 12.36(b)

Figure 12.36 Two patients with suspected recurrence of carcinoma of the cervix and frozen pelvis. Both had been treated with radiotherapy. (a) There is a well defined mass behind the bladder representing recurrent tumour. (b) Normal scan. No evidence of recurrent tumour. The patient remains alive and well two years later

Although CT can demonstrate *ovarian tumours and cysts*, ultrasound is a highly successful technique for diagnosing such lesions and for distinguishing cysts from tumours. CT is, therefore, likely to be reserved for those cases which are difficult to examine with ultrasound.

CT is also likely to have only a minor role in the staging of ovarian cancer, because this tumour spreads across the peritoneum, producing seedling metastases in various sites, such as the omentum, mesentery and diaphragm. These metastases may be too small to be identified with CT, and for this reason laparotomy will only be avoided in those patients in whom CT demonstrates extensive disease. Information can also be obtained regarding the size and the extent of the primary pelvic tumour, and in this way CT can be used to monitor the effect of therapy in patients with inoperable disease or in the detection of suspected recurrence.

At the present time, there is little information about the accuracy of CT staging compared to clinical staging in *prostatic cancer* (Price and Davidson, 1979), but in our experience it rarely provides information that affects management.

REFERENCES

Dixon, A. K., Nicholls, R. J., Mason, A. Y., Morson, B. C. and Fry, I. K. (1981). Preoperative computed tomography and clinical assessment of carcinoma of the rectum. Abstract. *European Seminar on Computed Tomography in Oncology*, London, February 1980

van Engelshoven, J. M. A. and Kreel, L. (1979). CT of the prostate. *Journal of Computer Assisted Tomography*, **3** (1), 45

Gosalbez, R. and Gil-Vernet, J. M. (1962). Bladder tomography: the use of air intra- and peri-vesically in the radiologic study of bladder tumours. *Journal of Urology*, **88**, 312

Hodson, N. J., Husband, J. E. and Macdonald, J. S. (1979). The role of computed tomography in the staging of bladder cancer. *Clinical Radiology*, **30**, 389–395

Husband, J. E. and Hodson, N. J. (1981). Computerised axial tomography in staging and assessing response to treatment in bladder cancer. In *Bladder Cancer — Principles of Combination Therapy*, eds. T. D. Oliver, W. F. Hendry and H. J. G. Bloom, Butterworths, Sevenoaks (in press)

Husband, J. E., Hodson, N. J. and Parsons, C. A. (1980). The role of computed tomography in recurrent rectal tumours. *Radiology*, **134**, 677–682

Kellett, M. J., Fry, I. K., Husband, J. E. and Oliver, T. D. (1980). CT scanning as an adjunct to bimanual examination for staging of bladder tumours. *British Journal of Urology*, **52**, 101–106

Lang, I. E., Nourse, M. H., Wishard, W. M., Jr. and Mertz, J. H. O. (1966). The accuracy of pre-operative staging of bladder tumours by arteriography: a five year study. *Journal of Urology*, **95**, 363

Morley, P. (1978). Clinical staging of epithelial bladder tumours by echotomography. In *Ultrasound in Tumour Diagnosis*, ed. C. R. Hill, V. R. McCready and D. O. Cosgrove, Pitman Medical, London, pp. 145–161

Price, J. M. and Davidson, A. J. (1979). Computed tomography in the evaluation of suspected carcinomatous prostate. *Urologic Radiology*, **1**, 39–42

Seidelmann, F. E., Cohen, W. N. and Bryan, P. J. (1977). Computed tomographic staging of bladder neoplasms. *Radiologic Clinics of North America*, **XV** (3), 419–440

Seidelmann, F. E., Cohen, W. N., Bryan, P. J., Temes, S. P., Kraus, D. and Schoenrock, G. (1978). Accuracy of CT staging of bladder neoplasms using gas-filled method: report of twenty-one patients with surgical confirmation. *American Journal of Roentgenology*, **130**, 735–739

UICC (1978). *TNM Classification of Malignant Tumours*, 3rd edn, Geneva

van Voorthuisen, A. (1980). Tumour staging and recurrence: rectum. Presented at the *International Symposium on Whole Body Computed Tomography, 5th CARVAT*, Rome, May 1980

Whitmore, W. F., Jr., Batata, M. A., Ghoneim, M. A., Grabstald, H. and Unal, A. (1977). Radical cystectomy with or without prior irradiation in the treatment of bladder cancer. *Journal of Urology*, **118**, 184–187

13

The Musculo-Skeletal System

Bones, muscles and other soft tissues are clearly demonstrated with CT and, because there are relatively large differences in contrast between these various tissues, interpretation is usually straight-forward. In spite of this, until recently, the use of CT has been somewhat neglected. This reflects the obvious application of the technique to the investigation of intra-abdominal masses and other lesions which are difficult to demonstrate using conventional radiology. There is, however, now increasing evidence that CT can often provide accurate

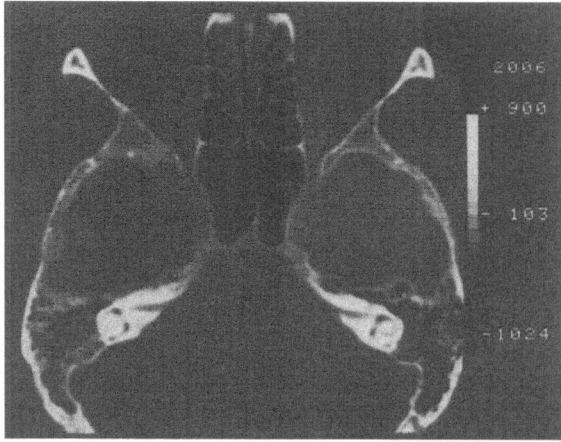

Figure 13.1 High-resolution scans: (a) vertebral body, (b) base of skull showing petrous bone. (Reproduced by kind permission of International General Electric and Siemens AG UB Med, respectively)

information regarding lesions of the musculo-skeletal system which is not otherwise readily available. This is particularly so in bones which can be difficult to demonstrate by conventional methods, such as the spine, sternum, scapula and sacrum. The development of high-resolution systems is already having an impact on the diagnosis of lesions in the musculo-skeletal system because of the fine detail that can be demonstrated (figure 13.1).

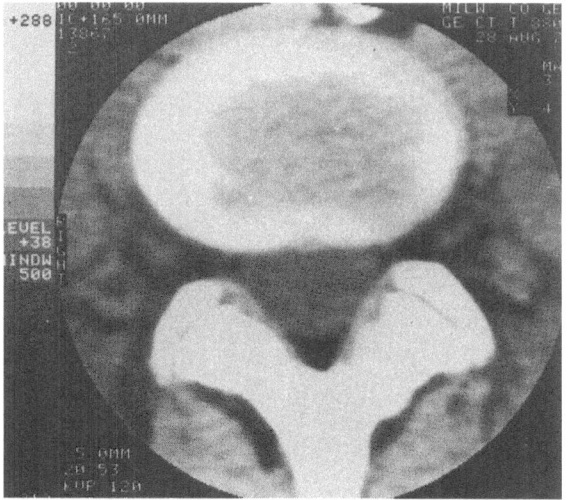

Figure 13.1(a)

TECHNIQUE OF EXAMINATION

No preparation is required for examination of the bones and surrounding soft tissues. The main difficulties at present are matching the precise level of the CT section to the anatomical level in the longitudinal plane, and providing a true cross-sectional image of the spine because of the natural spine curvature. With newer scanners, the gantry can be tilted and a scanogram is produced in which a cursor line demonstrates the plane of the proposed scan in both anteroposterior and lateral projections. The patient and gantry can then be arranged in the exact position required (*see* chapter 2).

For examination of bone, the CT image is viewed at a high window level and, more importantly, at a wide window width. This permits more latitude so that the cortex, medulla and adjacent soft tissues can be distinguished.

CT ANATOMY

It is beyond the scope of this text to provide a complete account of the cross-sectional anatomy of the musculo-skeletal system. Several anatomical atlases are now available which are ideally suited for this purpose (Carter *et al.*, 1977). The following description should be regarded only as an outline for easier understanding of the pathological processes demonstrated by CT.

The Spine

Lumbar Vertebrae

Scans through the middle of a typical lumbar vertebra show the vertebral body, the pedicles, transverse processes, laminae and spinous process (figure 13.2). The cortex is clearly distinguished from the medulla in which the trabecular pattern can be identified. As in other parts of the spine, the density of the medulla is often not uniform; there may be small areas of increased density representing

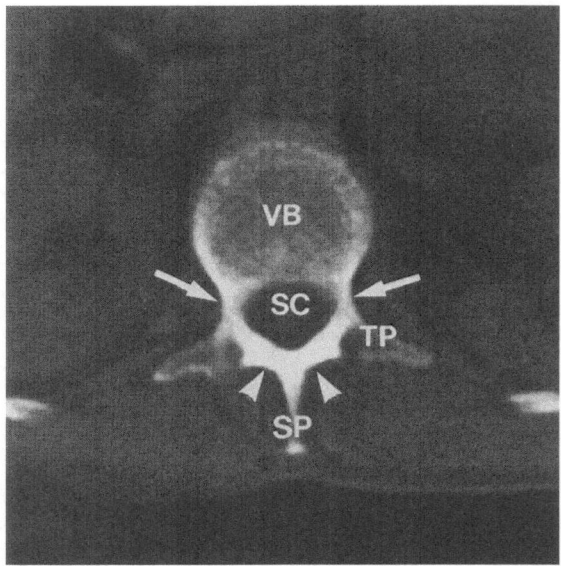

Figure 13.2   Scan through the middle of a typical lumbar vertebra. Vertebral body (VB), pedicles (arrowed), transverse process (TP), laminae (arrowheads), spinous process (SP). Note oval-shaped spinal canal (SC)

bone islands (figure 13.3) or small areas of increased lucency which are often seen centrally at the posterior aspect of the vertebral body (figure 13.4). The CT section may pass through the middle of one transverse process and only partly through the other, depending on the degree of spinal curvature

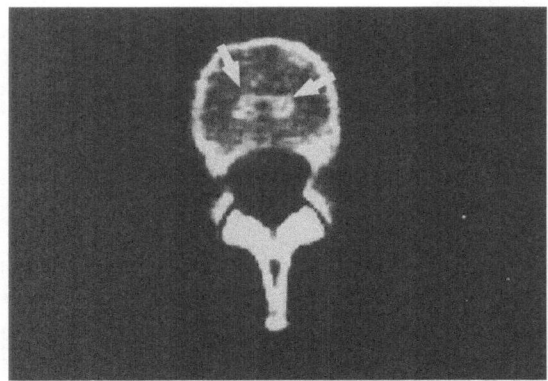

Figure 13.3   Scan through the fourth lumbar vertebra showing dense bone islands (arrowed)

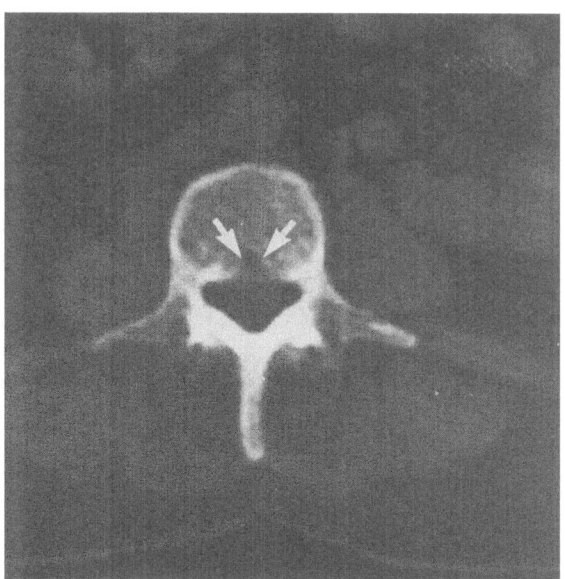

Figure 13.4 Normal fourth lumbar vertebra showing a central area of increased lucency within the vertebral body (arrowed). This represents the point of entry of the vascular plexus

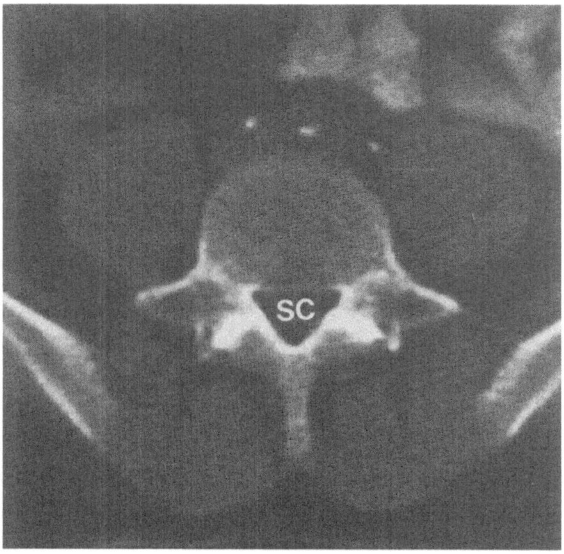

and on the patient's position. When this occurs, the scan may be difficult to interpret because the cortical margin is not clearly seen and may thus simulate cortical erosion. This phenomenon occurs at any site, but is a particular problem at the L5/S1 level where the lumbar lordosis is most marked.

The vertebral canal changes in shape through the lumbar region from oval at the level of the first lumbar vertebra to trefoil at the fifth lumbar vertebra (figure 13.5), and measurements for the dimensions of the normal canal seen with CT are now available (Lee *et al.*, 1978; Ullrich *et al.*, 1980).

Scans through the upper or lower margins of the vertebral body pass through the intervertebral foramina, the articular processes and part of the spinous process (figure 13.6). The cortical bone appears as a thick rim round the vertebral body.

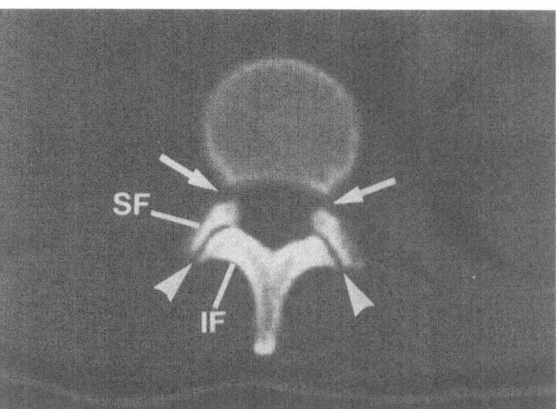

Figure 13.6 Scan through the lower part of a typical lumbar vertebra. Apophyseal joints (arrowheads), superior articular facet (SF), inferior articular facet (IF), intervertebral foramina (arrows)

Thoracic Vertebrae

The thoracic vertebrae show gradual increase in size caudally and are distinguished from the upper lumbar vertebrae by their articulations with the

Figure 13.5 Scan at the level of the fifth lumbar vertebra. Note trefoil-shaped spinal canal

heads and tubercles of the ribs (figure 13.7a). Only the proximal portion of each rib is seen because they pass laterally and obliquely out of the CT sections. Portions of several ribs are seen as they surround the chest wall in all scans through the thorax and upper abdomen (figure 13.7b).

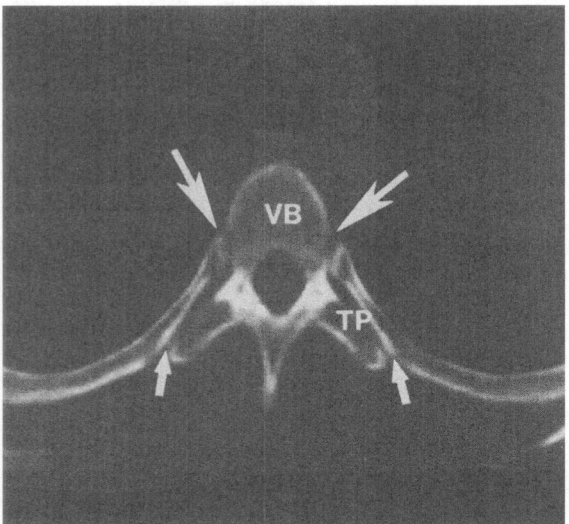

Figure 13.7(a)

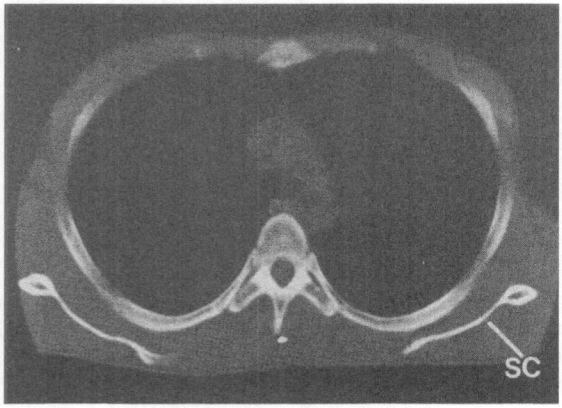

Figure 13.7(b)

Figure 13.7 (a) Scan through a typical thoracic vertebra showing the vertebral body (VB), transverse processes (TP), articular facets for the head of the ribs (large arrows) and tubercles of the ribs (small arrows). (b) Portions of several ribs are seen on each scan through the chest. Scapula (SC)

Cervical Vertebrae

The bodies of the cervical vertebrae usually appear more homogeneous than those in the lower thoracic and lumbar spine. The anatomical configuration of the cervical spine is more complex than other regions and the precise anatomical features shown are therefore highly dependent on the plane of the CT section in relation to the vertebral body. If a true cross section is obtained, it is possible to identify the foramen transversarium, the anterior and posterior tubercles, articular facets and the bifid cervical spinous process (figure 13.8). Sections through the

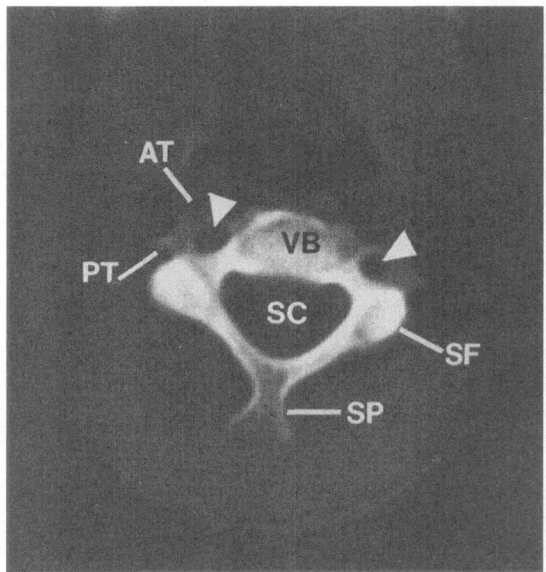

Figure 13.8 Scan through a typical cervical vertebra. Vertebral body (VB), spinal canal (SC), foramen transversarium (arrowheads), anterior tubercle (AT), posterior tubercle (PT), spinous process (SP), superior articular facet (SF)

atlas and axis demonstrate the anterior and posterior arches as well as the lateral masses containing the foramen transversarium. The odontoid process of the axis and its relation to the anterior arch of the atlas is also clearly shown (figure 13.9).

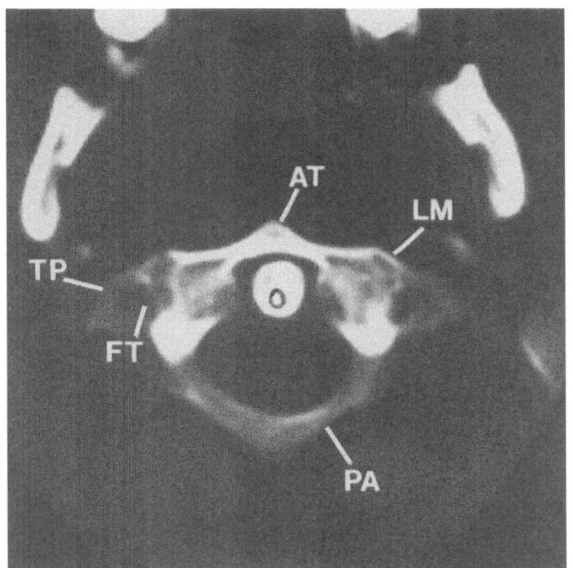

Figure 13.9 Scan through the atlas. Anterior tubercle (AT), odontoid peg (O), foramen transversarium (FT), transverse process (TP), lateral mass (LM), posterior arch (PA)

The Shoulder Girdle

Scans taken through the thoracic inlet pass through the upper part of the sternum, the sterno-clavicular joints, the anterior portions of the upper ribs (figure 13.10a) and the upper part of the scapulae. At this

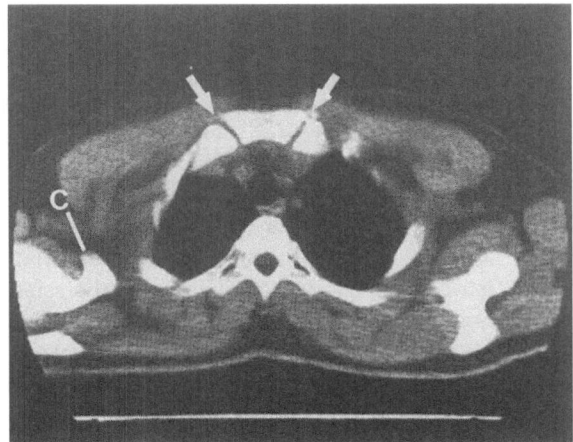

Figure 13.10(a)

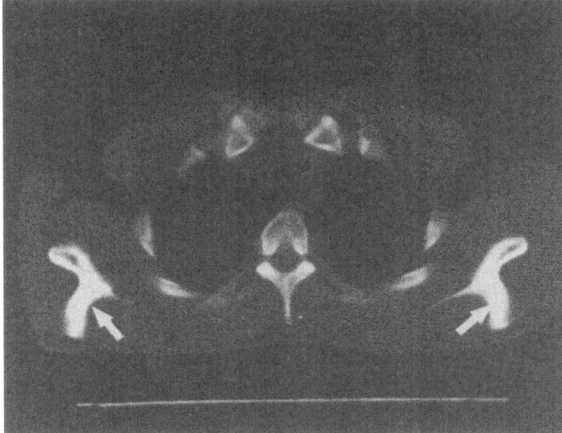

Figure 13.10(b)

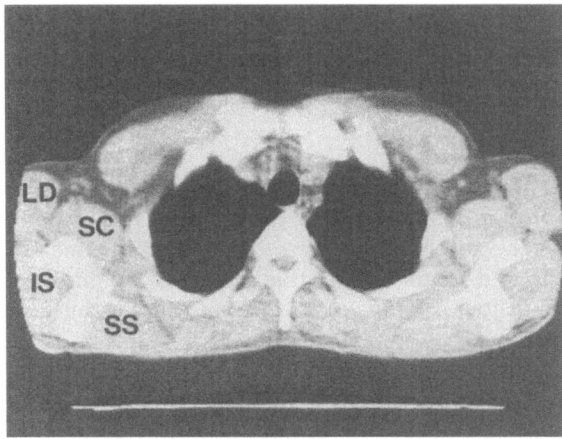

Figure 13.10(c)

Figure 13.10 Normal scans through shoulder girdle. (a) Sternoclavicular joints (arrowed), coracoid process (C). (b) Spine of scapula (arrowed). (c) Same slice as (b) to show soft tissues. Infraspinatus (IS), supraspinatus (SS), subscapularis (SC), latissimus dorsi (LD)

level, the spine of the scapula is seen as a short, thick process directed posteriorly from the dorsal surface (figure 13.10b). The muscles related to the scapula, including the infraspinatus, supraspinatus and subscapularis, are readily seen (figure 13.10c). Latissimus dorsi lies anterior and lateral to the scapular muscles.

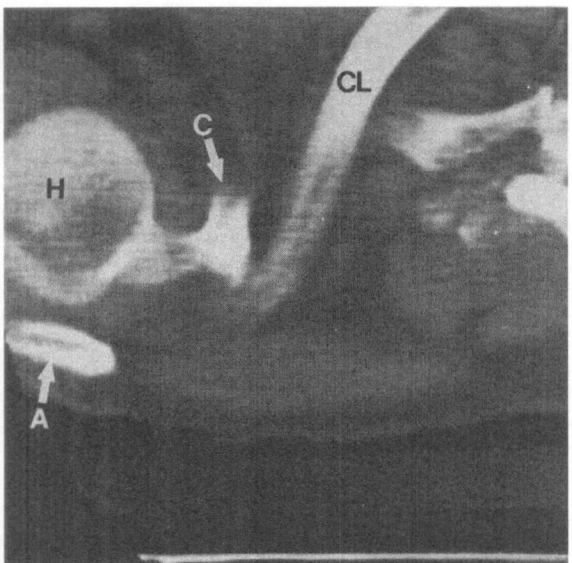

Figure 13.11   Scan through the normal shoulder girdle showing the humeral head (H), acromion (A), corocoid process (C), clavicle (CL)

Higher sections through the shoulder girdle often show the lateral third of the clavicle, the coracoid and the acromion processes as well as the humeral head and glenoid cavity (figure 13.11). At this level, the deltoid is now seen surrounding the humeral head as a C-shaped structure.

The Pelvis

Sections through the upper part of the bony pelvis show the iliac wings, the sacro-iliac joints and sacrum (figure 13.12a). As in other parts of the axial skeleton, the anterior cortex of the sacrum is frequently not seen, and scans through this area should be interpreted with caution. Because the sacrum is curved, the first two vertebrae are usually shown on the same CT image. Muscle groups identified in scans through the upper pelvis include the iliopsoas muscle on the medial aspect of the iliac bone, the gluteus minimus, gluteus medius and gluteus maximus laterally (figure 13.12b). Passing through the pelvis in a caudal direction, the space between the sacrum and iliac bone becomes increasingly

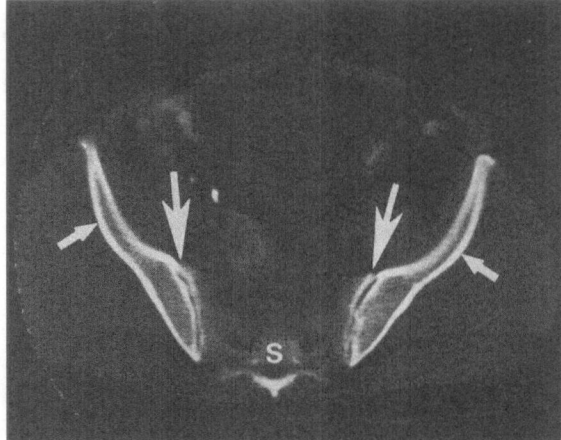

Figure 13.12(a)

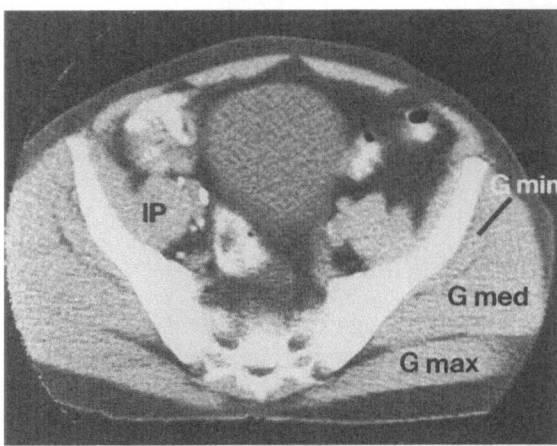

Figure 13.12(b)

Figure 13.12   Normal scan through the upper pelvis at different window settings. (a) To show bone. Iliac wings (small arrows), sacro-iliac joints (large arrows), sacrum (S). (b) To show soft tissues. Iliopsoas muscles (IP), gluteus maximus (G max), gluteus medius (G med), gluteus minimus (G min)

wide. This space, representing the greater sciatic notch, is occupied by pyriformis muscle, the sciatic nerve and inferior gluteal vessels. (These latter structures cannot usually be identified separately.)

CT sections through the middle of the hip joint show the acetabulum, the joint space and femoral head with the fovea which gives attachment to the ligament of the head of the femur (figure 13.13a).

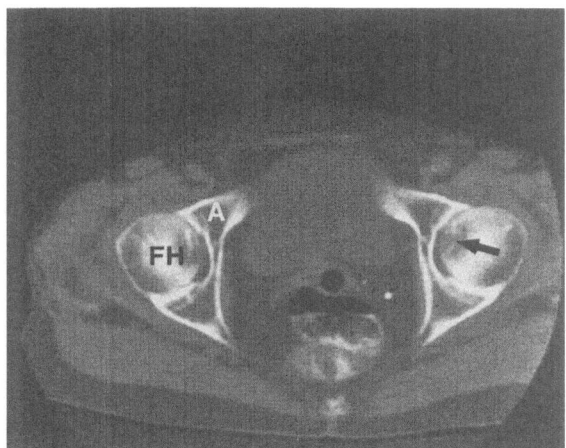

Figure 13.13(a)

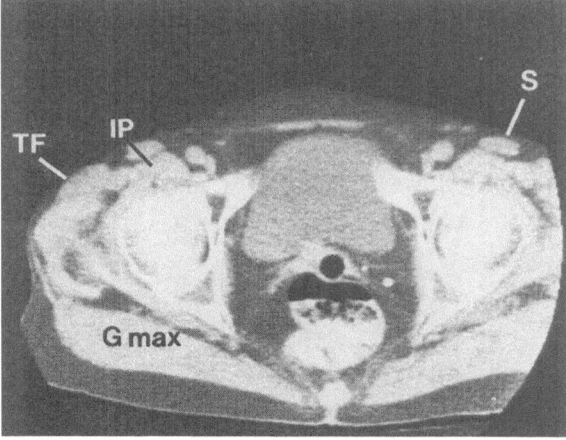

Figure 13.13(b)

Figure 13.13 Normal scans through the hip joint at different window settings. (a) To show bone. Femoral head (FH), acetabulum (A), fovea (arrowed). (b) To show soft tissues. Muscles include gluteus maximus (G max), sartorius (S), tensa fascia lata (TF), iliopsoas (IP)

The surrounding muscles include the iliopsoas, sartorius, rectus femoris, tensa fascia lata, gluteus medius and maximus and the gemelli muscles (figure 13.13b). Lower scans show the greater tuberosity of the femur, the superior pubic rami and the symphysis pubis. Immediately below this, the inferior pubic rami and ischial tuberosities are seen.

TUMOURS

Primary Tumours of Bone and Soft Tissues

Bone

CT sections through a primary bone tumour show areas of destruction, sclerosis and calcification depending on the histological type (figures 13.14, 13.15, 13.16, 13.17 and 13.18). CT can localise destruction and tumour formation more precisely

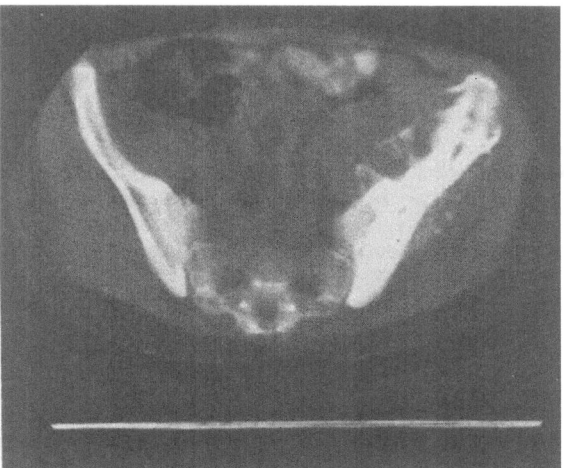

Figure 13.14(a)

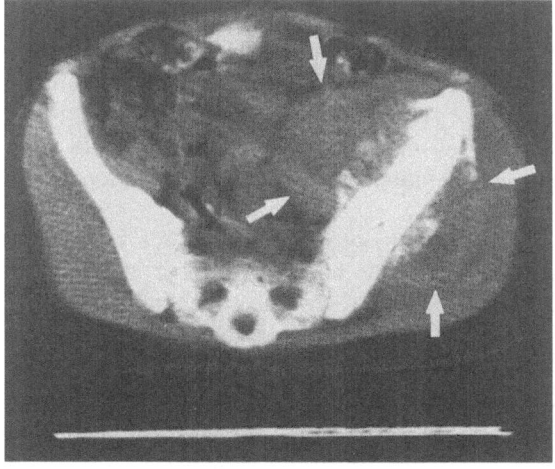

Figure 13.14(b)

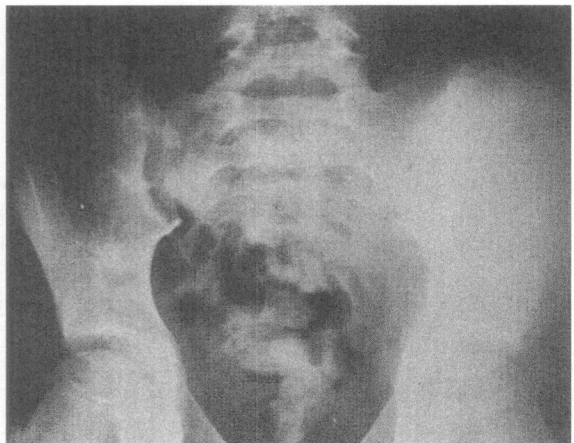

Figure 13.14(c)

Figure 13.14 Ewing's sarcoma of the left ilium. (a) The scan shows areas of bone destruction, sclerosis and new bone formation. (b) At the appropriate window level, the large soft-tissue mass associated with the tumour is clearly shown (arrowed). (c) The standard radiograph provides less information than the CT scan regarding the extent of the tumour

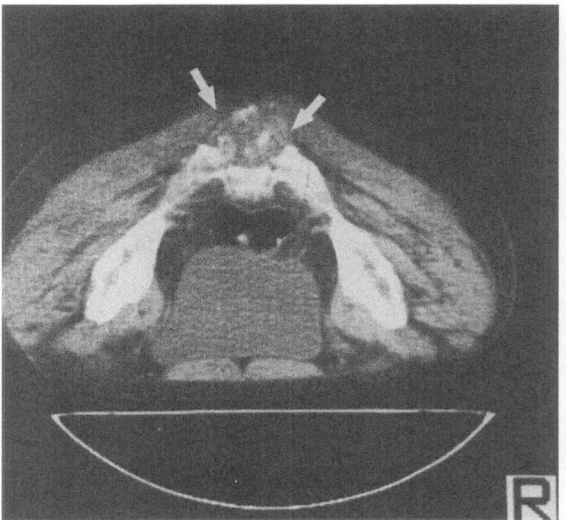

Figure 13.15(a)

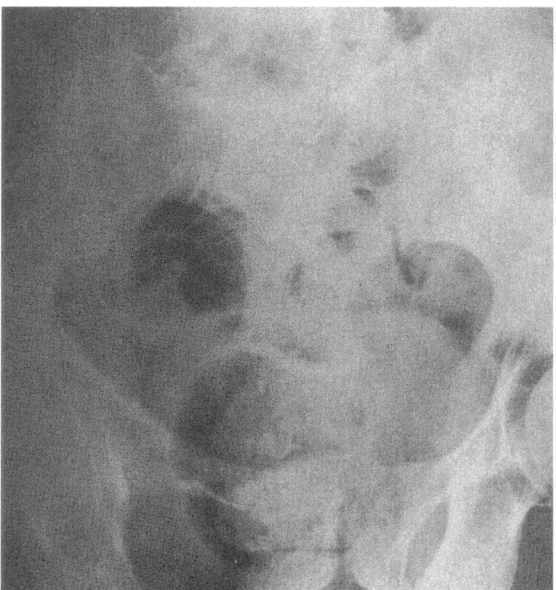

Figure 13.15(b)

Figure 13.15 Chondrosarcoma of the sacrum. (a) Scan shows gross destruction of the sacrum associated with a soft-tissue mass (arrowed). (b) The standard radiograph provides little information due to overlying bowel gas in the pelvis

than conventional radiographs, particularly regarding the extent of medullary involvement. In a series of 25 patients with histologically proven osteogenic sarcoma, de Santos *et al.* (1979) demonstrated that tumour tissue has a higher attenuation value than normal marrow (figure 13.16b). In a study of six patients with osteogenic sarcomas, Destouet *et al.* (1979) were able to distinguish cortical from medullary involvement in all cases. However, other processes such as inflammation, haematoma and reactive hyperplasia also have higher attenuation values than normal marrow, and this could lead to misinterpretation (I. Isherwood, personal communication).

One of the major advantages of CT in the assessment of primary bone tumours is the ability to demonstrate the extent of surrounding soft-tissue involvement (figure 13.14a and b). CT shows not only the size of the soft-tissue component but also the relationship of the mass to vital structures such as vessels and nerves and involvement of individual muscle groups. Intravenous contrast medium may be required to show the vessels and can also be

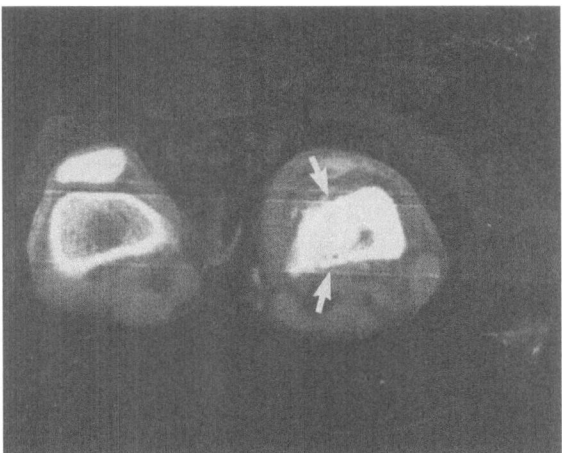

Figure 13.16(a)

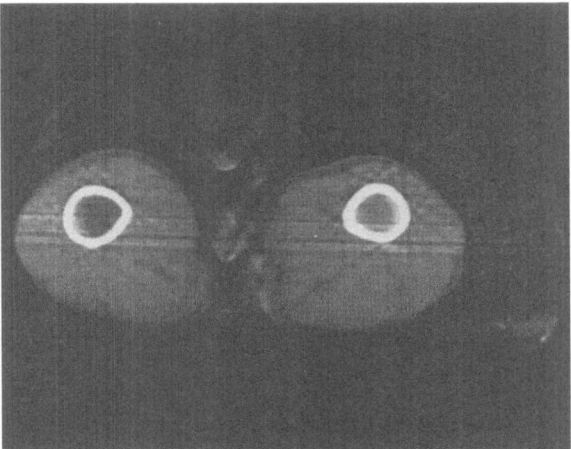

Figure 13.16(b)

Figure 13.16 Primary osteogenic sarcoma of the left femur. (a) New bone formation and sclerosis is clearly shown on the scan (arrowed). (b) A higher section through the femora shows higher attenuation values of the marrow on the left compared with that on the right. This may represent medullary extension

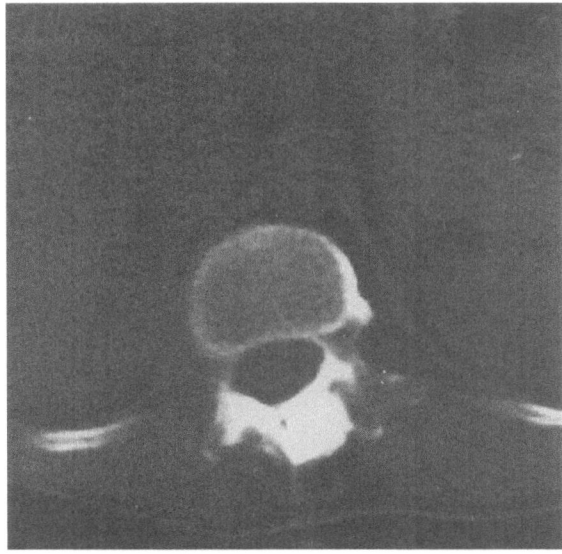

Figure 13.17 Osteoblastoma of the twelfth thoracic vertebra showing dense bone sclerosis

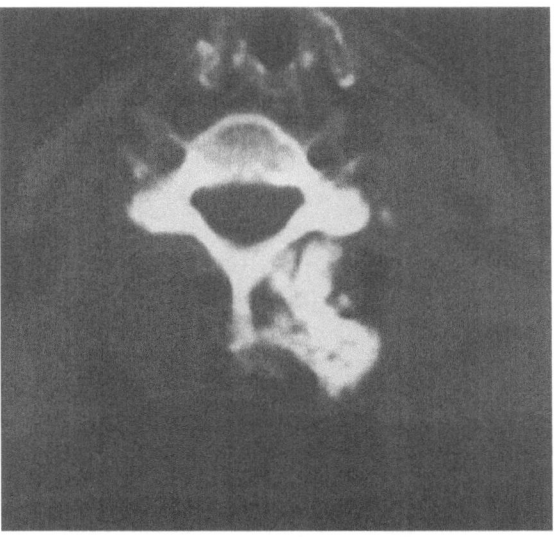

Figure 13.18 Benign chondroma arising from the cervical spine

helpful for assessing the limits of the soft-tissue component because the tumour itself may enhance. Muscle involvement is easy to diagnose if the muscle is completely surrounded by tumour or is enlarged. Lack of intervening fat between the tumour margin and adjacent muscles does not necessarily represent invasion (Heelan *et al.*, 1979). Overall, the information regarding the soft-tissue component of a bone tumour provided by CT seems to be superior to that obtained with standard radiography.

Soft Tissues

As with bone tumours, those arising primarily in soft tissues are well displayed with CT, providing accurate information regarding tumour extent (figures 13.19 and 13.20). Measurement of the attenuation values of a soft-tissue tumour may predict its nature; for example, a lipoma or a

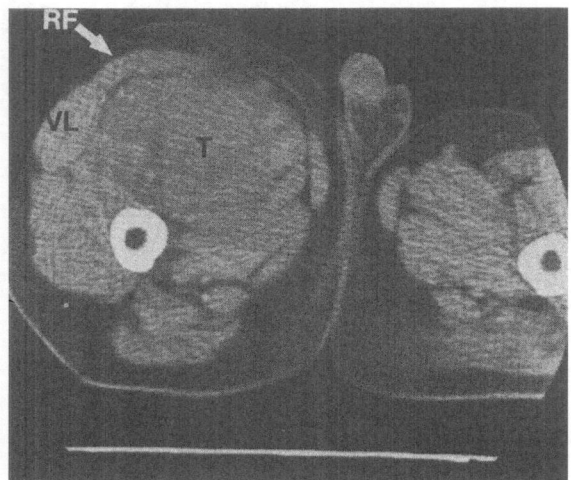

Figure 13.19(a)

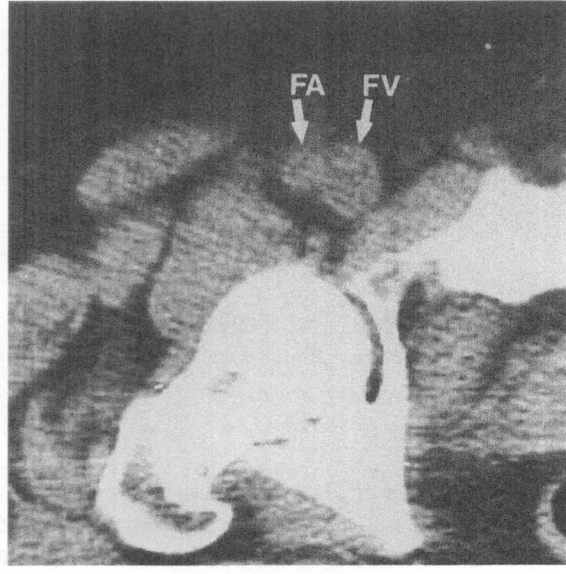

Figure 13.19(b)

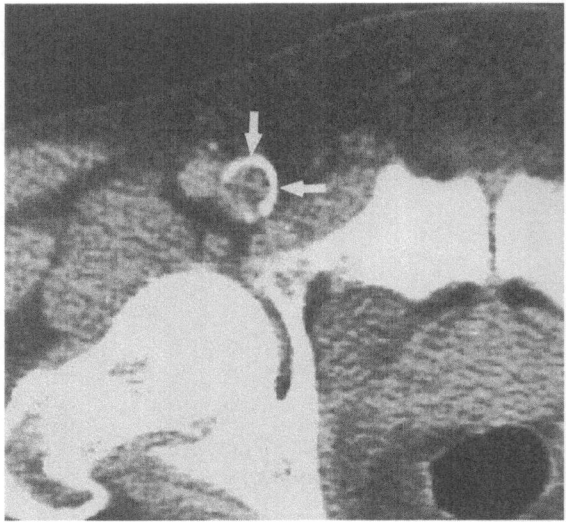

Figure 13.19(c)

Figure 13.19   Soft-tissue fibrosarcoma of the right thigh. (a) There is a clear fat plane between the tumour (T) and the rectus femoris (RF) and vastus lateraris (VL) muscles. The tumour is inseparable from the medial muscles of the thigh. (b) and (c) Scans at a high level taken before (b) and after (c) infusion of intravenous contrast medium into a vein in the foot. Femoral artery (FA), femoral vein (FV). After contrast, low-density thrombus is seen within the femoral vein. The contrast is seen as a thin C-shaped rim around the periphery of the occluded vessel (arrowed). The presence of thrombus was confirmed at operation

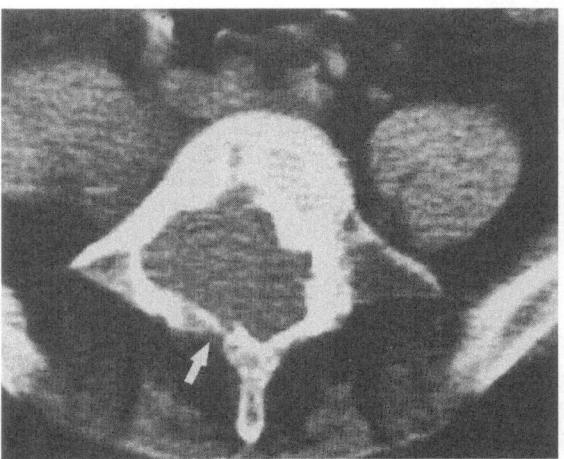

Figure 13.20   Neurofibroma showing gross destruction of the vertebral body and lamina on the right (arrowed)

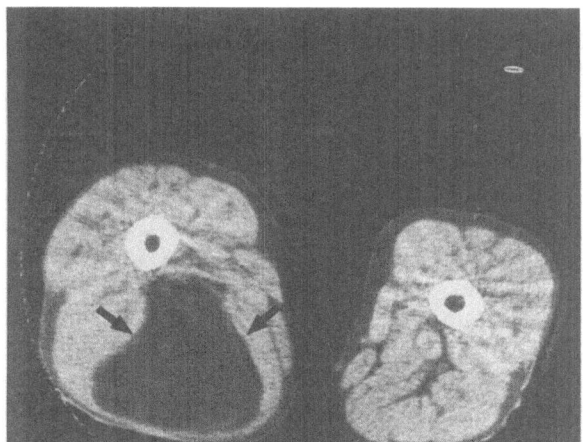

Figure 13.21   Liposarcoma of the right thigh. The mass (arrowed) has low attenuation values similar to fat but strands of soft tissue density are seen passing through it

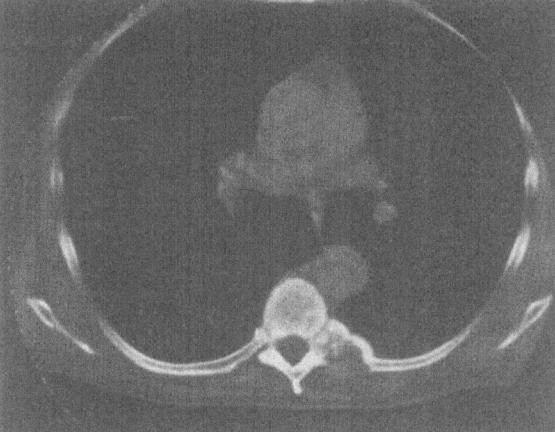

Figure 13.22(a)

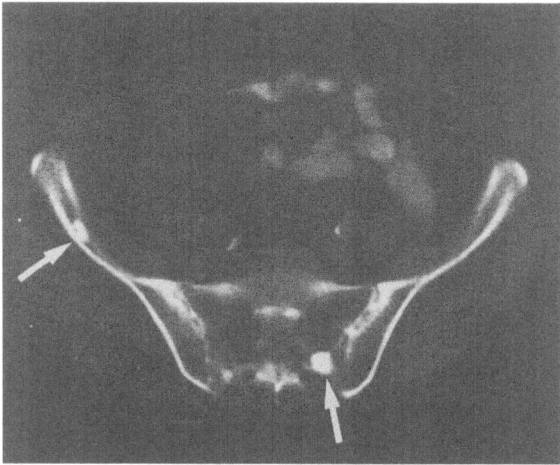

Figure 13.22(b)

Figure 13.22   Two patients with bone metastases. (a) Lytic bone metastases in the head of the eighth left rib due to carcinoma of the kidney. (b) Sclerotic bone metastases (arrowed) in a patient with carcinoma of the prostate

liposarcoma may be distinguished from a soft-tissue tumour, but benign and malignant tissue can rarely be differentiated (figure 13.21).

Secondary Tumours of Bone and Soft Tissues

Bone

As with conventional radiology, bone metastases appear as lytic or sclerotic lesions (figure 13.22). They can be identified down to the size of about 1 cm and are occasionally seen when the conventional radiographs appear normal. It is not, however, practicable to obtain a full CT scan of the skeletal system when screening for metastases. Such surveys are more effectively carried out using radioisotope scanning.

There is no difficulty in diagnosing a large area of bone destruction or sclerosis as representing metastatic disease if there are multiple lesions or if the patient has a known primary tumour. However, several difficulties are encountered in attempting to interpret minor abnormalities. Streak artefacts across bone give rise to an impression of increased or decreased density; this is particularly common in the thoracic spine due to movement of the heart.

Sclerotic metastases (figure 13.23a) have to be distinguished from bone islands (*see* figure 13.3) or Schmorl's nodes (figure 13.23b). Schmorl's nodes can usually be distinguished because they occur at the surfaces of the vertebral bodies, but, if doubt remains, review of the conventional radiographs will usually help to solve the problem (Roub and Drayer, 1979). A solitary sclerotic metastasis is rarely

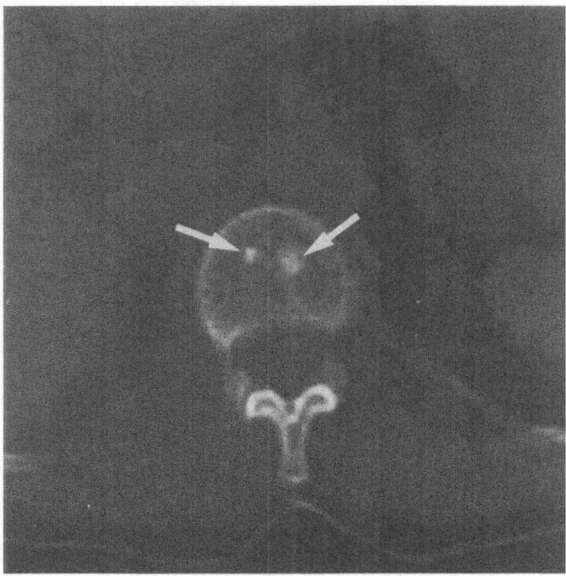

Figure 13.23(a)

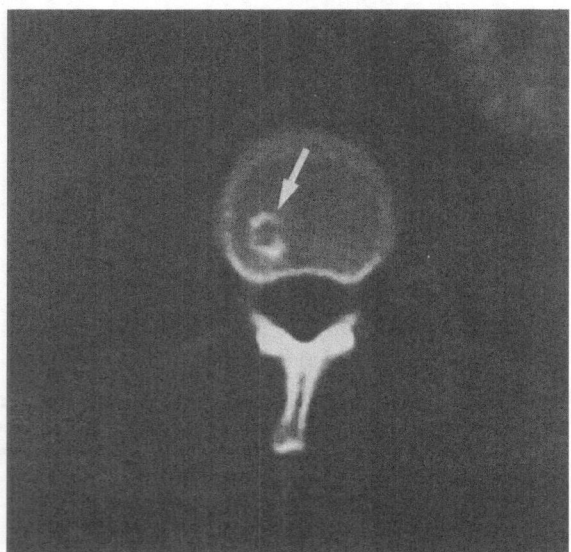

Figure 13.23(b)

Figure 13.23   Scan through the lower thoracic vertebrae in two patients. (a) Sclerotic metastases (arrowed) in a patient with carcinoma of the breast. These are indistinguishable from bone islands on a single examination. A follow-up examination in this patient showed that the lesions had increased in size. (b) Schmorl's node (arrowed)

diagnosed because this is usually indistinguishable from a bone island on the basis of CT.

Bone metastases may be associated with a soft-tissue mass and, as with primary tumours, CT defines the full extent of the soft-tissue component. If such a metastasis is in a vertebral body, extension of tumour into the spinal canal and intervertebral foramina can be shown (figure 13.24). Detection of spinal canal involvement, however, usually requires intrathecal contrast medium (metrizamide myelography) (Roub and Drayer, 1979). Secondary involvement of bone may occur by direct extension of a soft-tissue mass into the bony cortex (figure 13.25). Occasionally, CT may show cortical erosion not demonstrated by conventional radiology (figure 13.26).

Soft Tissues

Metastases in muscles and other soft tissue structures are occasionally seen with CT, particularly if the metastasis is surrounded by subcutaneous fat (figure 13.27).

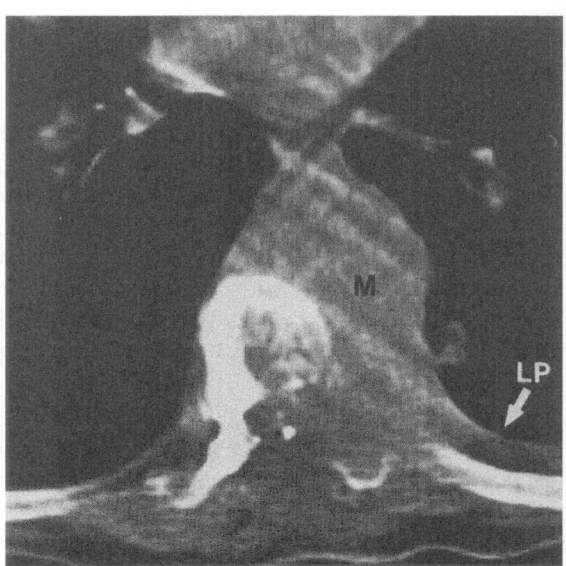

Figure 13.24   Vertebral body metastasis in a patient with an unknown primary tumour. The tumour extends into the spinal canal and has also produced a large soft-tissue mass (M). Note left pleural effusion (LP)

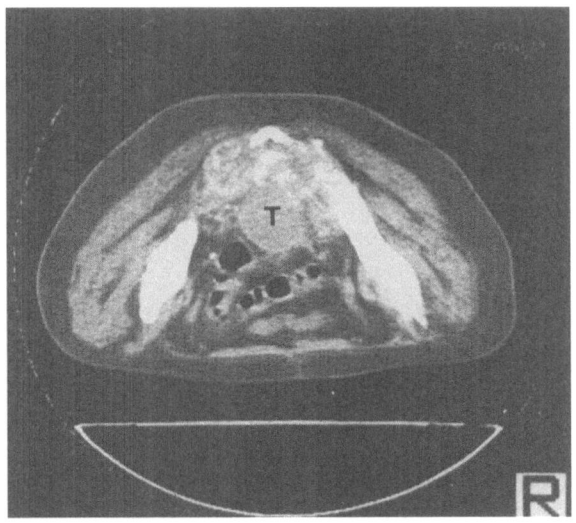

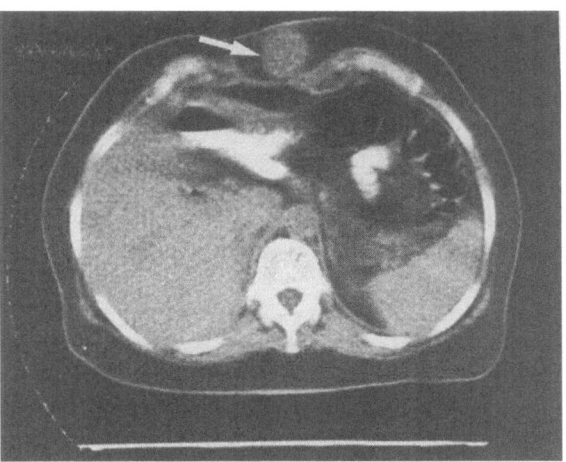

Figure 13.27 Metastasis in the subcutaneous soft tissues (arrowed) in a patient with carcinoma of the pancreas

Figure 13.25 Recurrent rectal tumour (T). The mass has spread into the sacrum which is almost completely destroyed

USE OF COMPUTED TOMOGRAPHY IN TUMOURS OF BONE AND SOFT TISSUES

CT does not replace conventional radiographic techniques, including tomography, in the assessment of musculo-skeletal tumours but should be regarded as complementary. Possibly, tomography may be used less frequently because CT can usually provide the same or more accurate information (Levine *et al.*, 1979). CT does not appear to have any advantage over standard radiography for determining the nature of a lesion in bone, and, indeed, the distinction between osteomyelitis and a malignant neoplasm may be impossible (Berger and Kuhn, 1978). CT does, however, have a place when planning surgery or defining portals for radiotherapy treatment planning. Thus, Levine *et al.* (1979) report that additional information which was useful in patient management was provided in 33 out of 50 patients with bone and primary soft-tissue tumours. In six patients suspected of having a soft-tissue mass, an unequivocally normal CT examination precluded the need for surgery. In the majority, the value of CT was in correctly defining the tumour extent, which permitted more complete tumour resection or more accurate radiotherapy treatment planning. In this study, angiography was compared

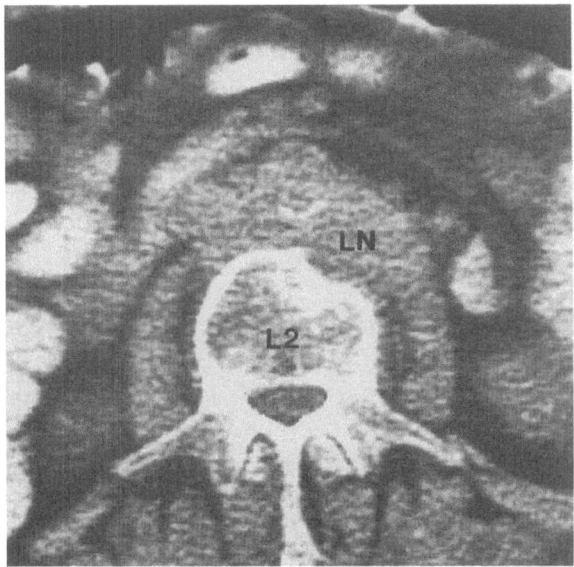

Figure 13.26 Lymph node enlargement in a patient with non-Hodgkin's lymphoma. The lymph node mass (LN) has eroded the anterolateral aspect of the second lumbar vertebra on the left

with CT in 22 of the patients. These investigations were compared with special reference as to whether certain malignant tumours should be treated by amputation or *en bloc* resection. The results showed that CT provided more information in the majority of cases. It seems likely, therefore, that angiography may be no longer necessary in such cases except when the major vessels are not well shown with CT and it is important to know whether they are involved.

In tumours not amenable to surgical resection, CT may be used to assess response to therapy (Berger and Kuhn, 1978). For example, at the Royal Marsden Hospital, if the soft-tissue component of the tumour is large, chemotherapy is used initially to reduce tumour bulk. CT scans are then repeated to define tumour regression and to assess whether radiotherapy is the next appropriate step (figure 13.28). It may also indicate that subsequent excision is feasible.

In patients with previous resected bone tumours, CT is a valuable method of detecting recurrence (McLeod *et al.*, 1978). In such patients, conventional radiology is of little use because the recurrence is usually within the soft tissues.

The major indication for using CT in the detection of bone metastases is in those patients in whom conventional radiographs appear normal but in whom there is a strong clinical suspicion of bone disease or

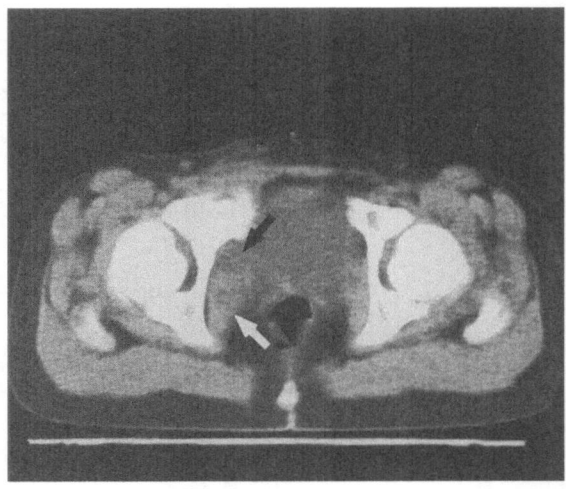

Figure 13.28(b)

Figure 13.28   Ewing's sarcoma of the right superior pubic ramus. (a) Before treatment, the scan shows a large soft-tissue mass (arrowed). The bladder (B) is compressed. (b) Repeat CT examination after three months treatment with chemotherapy shows considerable regression of the soft-tissue component of the tumour (arrowed)

in whom there is a positive radionuolide scan. Barlow and Goldman (1978) suggest that, in patients with known malignancy, CT may help to decide whether a vertebral fracture is pathological.

TRAUMA

One of the major advantages of CT in traumatised patients is that scans can be obtained with the minimum amount of manipulation and in the position in which the patient is most comfortable. In addition, the cross-sectional image can provide unique information. For these reasons, the method is likely to be used increasingly in the assessment of trauma as equipment becomes more widely available (figure 13.29).

In the assessment of spinal fractures, involvement of the posterior elements, which is difficult to show with conventional radiology, can be demonstrated. Bone encroachment on the spinal canal, the presence of loose fragments and the extent of soft-tissue

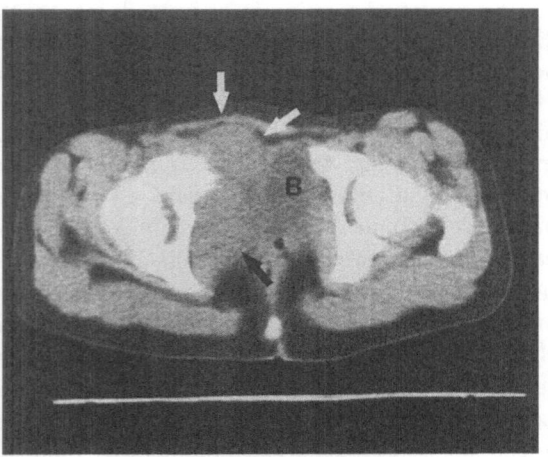

Figure 13.28(a)

haematoma can all be delineated (Keiffer, 1979; McInerney and Sage, 1979). CT has proved particularly valuable in the diagnosis of fractures of the anterior and posterior arches of the atlas (Kerschner *et al.*, 1977).

The pelvis is another region where the precise extent of trauma can be difficult to demonstrate, partly because the bone anatomy is complex and partly because patients are frequently in such severe pain that adequate positioning is extremely difficult.

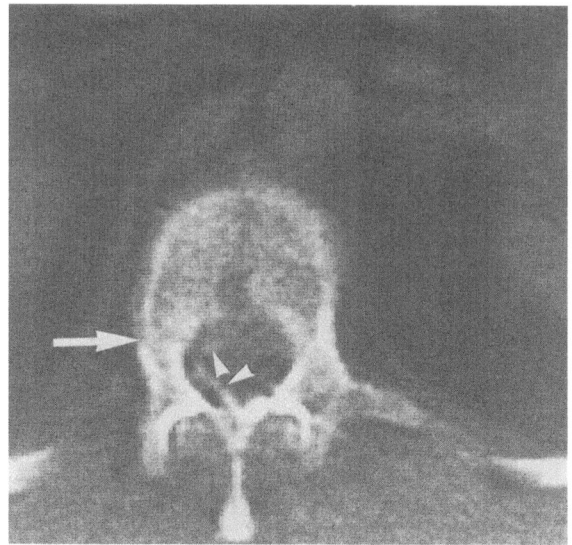

Figure 13.29(c)

Figure 13.29   Vertebral fractures. (a) Fracture of the sixth cervical vertebra. There is a sagittal fracture of the vertebral body (large arrow) and a comminuted avulsion fracture of the anterior cortical margin (small arrows). Note fracture of the lamina (arrowhead). These fractures have produced marked compression of the spinal canal. (b) Fracture of the right posterior arch of the atlas. (c) Comminuted fracture of the body and posterior elements of the first lumbar vertebra. There is a sagittal fracture through the body and a coronal fracture through the pedicle at its junction with the vertebral body (arrowed). Small bony fragments (arrowheads) are seen within the spinal canal. The fragments in the spinal canal were not shown on routine radiography. (Parts (a), (b) and (c) are reproduced by kind permission of Dr Naidich, Dr Sage and Dr Gilula, respectively)

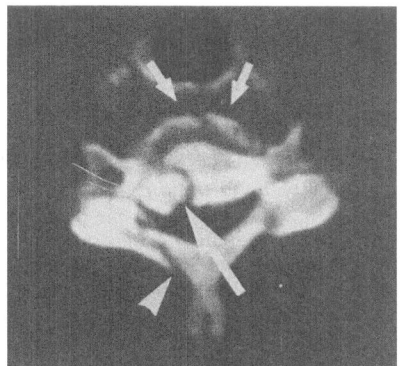

Figure 13.29(a)

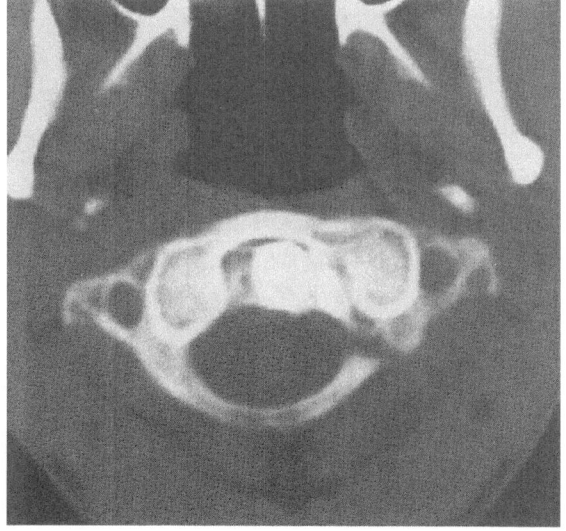

Figure 13.29(b)

In fractures around the hip joint, the number, size and position of fracture fragments can be seen as well as the presence of loose fragments within the joint itself (Lasda *et al.*, 1978; Gilula *et al.*, 1979; Blumberg, 1980) (figures 13.30 and 13.31).

Bones can be visualised through a plastercast, so that scans can be taken to assess the position of fractures if adequate visualisation cannot be obtained by other means (Gilula *et al.*, 1979).

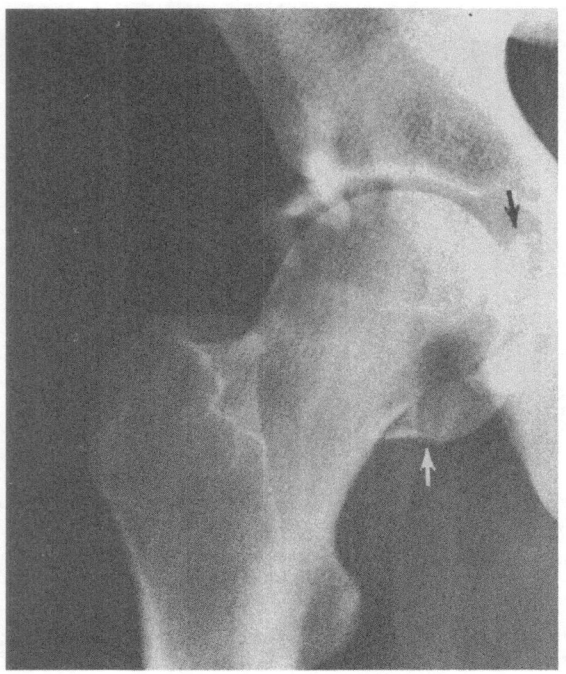

Figure 13.30(a)

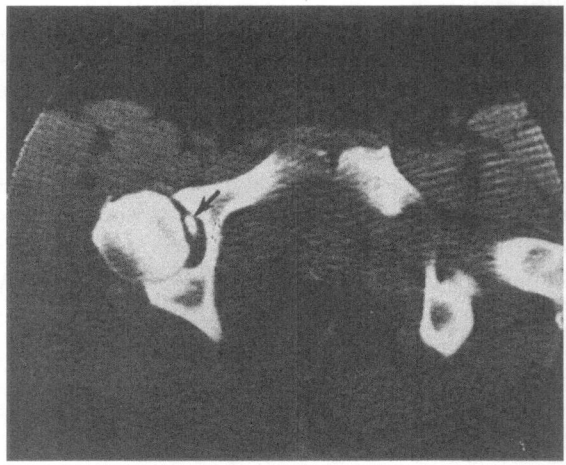

Figure 13.30(c)

Figure 13.30 Comminuted fracture of the right hip joint. (a) The conventional radiograph demonstrates the loose fragment (black arrow) and the displaced medial femoral head fracture fragment (white arrow). (b) Comminuted fracture (black and white arrowheads). (c) The fracture fragment within the joint space is clearly shown (arrow). (Reproduced by kind permission of Dr Gilula)

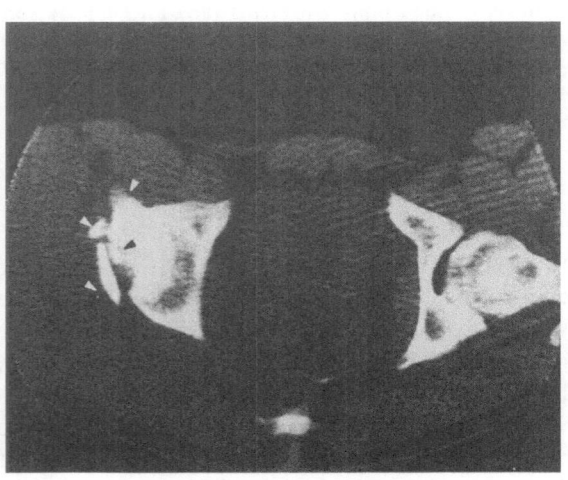

Figure 13.30(b)

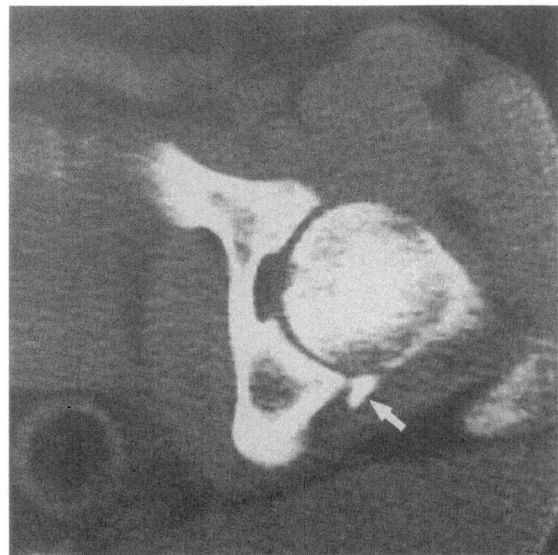

Figure 13.31 Loose fragment (arrowed) in a patient with a fracture of the left acetabulum

CONGENITAL AND DEVELOPMENTAL LESIONS

Useful information can be obtained with CT in congenital anomalies, particularly of the spine and hips. Congenital lesions of the spine are frequently complex, involving bone and soft-tissue elements. In spinal dysraphism, James and Oliff (1977) showed that CT gave unique information about bone anomalies as well as the nature of masses projecting out of the bony canal (meningocoele, lipoma, neural elements). In diastematomyelia, the size and nature of the bony spur and associated vertebral abnormalities can be clearly shown, simplifying the planing of surgical procedures (figure 13.32).

In congenital abnormalities of the hip, CT can accurately define the degree of anteversion both before surgery and during follow-up. It may also be useful in spondylolisthesis for demonstrating the nature of the lesion in the pars interarticularis (Sheldon *et al.*, 1977).

Initial studies of bone density using CT suggest that the technique may have important implications for the investigation of metabolic bone disease, such as osteoporosis and osteomalacia, but clinical studies confirming these views are not yet available (Bradley *et al.*, 1978; Pullan and Roberts, 1978). It is also possible that CT will come to have a place in the study of muscle diseases (Bulcke *et al.*, 1979) and perhaps in disorders of fat metabolism.

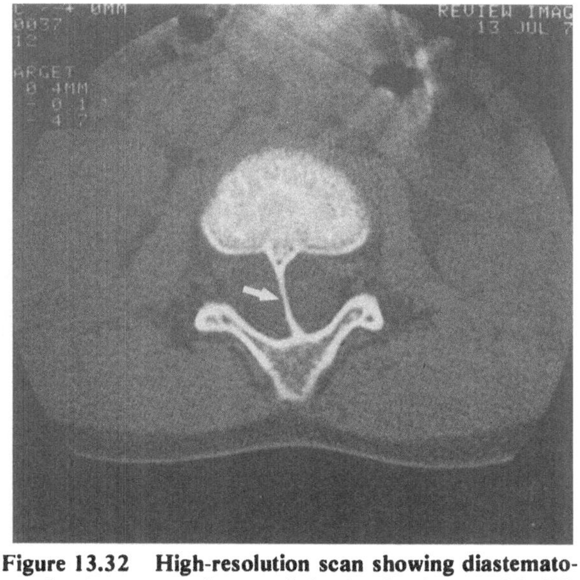

VERTEBRAL COLUMN AND SPINAL CORD

Spinal Stenosis and Disc Prolapse

CT provides a convenient and easy method for assessing the degree of stenosis of the lumbar and cervical spinal canal due to either congenital or acquired disease (Lee *et al.*, 1978; Ullrich *et al.*, 1980) (figure 13.33). It is important to remember when determining the shape of the spinal canal and measuring its size that the plane of the scan will not be perpendicular to the spinal canal unless the gantry can be appropriately tilted. In degenerative disease, the significance and extent of localised osteophytes is readily determined (figure 13.34). Narrowing of the intervertebral foramina and the relationship of osteophytes to the spinal cord can also be shown.

Figure 13.32 **High-resolution scan showing diastemato-myelia. Bony spur (arrowed) is clearly shown with CT. (Reproduced by kind permission of Dr Haughton)**

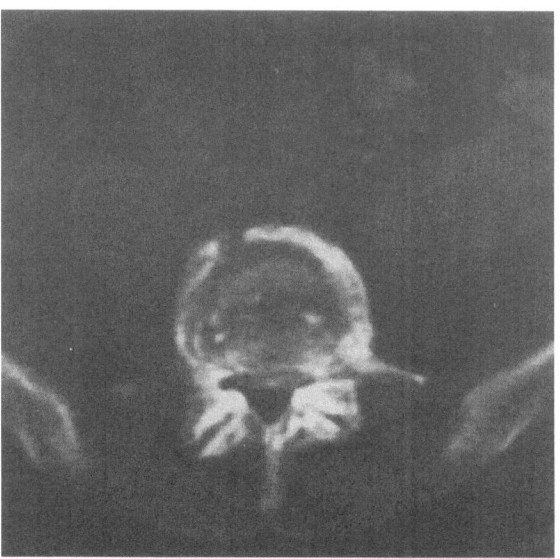

Figure 13.33(a)

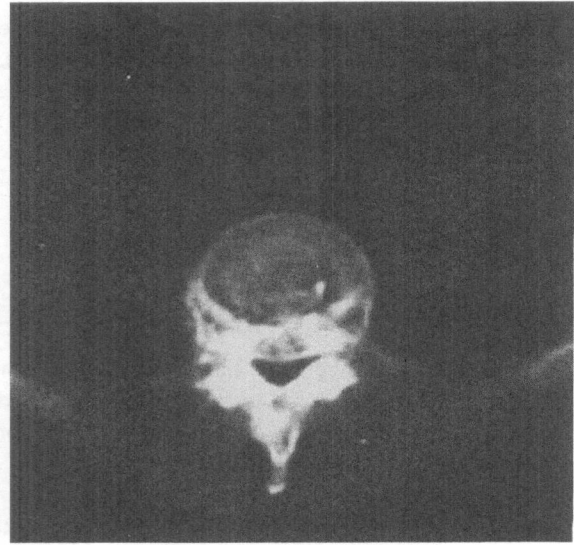

Figure 13.33(b)

Figure 13.33   (a) and (b) Traumatic spinal stenosis. The spinal canal is grossly narrowed and in addition there is sclerosis of the apophyseal joints

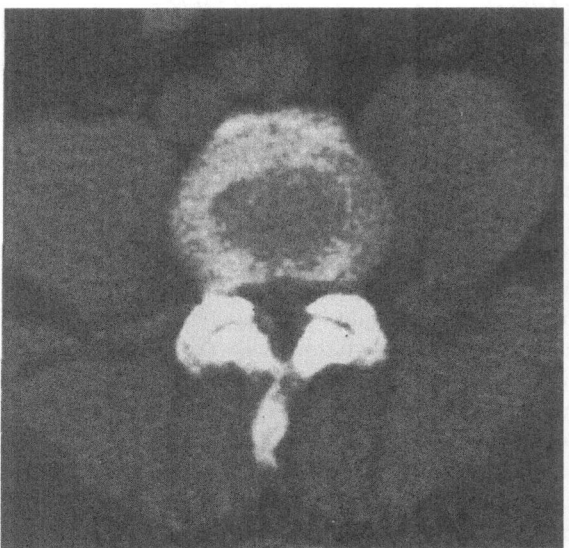

Figure 13.34(b)

Figure 13.34   Degenerative disease of the lumbar spine showing extensive osteophyte formation of the articular facets. (a) There is encroachment of the intervertebral foramina. (b) At a slightly higher level, the osteophytes encroach medially on the spinal canal

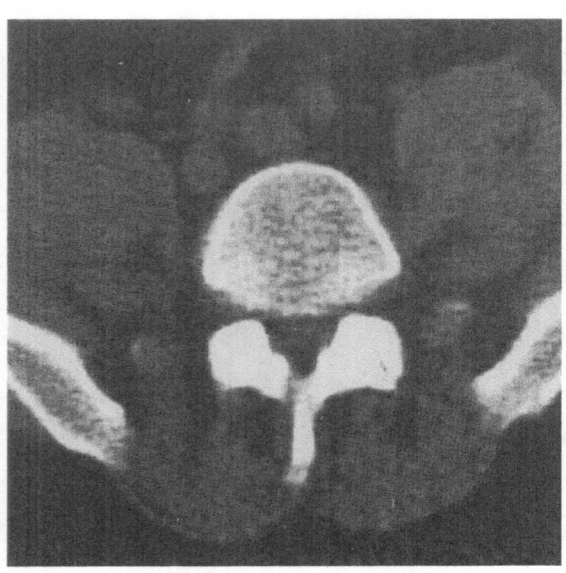

Figure 13.34(a)

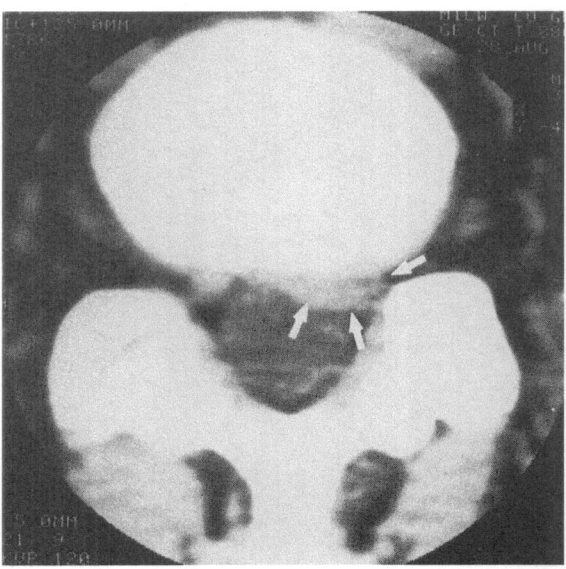

Figure 13.35   High-resolution scan showing posterior protrusion of intervertebral disc on the left (arrowed). (Reproduced by kind permission of Dr Haughton)

Visualisation of prolapsed intervertebral discs is more difficult but, with the latest generation of CT scanners, they can be seen without metrizamide (Syvertsen *et al.*, 1979; Glenn *et al.*, 1979) (figure 13.35). The demonstration of uncalcified prolapsed discs is favoured by a fast scanning speed with high resolution and a collimated x-ray beam of 5 mm or less, coupled with an adequate method of orientating the scan slices to the plane of the disc.

REFERENCES

Barlow, R. E. and Goldman, M. L. (1978). Computed tomography of the skeletal system. *Computerised Tomography*, **2**, 27–35

Berger, P. E. and Kuhn, J. P. (1978). Computed tomography of tumours of the musculo-skeletal system in children. *Radiology*, **127**, 171–175

Blumberg, M. L. (1980). Computed tomography and acetabular trauma. *Computerised Tomography*, **4**, 47–53

Bradley, J. G., Huang, H. K. and Ledley, R. F. (1978). Evaluation of calcium concentration in bones from CT scans. *Radiology*, **128**, 103–107

Bulcke, J. A., Termote, J.-L., Palmers, Y. and Crolla, A. D. (1979). Computed tomography of the human skeletal muscular system. *Neuroradiology*, **17**, 127–136

Carter, B. L., Moorhead, J., Wolpert, S. M., Hammerschlag, S. V., Griffiths, H. J. and Kahn, T. C. (1977). *Cross-sectional Anatomy – Computed Tomography and Ultrasound Correlation*, Englewood Cliffs, NJ, Appleton-Century-Croft

Destouet, J. M., Gilula, L. A. and Murphy, W. A. (1979). Computed tomography of long bone osteosarcoma. *Radiology*, **131**, 439–445

Gilula, L. A., Murphy, W. A., Tailor, C. C. and Patel, R. B. (1979). Computed tomography of the osseous pelvis. *Radiology*, **132**, 107–114

Glenn, W. V., Jr., Altschuler, E. A., Heishman, S. L., Wiltse, L. L. and Murphy, R. (1979). Multiplanar CT in diagnosis of lumbar disc disease. *Journal of Computer-Assisted Tomography*, **3** (4), 567

Heelan, R. T., Watson, R. C. and Smith, J. (1979). Computed tomography of lower extremity tumours. *American Journal of Roentgenology*, **132**, 933–937

James, H. E. and Oliff, M. (1977). Computed tomography in spinal dysraphism. *Journal of Computer Assisted Tomography*, **1**, 391–397

Keiffer, F. A. (1979). Computed tomography of the spine. *Computed Tomography (A Categorical Course)*, 65th Scientific Assembly and Annual Meeting, The Radiological Society of North America

Kershner, M. S., Goodman, G. A. and Perlmutter, G. S. (1977). Computed tomography in the diagnosis of an atlas fracture. *American Journal of Roentgenology*, **128**, 688–689

Lasda, N. A., Levinson, E. N., Yuan, H. A. and Bunnell, W. P. (1978). Computerised tomography in disorders of the hip. *Journal of Bone and Joint Surgery*, **60**-A, 1099–1102

Lee, B. C. P., Kazam, E. and Newman, A. D. (1978). Computed tomography of the spine and spinal cord. *Radiology*, **128**, 95–102

Levine, E., Lee, K. R., Neff, J. R., Maklad, N. F., Robinson, R. T. and Preston, D. F. (1979). Comparison of computed tomography and other imaging modalities in the evaluation of musculo-skeletal tumours. *Radiology*, **131**, 431–437

McInerney, D. P. and Sage, M. R. (1979). Computer-assisted tomography in the assessment of cervical spine trauma. *Clinical Radiology*, **30**, 203–206

McLeod, R. A., Stephens, D. H., Beabout, J. W., Sheedy, P. F., II, and Hattery, R. R. (1978). Computed tomography of the skeletal system. *Seminars in Roentgenology*, **13**, 235–247

Pullan, B. R. and Roberts, T. E. (1978). Bone mineral measurement using an EMI scanner and standard methods: a comparative study. *British Journal of Radiology*, **51**, 24–28

Roub, L. W. and Drayer, B. P. (1979). Spinal computed tomography: limitations and applications. *American Journal of Roentgenology*, **133**, 267–273

de Santos, L. A., Bernardino, M. E. and Murray, J. A. (1979). Computed tomography in the evaluation of osteosarcoma: experience with 25 cases. *American Journal of Roentgenology*, **132**, 535–540

Sheldon, J. J., Sersland, T. and Leborgne, J. (1977). Computed tomography of the lower lumbar vertebral column. *Radiology*, **124**, 113–118

Syvertsen, A., Haughton, V. and Williams, A. (1979). CT anatomy of the spine. *Journal of Computer Assisted Tomography*, **3** (4), 567

Ullrich, C. G., Binet, E. F., Sanecki, M. G. and Kieffer, S. A. (1980). Quantitative assessment of the lumbar spinal canal by computed tomography. *Radiology*, **134**, 137–143

14

The Spinal Cord

by P. Pullicino

TECHNIQUE OF EXAMINATION

The spinal canal has until recently been a 'blind spot' in computed tomography. Initial attempts at visualisation of the spine and spinal cord with the body scanner (Isherwood *et al.*, 1977; Stephens *et al.*, 1976) showed that, whilst vertebral bodies could be clearly demonstrated, structures within the spinal canal could only be poorly and inconsistently visualised, especially in the dorsal and lumbar regions. Four factors are responsible for this. First, movement artefacts often obscure the detail within the spinal canal, especially in the thoracic spine adjacent to the heart. Minimisation of all types of patient movement is therefore important but difficult with the longer scanning times of the early body scanners. Secondly, the width of the cerebrospinal fluid space around the spinal cord is critical for its visualisation. The spinal cord is only seen as a distinct structure by virtue of the low-attenuation cerebrospinal fluid surrounding it. With normal-resolution scanners, the cord will not be identified if the cerebrospinal space is less than about 2 mm. Thirdly, scanning through the dense bone of the vertebral bodies gives rise to beam hardening which decreases the contrast resolution within the spinal canal and also results in an artefact, a zone of increased density immediately inside the bone as has been seen on head scans (Gado *et al.*, 1975a,b). Partial volume averaging is a further factor which can cause the margins of the spinal cord to appear indistinct and may give rise to apparent narrowing of the spinal canal. This will occur if the spine is not scanned at right angles to its axis and will be most marked when scans are taken with a slice thickness collimator of 13 cm. It can be minimised by using a collimator of 5 mm or less. Despite these difficulties, the spinal cord can often be clearly seen with CT, especially in the cervical region. Patient cooperation, correct positioning and the use of short scan speeds and thin slices will all increase the frequency of visualisation but it will still be difficult in the dorsolumbar region in some patients.

The difficulties outlined above have up to now severely restricted the use of CT for the diagnosis of spinal cord lesions. However, the use of techniques to produce contrast enhancement of the cord has widened this application of CT. There are two agents which may be used for enhancing the spinal cord: (1) intravenous organic iodine and (2) xenon gas (Pullicino *et al.*, 1979). Intravenous contrast medium causes slight enhancement of the normal spinal cord up to approximately 5 EMI units and is now used routinely. Enhancement is due to an increase in the attenuation of areas perfused by blood vessels. The fact that xenon gas enhancement induces anaesthesia limits its use.

INTRAMEDULLARY LESIONS

CT can be a useful non-invasive method of first-line investigation in patients presenting with symptoms referable either to cervical spinal cord or to any other spinal level if this can be precisely defined on clinical examination. If the margins of the cord are clearly seen, demonstration of its diameter may be helpful in the initial differential diagnosis. An enlarged isodense cord indicates an intramedullary tumour, whereas an atrophic cord suggests previous damage by trauma, inflammation, degeneration or infarction. Whilst the specificity of diagnosis is rather low, demonstration of atrophy suggests a lesion that is not amenable to surgery.

The use of intravenous contrast enhancement is helpful in the differential diagnosis of spinal cord lesions. For example, enhancement occurs with an arteriovenous malformation (Di Chiro *et al.*, 1977) and with certain tumours. Thus, gliomas of the spinal cord frequently show marked enhancement. Enhancement of a tumour nodule adjacent to a syrinx may establish the diagnosis.

CT has been found to be most reliable in the diagnosis of syringomyelia (figure 14.1) (Bonafe *et al.*, 1980). In this condition, the CT scan shows an area of low attenuation within the spinal cord and the cord may be swollen, atrophic or of normal size. Cerebellar tonsillar herniation can be shown by axial or coronal scans of the foramen magnum if the condition is severe but is more reliably seen using an intrathecal injection of metrizamide.

The main differential diagnosis of syringomyelia on CT is that of a spinal cord tumour with an associated syrinx or cyst revealed as a well defined low-attenuation centre to the cord. Intramedullary tumours without a cyst or syrinx are seen either as a generally less well defined area of low attenuation within an expanded cord (figure 14.2) or as an

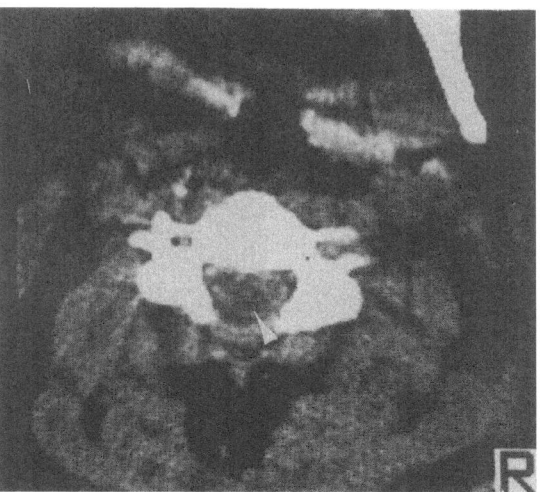

Figure 14.2 Post-contrast scan at C4 level, showing an irregular low-attenuation area (arrowhead) within the cord. It proved to be a cystic tumour at operation

isodense expansion. Features which favour syrinx are accompanying atrophy of the spinal cord as well as flattening of its anterior margin (Bonafe *et al.*, 1980).

INTRADURAL EXTRAMEDULLARY LESIONS

Intradural extramedullary lesions such as meningiomas are more difficult to identify than intramedullary lesions because they decrease the volume of the low-attenuation contrast of the

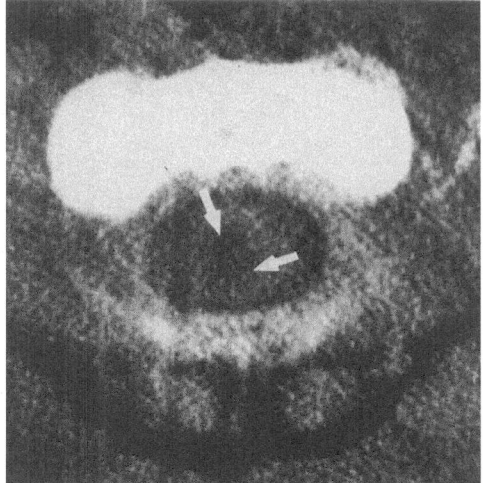

Figure 14.1 Unenhanced scan at C2 level showing syringomyelia (arrowed)

cerebrospinal fluid space by which the cord is normally seen. However, meningiomas may show
marked enhancement (figure 14.3) which not only
helps to identify them but also distinguishes them
from other tumours such as neurofibromas which
show minimal enhancement (figure 14.4).
Occasionally tumours have an intrinsically high or

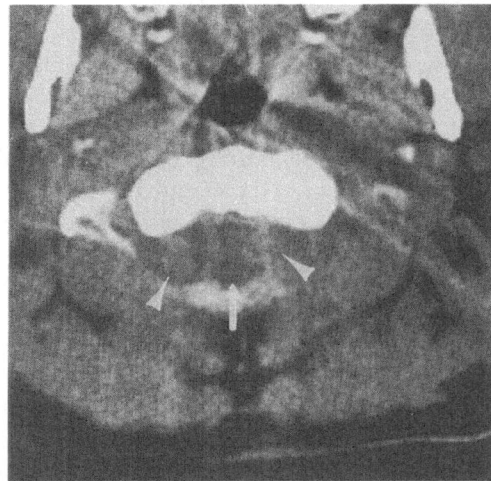

Figure 14.4   Post-contrast scan at C2 level showing two
enhancing neurofibromata (arrowheads) with the spinal
cord lying posteriorly (arrow). Multiple neurofibromata
confirmed at operation

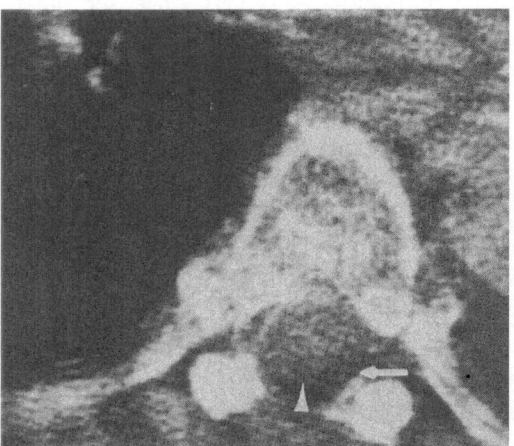

Figure 14.3(a)

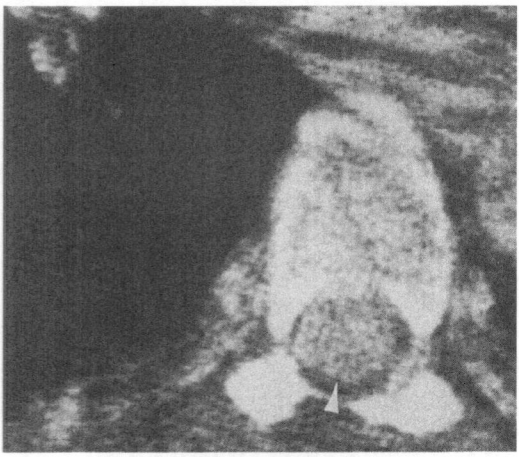

Figure 14.3(b)

Figure 14.3   Meningioma. (a) Pre-contrast scan at D5
level showing relatively dense soft-tissue mass
(arrowhead). The spinal cord is indented posteriorly and to
the left (arrowed). (b) After intravenous contrast medium,
there is dense enhancement of the lesion. Meningioma
was confirmed at operation

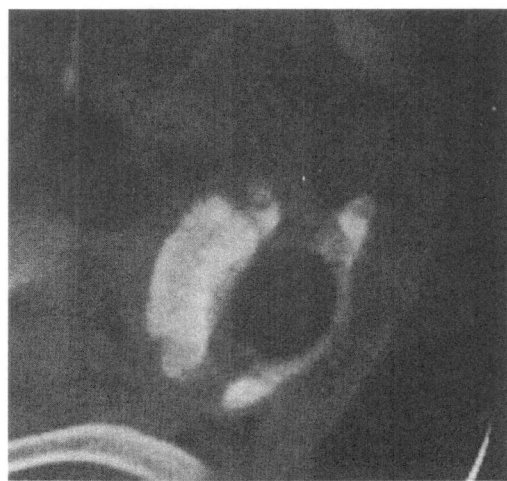

Figure 14.5   Unenhanced scan at L5 level in a six-
month-old child showing a lipoma with characteristically
low attenuation value

low attenuation, and in this situation CT is helpful in
predicting the nature of the lesion. For example, a
meningioma may be calcified and a lipoma has a low
attenuation value (figure 14.5).

EXTRADURAL LESIONS

Extradural lesions encroaching on the subarachnoid space are usually easy to recognise because the bone is often involved (figure 14.6). Relationship of the spinal cord to the lesion and the presence or absence of compression may also be noted.

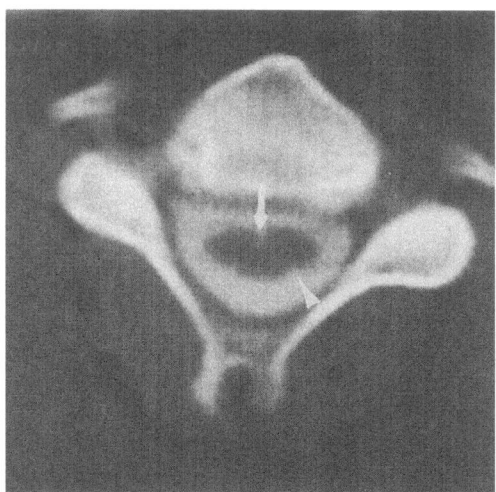

Figure 14.7 Scan of the upper cervical cord with intrathecal metrizamide showing atrophy after a traumatic injury to the cord at a lower level. The anterior median fissure (arrow) and posterolateral sulci (arrowhead) can be seen

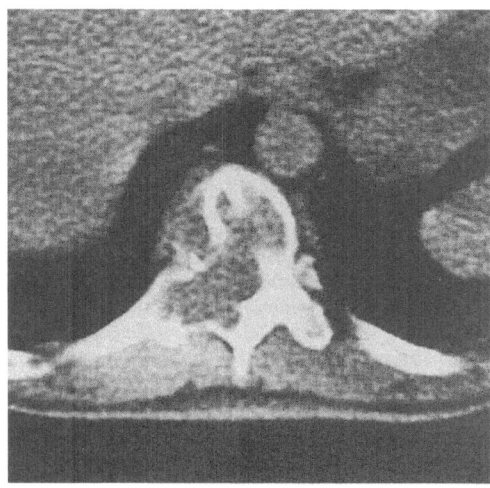

Figure 14.6 Multiple myeloma. Enhanced scan at D10 level. There is destruction of the body of the vertebra and of the right pedicle. Tumour extends into the spinal canal. The spinal cord cannot be seen as a separate structure

METRIZAMIDE CT MYELOGRAPHY

CT scanning of the spinal cord after injection of intrathecal metrizamide can be performed either as an adjunct to myelography or as a single investigation. The proponents of CT metrizamide myelography as an elective procedure point out the negligible incidence of side-effects with the low concentration of metrizamide needed. At the National Hospital for Nervous Diseases, CT is used as a complementary procedure to conventional myelography to clarify points that are unclear on the initial film (figures 14.7 and 14.8).

The major advantage of CT metrizamide myelography over conventional myelography is that the spinal cord can be clearly outlined even when the concentration of metrizamide has decreased below the level at which it can be demon-

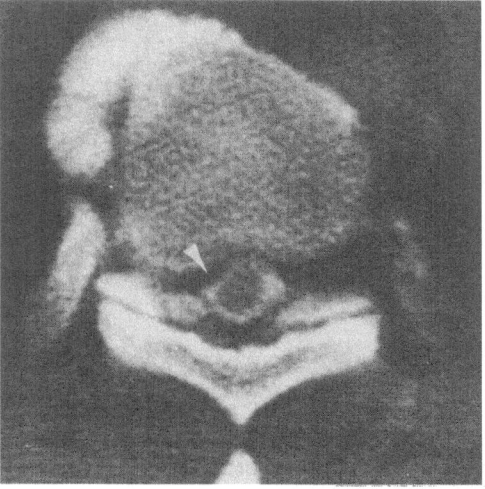

Figure 14.8 Metrizamide scan in the mid-dorsal region showing an anterolateral disc protrusion (arrowhead) which slightly deforms the spinal cord

strated by conventional radiography. Thus, CT can be performed up to about 4 to 6 h after the metrizamide myelogram. Marking the level of the lesion outlined at myelography on the patient's skin facilitates scanning.

CT is likely to complement the conventional metrizamide myelogram in the following situations.

(1) Lesions which have produced an apparent complete block on the metrizamide myelogram: when this occurs, CT scanning frequently shows that metrizamide has in fact passed beyond the lesion and this may obviate the need for cervical puncture.

(2) Extradural compression of the subarachnoid space, e.g. by osteophytes: a small localised lesion can be missed on conventional myelography or its true relation to the cord may not be apparent (figure 14.9).

(3) Syringomyelia: scans repeated after an interval of several hours may show a communication of the syrinx with the fourth ventricle or subarachnoid space.

(4) Lumbar canal stenosis: the trefoil appearance

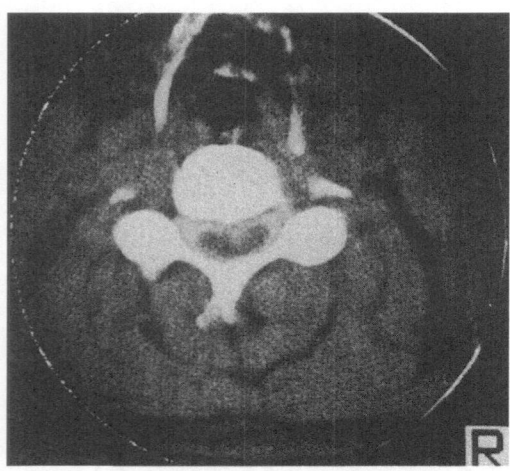

Figure 14.9 Scan in the midcervical region with intrathecal metrizamide. The cord is indented anteriorly. This localised abnormality was not apparent on myelography

of the lumbar canal may be masked on conventional metrizamide myelography and the full significance of the abnormality is missed.

The introduction of modern high-resolution scanning has resulted in more accurate demonstration of the cord, and its increasing availability has already made a major impact on the examination of lesions of the spinal cord.

REFERENCES

Bonafe, A., Ethier, R., Melancon, D., Belanger, G. and Peters, T. (1980). High resolution computed tomography in cervical syringomyelia. *Journal of Computerised Axial Tomography*, **4**, 42–47

Di Chiro, G., Doppman, J. L. and Wener, L. (1977). Computerised tomography of spinal arteriovenous malformation. *Radiology*, **123**, 351–354

Gado, M. H., Phelps, M. E. and Coleman, R. E. (1975a). An extravascular component of contrast enhancement in cranial computed tomography. I. The tissue–blood ratio of contrast enhancement. *Radiology*, **117**, 621–626

Gado, M. H., Phelps, M. E. and Coleman, R. E. (1975b). An extravascular component of contrast enhancement in cranial computed tomography. II. Contrast enhancement and the blood–tissue barrier. *Radiology*, **117**, 595–597

Isherwood, I., Fawcitt, R. A., Nettle, J. R. L., Spencer, J. W. and Pullan, B. R. (1977). In *Computer Tomography of the Spine – A Preliminary Report*, First European Seminar on Computerised Axial Tomography in Clinical Practice, eds. G. H. du Boulay and I. F. Moseley, Springer-Verlag, Berlin, pp. 322–335

Pullicino, P., du Boulay, G. H. and Kendall, B. E. (1979). Xenon enhancement for computed tomography of the spinal cord. *Neuroradiology*, **18**, 63–66

Stephens, D. H., Hattery, R. R. and Sheedy, P. F., II (1976). Computerised tomography of the abdomen. *Radiology*, **119**, 331–335

15

The Head and Neck

with C. A. Parsons

Although the anatomy is complex, lesions of the head and neck are relatively easily visualised both by direct vision and by conventional radiology (Fletcher and Jing, 1972; Dodd and Jing, 1977). Furthermore, biopsy within the pharynx and paranasal sinuses is a minor procedure, so that the process of diagnosis and staging in this region is more straightforward than in the thorax and abdomen. The main advantage of CT scanning for lesions of the head and neck is the ability to demonstrate inaccessible soft-tissue structures and bone detail which may be difficult to evaluate by conventional techniques.

PARANASAL SINUSES

Technique of Examination

Scans should begin at the hard palate and proceed cranially to include the frontal sinuses. The scans should be parallel to the anthropomorphic baseline which connects the infra-orbital margin with the upper border of the external auditory meatus. Using a slice thickness of 13 mm, scans are usually taken at 1 cm intervals. After the initial series of scans is viewed, it may be necessary to repeat the examination in the coronal plane. This is useful for showing

bone destruction in the floor of the orbit or in the hard palate and extension through the skull base into the cranial cavity. Coronal scans are taken with the patient lying prone and the chin hyperextended. The facility to angle the gantry (now available on many machines) has helped considerably in obtaining true coronal sections.

Enhancement is not required routinely because lesions within the paranasal sinuses are surrounded by air and bone which provides natural contrast. It is, however, indicated if intracranial extension of tumour is suspected.

CT Anatomy

Bones

The bones in the region of the sinuses are elegantly demonstrated with CT (figure 15.1) and several features are worth emphasising. The opening of the maxillary antrum into the nasal cavity varies considerably in size, and the whole of the medial wall of the antrum may be absent. The sigmoid shape of the posterior wall of the antrum is well shown. The pterygoid processes lie medially behind the antrum arising from the roots of the greater wings of the sphenoid. Each process consists of a medial and a

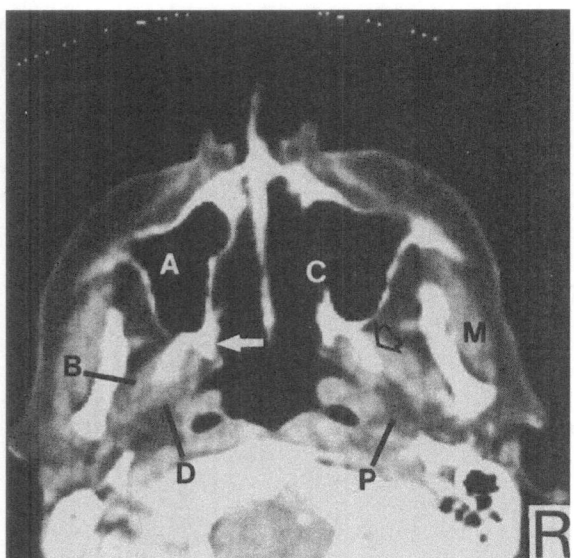

Figure 15.1 Transverse section through the maxillary antra. Left antrum (A), lateral pterygoid muscle (B), ostium to right antrum (C), medial pterygoid muscle (D), medial pterygoid plate (white arrow), lateral pterygoid plate (open arrow), masseter muscle (M), parapharyngeal space (P)

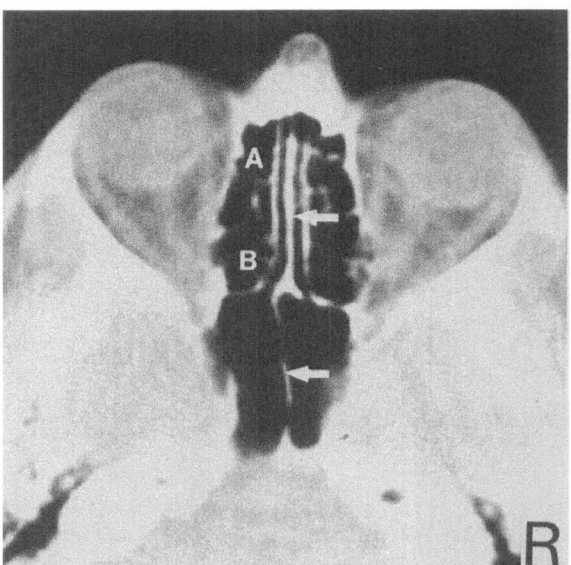

Figure 15.2 Transverse section through the orbits and ethmoid and sphenoid sinuses. The anterior (A) and posterior (B) groups of ethmoid cells are shown without overlapping structures. The nasal septum (upper arrow) and median plate of bone (lower arrow) separating the two halves of the sphenoid sinus are shown

lateral lamina which together form the boundaries of the pterygoid fossa.

Scans through the ethmoid sinuses permit distinction between the anterior and posterior group of cells (figure 15.2). The two halves of the nasal cavity and intervening septum can be traced upwards between the ethmoid sinuses to the cribriform plate. The anterior wall of the sphenoid sinus and the median plate of bone separating the two halves of the sinus are also well demonstrated by CT, both in the transverse and coronal planes (figures 15.2, 15.3 and 15.4).

Soft Tissues

One of the unique features of CT is the ability to demonstrate soft-tissue structures in relation to the bony walls of the sinuses (*see* figures 15.2 and 15.3). Immediately posterior to the maxillary antrum there is a fat-containing space which extends posteriorly as far as the anterior surface of the lateral pterygoid

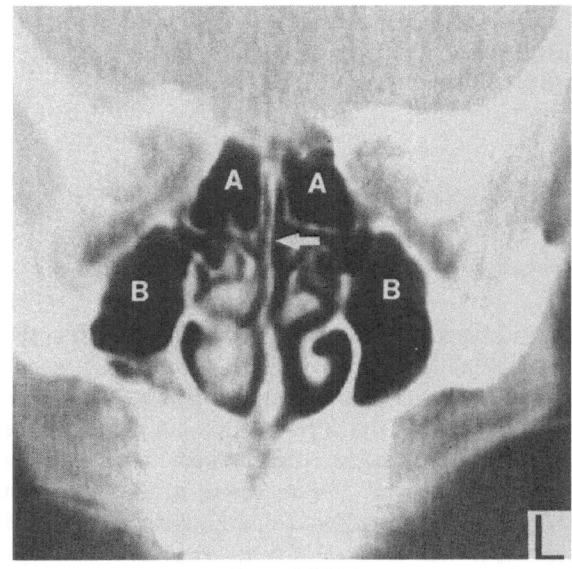

Figure 15.3(a)

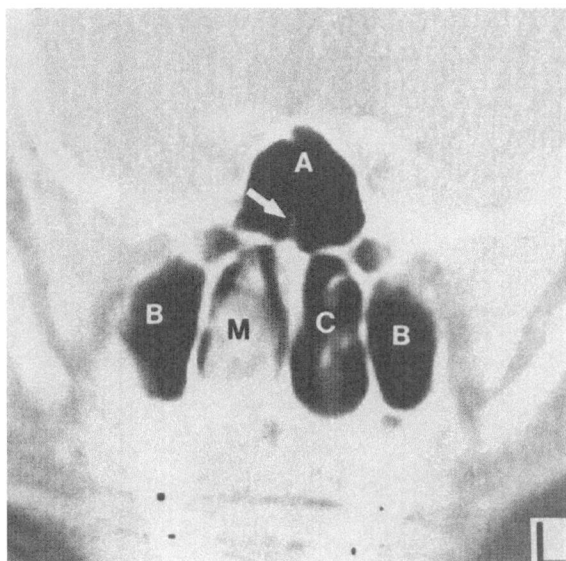

Figure 15.3(b)

Figure 15.3 Coronal sections through the ethmoid and sphenoid sinuses. (a) Through the posterior ethmoid air cells (A), maxillary antra (B), the nasal septum (arrow). Note mucosal swelling overlying the turbinate bones on the right. (b) Through a normal sphenoid sinus (A) showing the median plate of bone (arrow) and adjacent maxillary antra (B) and nasal cavity on the left (C). Note mucosal swelling (M) of overlying turbinate bones on the right

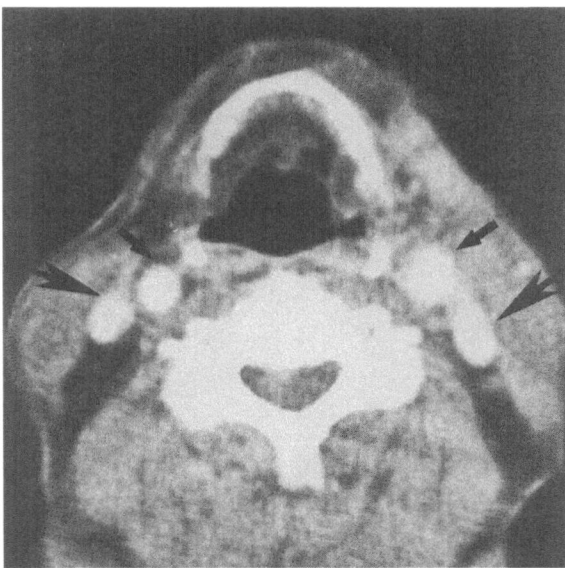

Figure 15.4 CT scan at the level of the hyoid showing carotid arteries (small arrows) and jugular veins (large arrows) opacified with intravenous contrast medium

muscle. This muscle arises by two heads, one from the greater wing of sphenoid and the other from the lateral surface of the lateral pterygoid lamina. The muscle passes laterally and backwards to be inserted into the front of the neck of the mandible. The lateral pterygoid muscle can easily be distinguished from the medial pterygoid muscle because the latter arises from the medial surface of the lateral pterygoid plate and is inserted into the mandible close to its angle. The masseter muscle is shown covering the superficial surface of the vertical ramus of the mandible. Between the pterygoid muscles and the constrictor muscles of the pharynx lies the parapharyngeal space, which contains and transmits the styloid muscles and the great vessels. These are best shown after an injection of intravenous contrast medium (figure 15.4).

Tumours

The majority of CT examinations of the paranasal sinuses are undertaken to assess the extent of disease in patients with known malignant tumours (Parsons and Hodson, 1979). The tumour appears as a soft-tissue mass either partially or completely filling the sinus (figure 15.5). The attenuation values range from 15 to 45 EMI units and fall within the same range as those of benign mucosal swelling and antral fluid. It may, therefore, be impossible to distinguish tumour from associated inflammatory changes.

Malignant tumours of the paranasal sinuses spread through the adjacent sinus walls into the surrounding structures. The most common finding is erosive bone destruction in part of the sinus wall, pterygoid plate or skull base. The accuracy of CT in the detection of such erosion is comparable to polytomography (Thawley *et al.*, 1978). Long-standing, slowly growing tumours arising in the

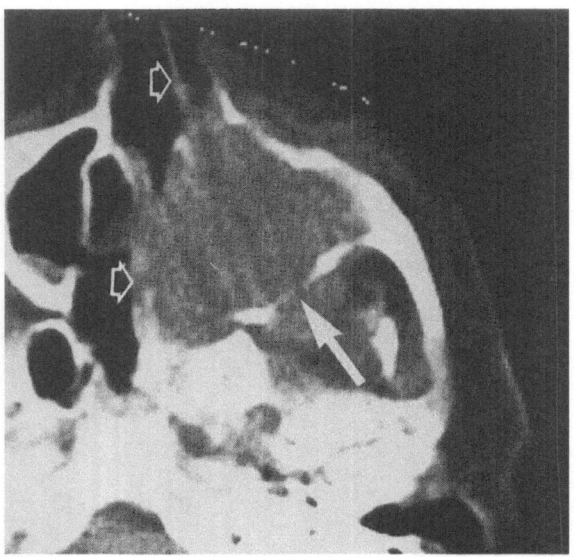

Figure 15.5 Advanced carcinoma of right maxillary antrum extending through the posterior wall (large arrow) and medial wall (lower open arrow) destroying the posterior part of the nasal septum (upper open arrow)

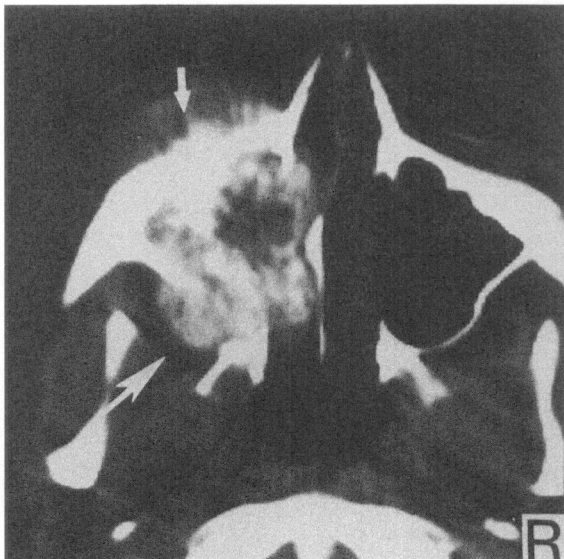

Figure 15.6 Osteosarcoma of left maxillary antrum showing spicular new bone formation (small arrow) extending forwards into the cheek. There is limited soft-tissue extension posteriorly into the pterygoid region (large arrow)

antrum may cause displacement of the sinus wall and of the nasal septum. Such tumours also frequently produce areas of sharply defined bone destruction.

Primary osteogenic sarcomas of the sinuses may be associated with new bone formation which may be spicular, homogeneous or irregularly distributed throughout the tumour mass (figure 15.6). Although the bone component of such tumours may be very sharply defined, there is often an associated diffuse soft-tissue mass. Bone sclerosis, particularly of the pterygoid plates, may be seen when there is associated infection or following neutron therapy.

Paranasal sinus tumours are frequently advanced at the time of presentation. The soft tissue mass can often be seen extending beyond the bony confines of the sinus. When the maxillary antrum is primarily involved, tumour extension may be seen passing through the anterior wall into the cheek or medially into the nasal cavity. Such findings are usually obvious on clinical examination and CT provides little, if any, additional information. However, the demonstration of tumour spread posteriorly by CT

is much more important because such information is often difficult or impossible to obtain by other methods. Thus, maxillary sinus tumours may spread into the infratemporal fossa or superiorly into the ethmoid air cells and orbit. Since malignant tumours commonly spread from one sinus to the other, it is important to include all paranasal sinuses in the area investigated. However, opacification of an adjacent sinus may be caused by an accumulation of fluid as the result of occlusion of the ostium by tumour in the nasal cavity. Soft-tissue tumour extending into the region of the pterygoid muscles may be evident as a mass or as a loss of tissue planes due to soft-tissue tumour infiltrating the surrounding fat (figure 15.7).

Extension of tumour from the ethmoid air cells through the medial wall of the orbit may be recognised as a soft-tissue mass which, if large, may displace the optic nerve and globe causing proptosis (figure 15.8). Lesser degrees of tumour invasion cause an increase in the density of the retro-orbital fat lying between the medial wall of the orbit and the medial rectus muscle (figure 15.9). Extension of

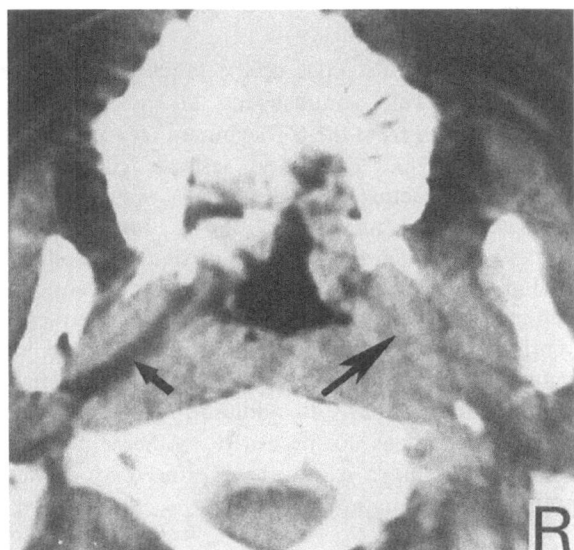

Figure 15.7   Loss of fat plane on the right due to infiltration by tumour (large arrow). The normal fat plane posterior to the left pterygoid muscles is clearly shown (small arrow)

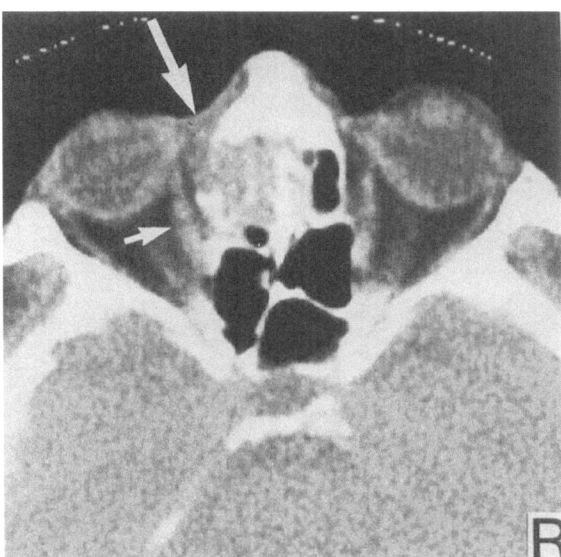

Figure 15.9   Tumour (large arrow) extending from ethmoid through the medial wall of orbit to replace the fat which lies medial to the medial rectus muscle (small arrow)

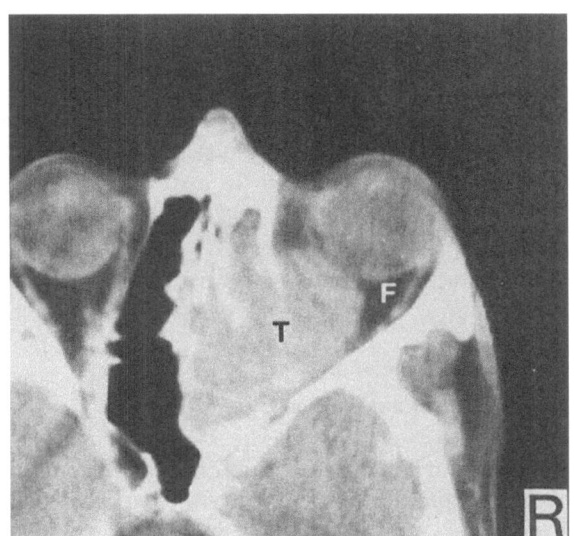

Figure 15.8   Carcinoma of the ethmoid (T) extending into the retro-orbital fat (F) displacing the globe laterally and causing proptosis

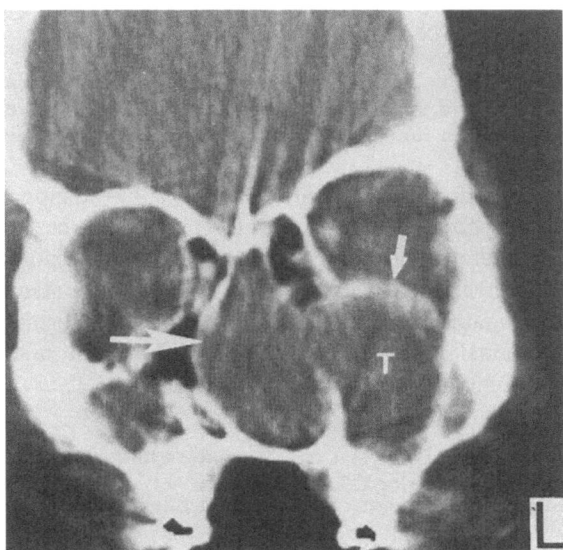

Figure 15.10   Elevation of the floor of the left orbit (small arrow) due to a large antral tumour (T) which has also spread into the nasal cavity displacing the septum (large arrow)

maxillary antral tumours through the floor of the orbit may be difficult to recognise on scans taken in the transverse plane. If this situation is suspected, coronal slices should also be taken (figure 15.10). Intracranial extension occurs in advanced disease; the intracranial part of the tumour enhances after injection of intravenous contrast medium (figure 15.11).

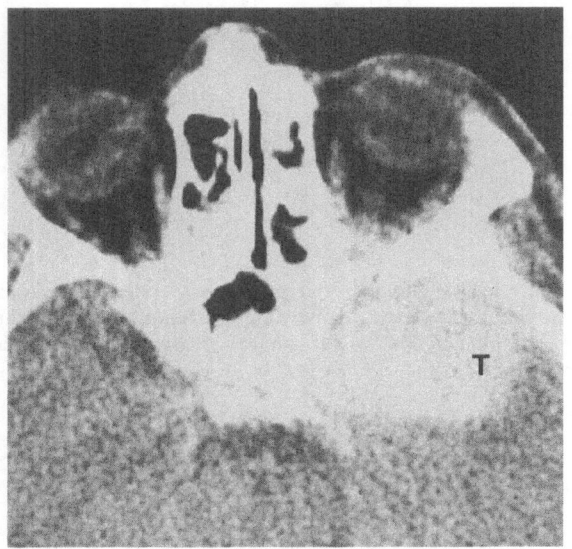

Figure 15.11 Tumour (T) extending into the middle cranial fossa and shown only after intravenous contrast medium. The tumour originated in the maxillary antrum

Tumour spread posteriorly into the infratemporal or pterygopalatine fossa or into the orbit can be seen in a high proportion of patients when not identifiable by conventional radiology. In a series of patients investigated at the Royal Marsden Hospital, additional information was provided by CT in 15 out of 32 patients (Parsons, 1981) (table 15.1).

Table 15.1   Paranasal sinus tumours: additional information obtained using CT on 32 patients

CT findings	No. of patients
Extension into pterygoid region	11
Orbital involvement	3
Sphenoid sinus involvement	1

Benign Conditions

Congenital abnormalities of the facial skeleton are particularly well demonstrated in the transverse plane obtained from the CT scanner (Wortzman and Holgate, 1976). Traumatic lesions, particularly impacted fractures and small amounts of intracranial air, can be well shown. Inflammatory disease involving the paranasal sinuses produces similar radiological appearances to conventional methods (Forbes *et al.*, 1978). Both in CT and conventional radiography, polypoid mucosal thickening may represent early neoplastic rather than benign inflammatory disease. In addition, the presence of bony erosion does not necessarily indicate a malignant process since it may be produced by inflammatory granulomata.

PHARYNX

Clinical examination of the nasopharynx is usually easy and accurate. However, it may be difficult to recognise that the posterior wall of the nasopharynx is uniformly displaced forwards or that the lateral wall on one side is displaced medially. In addition, extension of a disease process laterally into the parapharyngeal space cannot accurately be identified. Similarly, in the oropharynx the true upper and lower extent of tumour and degree of spread laterally into the pterygoid region cannot be defined accurately by physical examination. Likewise, it may be difficult to distinguish between fixation of the faucial pillars due to tumour extension and immobility caused by paresis.

In all these situations, CT can provide valuable information.

Technique of Examination

When examining the oropharynx, scans should be obtained from the level of the thyroid cartilage to the level of the skull base. When examining the nasopharynx, scans from the level of the hyoid bone are sufficient. Should the base be eroded, the investigation must be continued to include the brain.

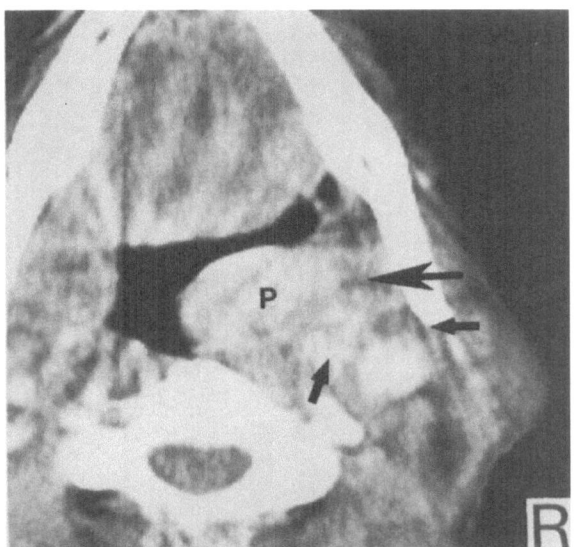

Figure 15.12 Plasmacytoma (P) of the tonsil showing enhancement which demonstrated its lateral extent (large arrow). The opacified great vessels are seen lateral to the tumour (small arrows)

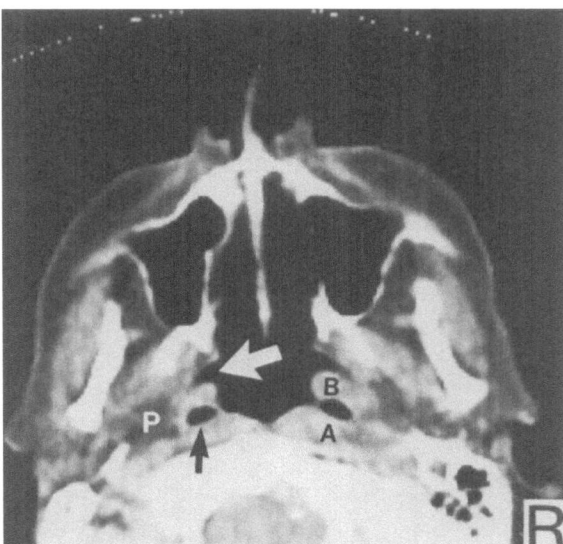

Figure 15.13 Normal nasopharynx. The Eustachian orifice (large arrow) and fossa of Rosenmuller (small arrow) are separated by the salpingo-pharyngeal fold (B). The prevertebral muscles (A) produce a symmetrical undulating posterior wall. The fat of the parapharyngeal space (P) is clearly distinguished from surrounding soft tissue

Tumours of this region may show enhancement and scans should be repeated after intravenous contrast medium (figures 15.11 and 15.12).

Lymph node involvement by nasopharyngeal and oropharyngeal tumours is best shown after infusion of intravenous contrast medium because this helps to distinguish large nodes from vessels.

CT Anatomy

Nasopharynx

The majority of CT examinations of the naso-pharynx are undertaken to assess malignant tumours. A knowledge of the anatomical boundaries which determine local routes of spread is essential if the radiological investigation is to be tailored to the patient's disease and the information obtained is to be interpreted accurately. The soft tissues of the posterior wall of the nasopharynx are thinnest in the midline but the prevertebral muscles produce sym-metrical thickening 1 to 2 cm laterally to this (figure 15.13). The lateral and posterior walls join at the

pharyngeal recess of Rosenmuller. Anterior to this and on the lateral wall lies the salpingo-pharyngeal fold of mucous membrane covering the vertically running muscle of the same name. This forms the posterior boundary of the Eustachian orifice. Air may be seen lying within the cartilaginous part of the tube as it passes upwards and backwards towards the tympanic cavity. The parapharyngeal space lies laterally, extending from the skull base down to the level of the hyoid bone (figure 15.13). The lateral boundary of this space is the posterior surface of the pterygoid muscle, the parotid gland (*see* figure 15.24) and investing layer of the deep cervical fascia. The posterior boundary is the prevertebral fascia. Tumour extending into the parapharyngeal space may extend from the skull base down to the hyoid within these limits.

Oropharynx

Several of the anatomical features of the oropharynx are similar to those seen in the nasopharynx (figure

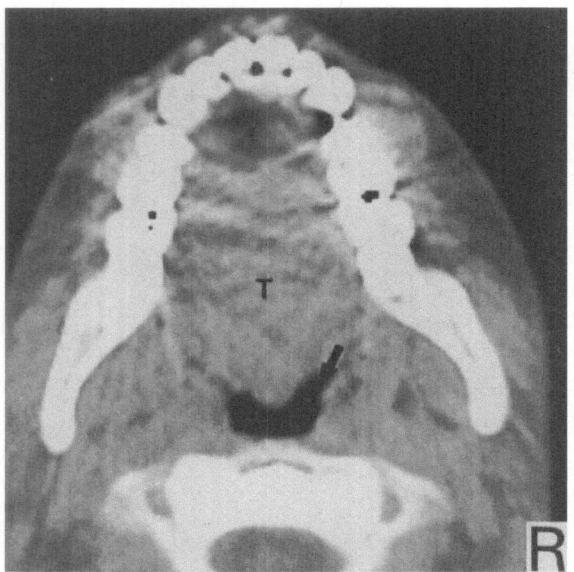

Figure 15.14   Normal oropharynx showing the glosso-tonsillar recess (arrowed). Tongue (T)

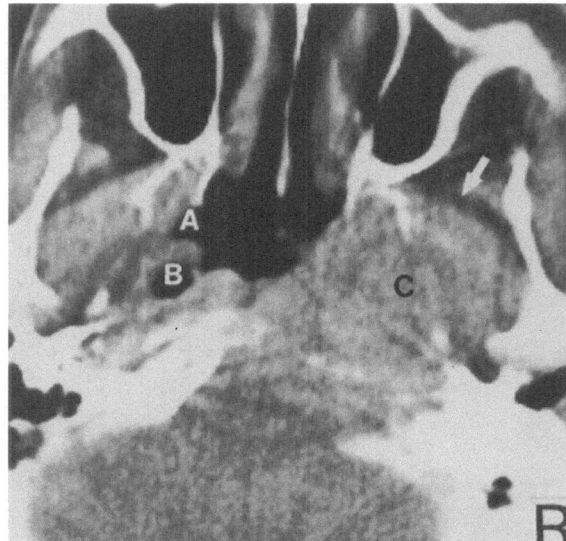

Figure 15.15   Normal Eustachian orifice (A) and fossa of Rosenmuller (B) on the left. These have been obliterated by a large nasopharyngeal carcinoma (C) on the right where the tumour occupies the parapharyngeal space displacing the lateral pterygoid muscle anteriorly (arrowed)

15.14). The normal posterior wall is symmetrically undulating due to the bulge caused by the pre-vertebral muscles. On the lateral wall, however, the pillars of the fauces with the intervening tonsil are not as prominent as the recesses and tubal elevation seen in the nasopharynx. This wall terminates anteriorly in the glosso-tonsillar recess and is continuous with the lateral pharyngo-epiglottic fold and base of tongue. An immediate lateral relation of this region remains the parapharyngeal space.

Tumours

Tumours of the nasopharynx are usually recognised as an obvious mass. Most commonly, they arise on the lateral wall, either in the fossa of Rosenmuller or adjacent to the Eustachian orifice. Tumours of the posterior wall and roof are also common, but tumours arising on the nasopharyngeal surface of the soft palate are rare. The mass may be so large at the time of presentation that the precise site of origin cannot be identified. Local tumour extension usually follows anatomical planes (figure 15.15). Anteriorly, the nasal cavity and hard palate may be invaded

with extension of larger tumours into the maxillary and ethmoid sinuses. Spread may also occur superiorly through the cribriform plate into the anterior cranial fossa or into the sphenoid sinus with destruction of the adjacent middle fossa floor. Orbital involvement will be visible as soft-tissue tumour lying within the retro-orbital fat, or as bone destruction or as widening of the optic canal. Tumour which spreads laterally replaces the fat of the parapharyngeal space and may encompass the great vessels. The limits of tumour in this space can be clearly identified when it is surrounded by fat, but, once the tumour has spread into muscle, precise delineation of its extent within the muscle cannot be identified (figure 15.15). The lateral pterygoid muscle is most commonly involved, and the bony pterygoid plates which give origin to this muscle may be destroyed. Tumour on the roof of the naso-pharynx or superior surface of the soft palate may be difficult to identify unless coronal slices are taken (figure 15.16).

Involvement of the retropharyngeal lymph nodes

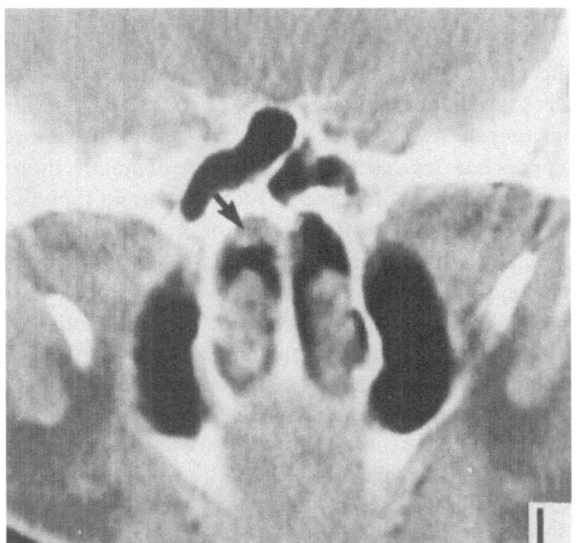

Figure 15.16   Residual tumour in the roof of the nasal cavity (arrowed) shown only on the coronal view. The turbinates are also shown. There is no erosion of bone

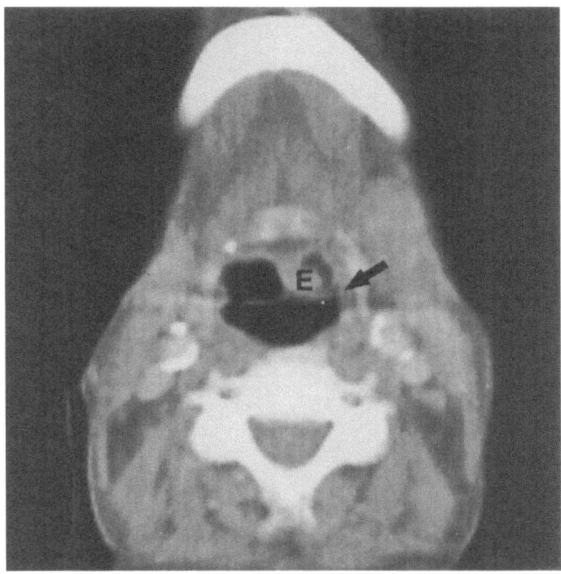

Figure 15.17(b)

Figure 15.17   Carcinoma of the right tonsil. (a) The tumour (A) is shown to extend forwards into the tongue (T) by enhancement after intravenous contrast medium. The common carotid artery and jugular vein are opacified (arrowed). (b) A lower section shows the tumour extending into the epiglottis which is thickened (E). The pharyngo-epiglottic fold is also thickened (arrowed)

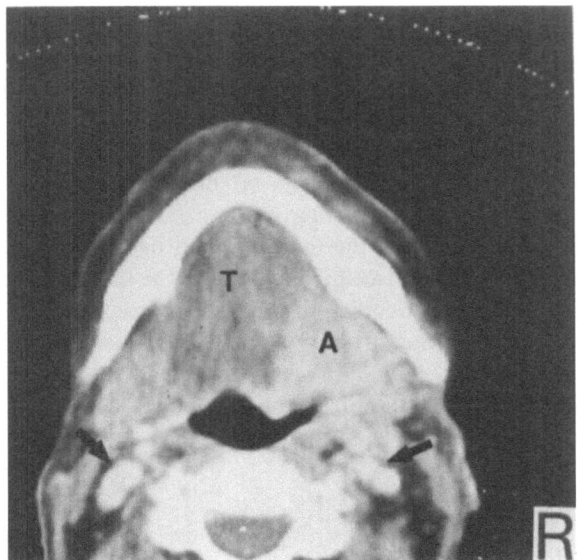

Figure 15.17(a)

of Rouvier will be evident as a soft-tissue mass extending forwards into the fossa of Rosenmuller and may cause erosion of the lateral mass of the atlas. Lymph node involvement in the internal jugular chain may be evident as discrete soft-tissue densities or as obliteration of the fat plane lying deep to the sterno-mastoid muscle.

Tumours of the oropharynx appear as a soft-tissue mass which most frequently arises from the tonsil and may extend forwards into the base of the tongue. The vallecula may be obliterated and the lateral pharyngo-epiglottic fold and the epiglottis may be thickened (figure 15.17). Extension superiorly causes thickening and irregularity of the nasopharyngeal walls. The normal increase in density which occurs in the submandibular salivary gland following intravenous contrast injection should not be confused with tumour enhancement (figure 15.18).

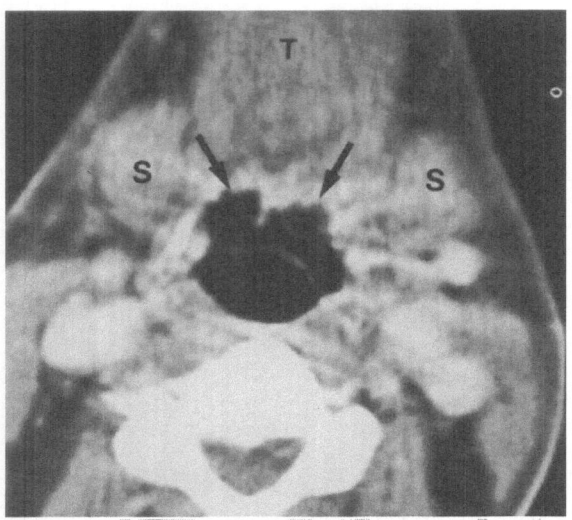

Figure 15.18(a)

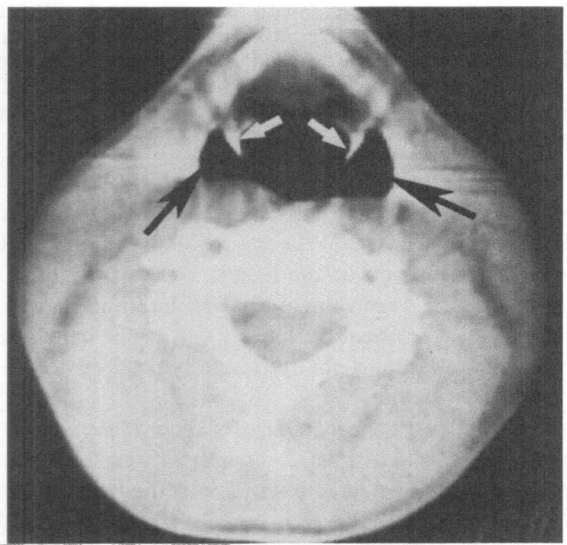

Figure 15.18(b)

Figure 15.18 Normal anatomy of the oropharynx. (a) The floor of the mouth showing the normal sub-mandibular glands (S) on each side of the base of the tongue (T). These have enhanced following intravenous injection of contrast medium. The valleculae (black arrows). (b) At a lower level the ary-epiglottic folds (small arrows) are seen running postero-inferiorly and separate the oropharynx from the pyriform fossae (large arrows)

LARYNX

There is a considerable variety of operative procedures applicable to management of patients with laryngeal cancer. In order to select the most appropriate procedure, the surgeon demands more detailed information about tumour extent than he has required previously. The combination of clinical examination including direct laryngoscopy, conventional tomography and laryngography can provide many of the answers, but these methods fail to show the submucosal extent of tumour, do not provide a satisfactory assessment of cartilage involvement nor show the extent of spread into the adjacent soft tissues. CT can provide much of the additional information which is now essential for planning surgery.

Technique of Examination

CT examination of the larynx is undertaken with the supine patient breathing quietly and with the neck hyperextended. There must be no movement of the tongue and no swallowing throughout the scan. It is helpful if the tongue is slightly protruded to open up the valleculae. The whole of the potential tumour-bearing area must be included in the examination so that scanning should begin at the level of the cricoid cartilage and proceed upwards to the hyoid bone. Narrow collimation (e.g. 6 mm) is an advantage and scans should overlap so that the true and false cords may be distinguished from one another. If wider collimation is used, partial volume averaging may merge the images of the true and false cords. It is helpful to opacify the thyroid gland by injection of intravenous contrast medium before the scan. In this way, tumour extending through the thyroid cartilage can be separated from the gland. Enhancement will also identify the major vessels and allow them to be separated from tumour and lymph nodes.

CT Anatomy

A great deal of anatomical information is available with CT which cannot be obtained by conventional methods. The suprahyoid epiglottis forms the posterior boundary of the valleculae and the anterior boundary of the laryngeal vestibule. The normal epiglottis is uniform in width (2 to 3 mm), and from its anterior surface the median glosso-epiglottic fold runs forwards to the tongue (figure 15.18a). At a slightly lower level, fibro-fatty tissue fills the space between the anterior surface of the epiglottis and the hyoid bone. Extending downwards and posteriorly from the epiglottis, the aryepiglottic fold can be recognised on each side (figure 15.18b). The body of the thyroid cartilage on each side is composed of two cortical layers (figure 15.19). The cartilages for each side unite anteriorly, and this junction is commonly notched. This must not be confused with an area of cartilage destruction. The anterior thyroid angle gives attachment to the vestibular folds or false vocal cords. The folds and vestibular ligaments are inserted posteriorly into the anterolateral surface of the arytenoid cartilage. The airway between the false cords is wider than at the level of the true vocal cords, so that it may be possible to identify both sets of folds on a particularly thick CT slice. The true vocal cords are attached in front to the angle of thyroid cartilage and behind to the vocal processes of the arytenoid cartilages (figure 15.20). The medial margins of the true cords have a particularly clearcut outline. Posteriorly, the upper margin of the cricoid cartilage can be identified medially to the arytenoid cartilage. In the transverse plane, the laryngeal ventricle cannot usually be identified, but Mancuso *et al.* (1978) do not share this view. In the immediate subglottic region, the cricoid cartilage can be identified circumferentially.

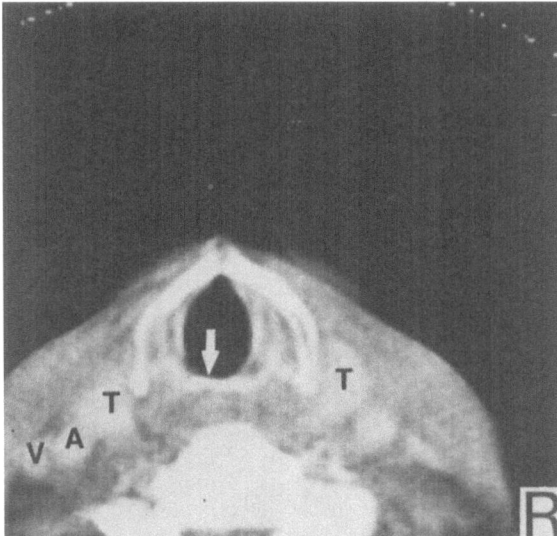

Figure 15.20 **Normal true vocal cords. Note the sharp medial border, attachment to the arytenoid cartilages (arrow) and dense upper pole of thyroid gland (T); common carotid artery (A) and jugular vein (V)**

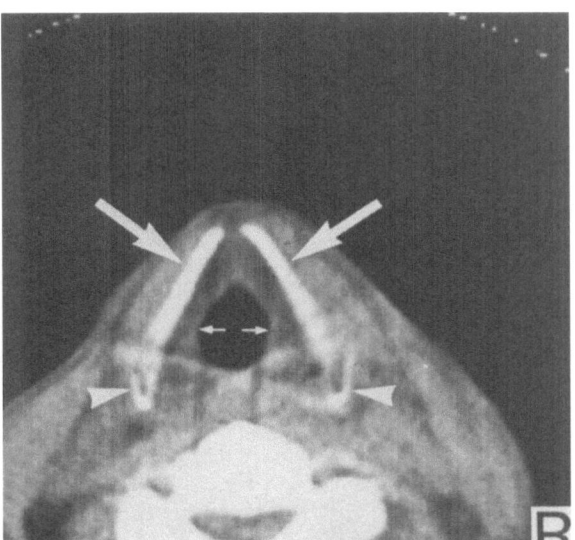

Figure 15.19 **Normal false cords with sharp medial border (small arrows). The ala of thyroid cartilage (large arrows) fail to meet anteriorly at this level leaving a notch. The double cortex of the thyroid cartilage is evident in the superior cornua (arrowheads)**

Tumours

The transverse plane allows the thickness of the *epiglottis* to be assessed throughout its width, so that the right and left halves can be compared. Forward extension of epiglottic tumours into the valleculae is readily seen because soft tissue replaces the air normally contained within them. Saliva filling the valleculae may cause exactly similar appearances and lead to a false positive diagnosis of tumour.

Although the clinician can usually assess epiglottic tumours easily, a large exophytic mass may prevent inspection of the infrahyoid region. Soft-tissue tumour extending into the fibro-fatty pre-epiglottic space produces an increase in density of this region (figure 15.21). Delineation of this area is more accurate using CT than conventional methods. Tumour extension into the pre-epiglottic space and valleculae is important because it makes laryngectomy technically difficult. The more massive epiglottic tumours may be shown to encircle the hyoid bone.

The *aryepiglottic folds* may rarely be the primary site of tumour. Detection of minor degrees of thickening is possible with CT because fold thickness may be compared between the two sides. Assessment of the pyriform sinus, however, is difficult, since it is impossible to distinguish between soft-tissue tumour filling the sinus, a pool of saliva, or simply a collapsed sinus containing no air. For this reason, a barium swallow remains a complementary and essential investigation.

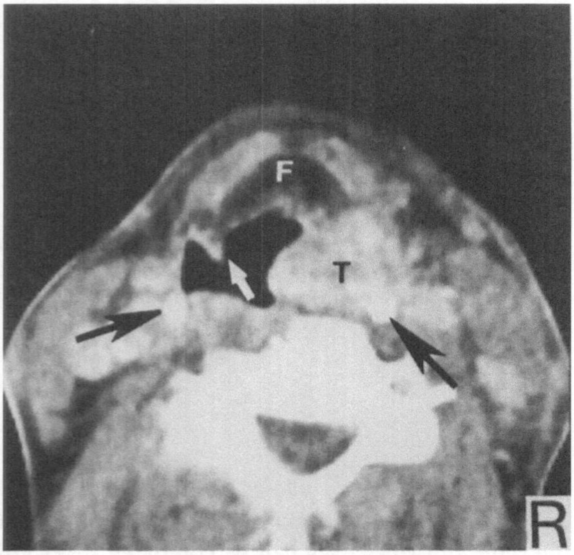

Tumours of the false and true cords may produce a number of abnormalities. The most useful sign is irregularity of the medial border of the cord. Quite small lesions (2 to 3 mm) may be detected in this way. Much larger tumours occupying the superior or inferior surface but sparing the medial border may not be demonstrated (figure 15.22). Tumour invasion may cause enlargement of the vocal cord, but this is indistinguishable from oedema associated with adjacent tumour or radiotherapy.

Patients with advanced tumours show profound transglottic oedema, so that the precise limits of the tumour itself cannot be defined. However, it is usually possible with tumours of moderate size to determine whether they extend forwards as far as the anterior commissure or cross it.

Evaluation of the *thyroid cartilage* may be difficult in those patients in whom there is patchy ossification because this may simulate erosion by tumour or necrosis following radiotherapy. When necrosis occurs, the cartilage may collapse inwards so that the vocal cord is displaced medially. A similar appearance of the cord may be found in

Figure 15.21 Suprahyoid laryngeal tumour (T) extending forwards into the fat of the pre-epiglottic space (F). The tumour involves the aryepiglottic fold and pyriform sinus, the normal aryepiglottic fold is shown on the left (small centre arrow). The superior cornua of the thyroid cartilage are arrowed

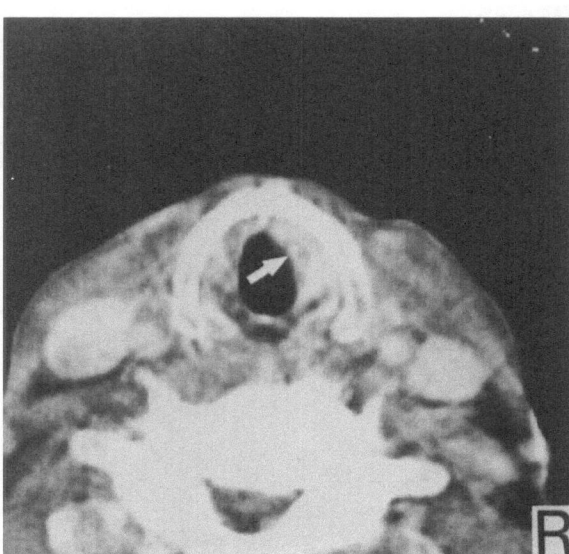

Figure 15.22 Very large tumour of the right true vocal cord appearing to be quite small since it involves the medial border of the cord to only a minor degree (arrowed)

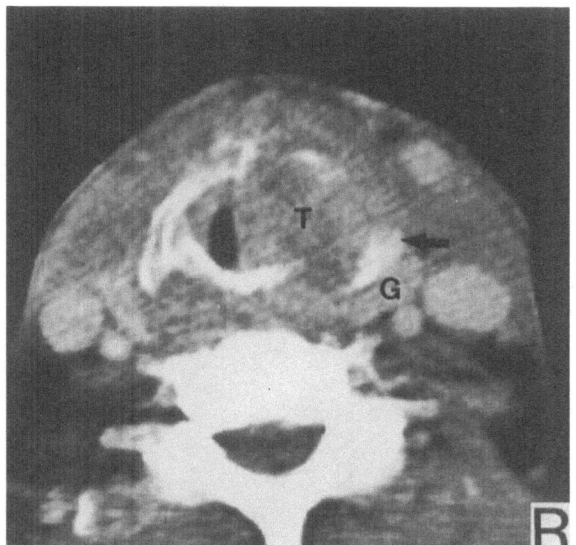

Figure 15.23 Large tumour (T) of right true cord which has destroyed the thyroid ala (arrow). The upper pole of the thyroid gland (G) and the major vessels have been opacified

recurrent laryngeal nerve palsy when there is failure of the cord to retract during breathing. This must be distinguished from a thick cord due to oedema or tumour. Perforation of the thyroid cartilage and displacement of the thyroid gland are not uncommon and may not be realised clinically (figure 15.23). Tumours involving the posterior part of the cords may displace the arytenoid cartilage medially and invade the cricoid. All these features are important in preoperative assessment.

PAROTID GLAND

The main advantage of CT over clinical examination and sialography in examination of tumours of the parotid gland is the ability to detect extension of tumour from the deep part of the gland into surrounding tissue. It is, therefore, useful in the preoperative assessment of tumours and also for demonstrating recurrence following previous incomplete resection.

Technique of Examination

The parotid gland should be examined both before and after infusion of intravenous contrast medium because there is general enhancement both of the parenchyma and adjacent blood vessels. The examination should begin below the angle of the mandible and extend as high as the zygomatic arch or beyond this if a lesion is shown to extend further.

CT Anatomy

The unenhanced parotid gland has a lower density (−5 to −15 EMI units) than the surrounding muscles, but, after injection of intravenous contrast medium, the gland appears much denser than the surrounding muscles, even though they may also show enhancement. The parotid can be recognised just below the level of the temporo-mandibular joint occupying a more or less triangular space (figure 15.24). The anterior surface of this space is bounded by the mandible and flanked by the masseter muscle

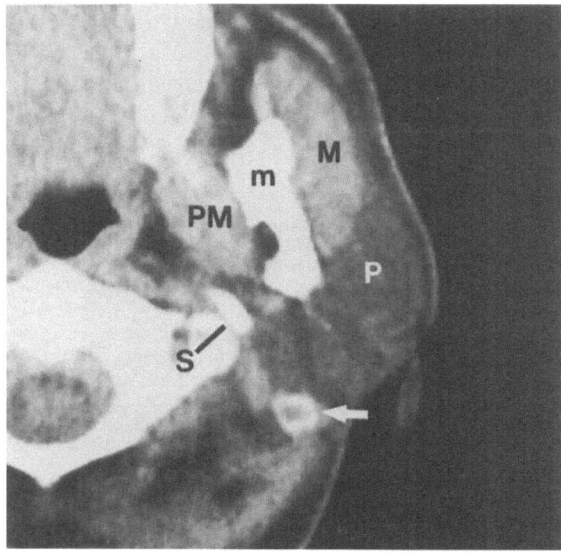

Figure 15.24 The normal parotid (P) is low in density and bounded by the masseter (M), mandible (m) and lateral pterygoid muscle (PM) anteriorly, the styloid process (S) medially and mastoid tip (white arrow) posteriorly

superficially and the lateral pterygoid muscle medially. The sterno-mastoid muscle is the posterior boundary of this space; deep to this lie in turn the posterior belly of digastric muscle, the styloid process and its attached muscles. The great vessels lie medially, the internal jugular vein separating the parotid from the body of the atlas. The low-density, deep lobe of parotid can be identified because it has a triangular shape with its apex passing medially and forwards (figure 15.24). The gland is enveloped in a sheet of deep cervical fascia so that its boundaries are moderately well defined. This fascial sheet is attached above to the zygomatic arch and below separates the lower pole of the parotid gland from the more deeply lying submandibular salivary gland.

Tumours

Parotid gland tumours are recognised as soft-tissue masses which may remain superficial (figure 15.25a) or extend deeply into the parapharyngeal space (figure 15.25b). The deep extent at first lies anterior to the styloid muscles but, as the tumour becomes larger, these muscles are invaded and the lateral pharyngeal wall is displaced medially (figure 15.26). The fat lying against the posterior surface of the pterygoid muscles may be replaced, and, if the muscle itself is invaded, it will be bulkier than its

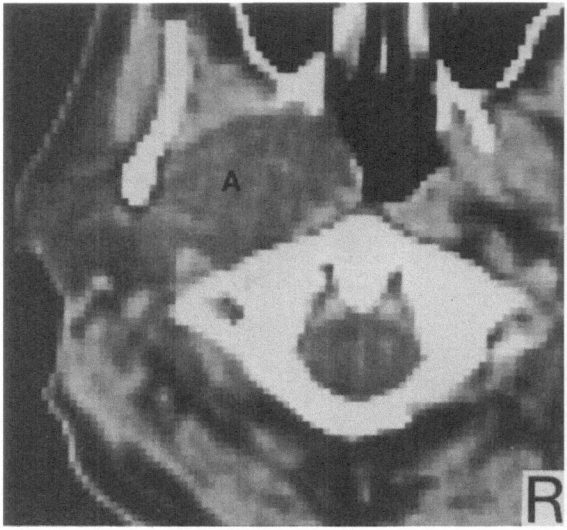

Figure 15.25(b)

Figure 15.25 Tumours of the parotid gland. (a) Carcinoma of the right parotid (P) which has extended superficially into the subcutaneous tissues of the cheek. (b) Mixed salivary adenoma of the left parotid gland (A) extending into the parapharyngeal space. (By kind permission of Dr Hoare)

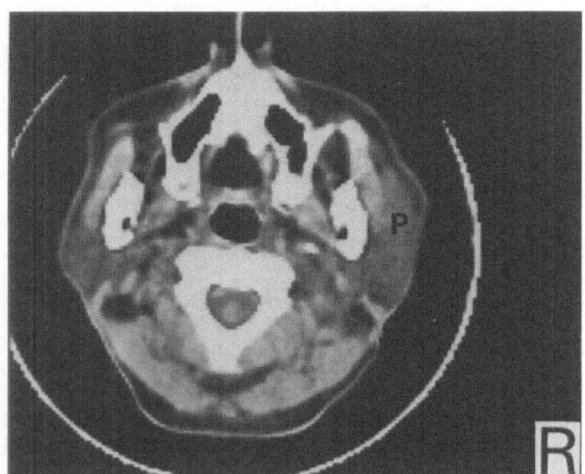

Figure 15.25(a)

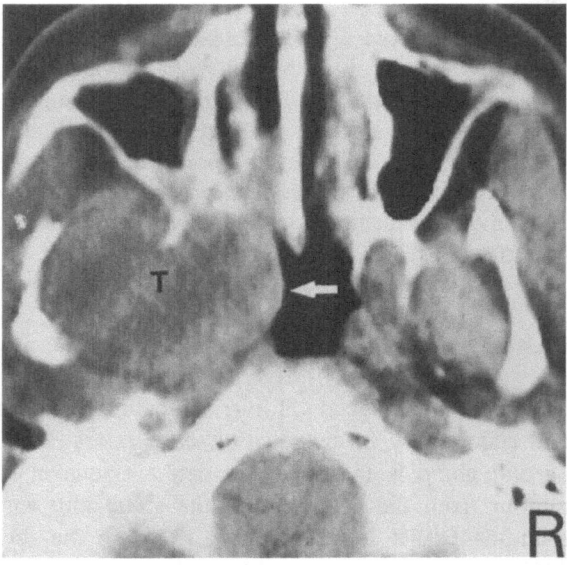

Figure 15.26 Large recurrent tumour of the left parotid (T) filling the parapharyngeal space and displacing the lateral wall of nasopharynx medially (arrow)

fellow on the normal side. The route of forward extension of deep parotid tumours is determined by the bone of the mandible lying laterally and the alveolus medially, so that tumour extends forwards to the cheek between these bony limits. The soft-tissue mass may be ill-defined and irregular in outline or very well defined and more or less spherical. Destruction of the pterygoid plates and posterior wall of the maxillary antrum may occur or the tumour may spread upwards through the parapharyngeal space to erode the skull base. Enhancement of parotid tumours is unpredictable, but, when it occurs, can be a great help in accurately defining tumour limits. Larger parotid tumours may encircle the great vessels; an important feature when attempting removal (figure 15.27).

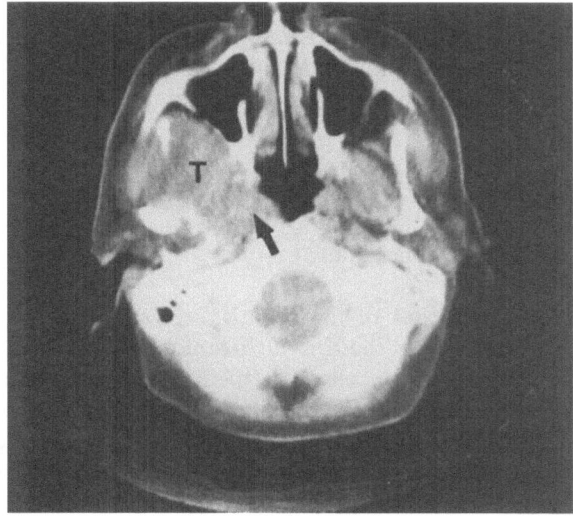

Figure 15.27 Large parotid tumour (T) filling the parapharyngeal space with destruction of normal tissue planes. The tumour involves the prevertebral muscles (arrow)

Although CT is rarely required for the examination of the submandibular salivary gland, normal glands should be recognised so that they are not confused with other structures, particularly enlarged lymph nodes. The glands are symmetrical, ovoid and measure 2.5 cm × 2.5 cm × 1 cm. They lie immediately lateral to the junction of the tongue and hyoid bone. They show a high degree of enhancement (*see* figure 15.18).

REFERENCES

Dodd, G. D. and Jing, B. S. (1977). *Radiology of the Nose, Paranasal Sinuses and Nasopharynx*, Williams and Wilkins Co., Baltimore

Fletcher, G. H. and Jing, B.-S. (1972). *The Head and Neck. An Atlas of Tumour Radiology*, Year Book Medical Publishers, Chicago

Forbes, W. St C., Fawcitt, R. A., Isherwood, I., Webb, R. and Farrington, T. (1978). Computed tomography in the diagnosis of the paranasal sinuses. *Clinical Radiology*, **29**, 501–511

Mancuso, A. A., Calcaterra, T. C. and Hanafee, W. N. (1978). Computed tomography of the larynx. *Radiologic Clinics of North America*, **XVI** (2), 195–208

Parsons, C. A. (1981). Delineation of tumours in the head and neck. In *Computerised Axial Tomography in Oncology*, eds. J. E. Husband and P. A. Hobday, Churchill Livingstone, Edinburgh, pp. 69–80

Parsons, C. A. and Hodson, N. (1979). Computed tomography in paranasal sinus tumours. *Radiology*, **132**, 641–645

Thawley, S. E., Gado, M. and Fuller, T. R. (1978). Computerised tomography in the evaluation of head and neck lesions. *The Laryngoscope*, **88**, 451–459

Wortzman, G. and Holgate, R. C. (1976). Computerised tomography (CT) in otolaryngology. *The Laryngoscope*, **86**, 1552–1562

16

The Orbits

by G. A. S. Lloyd

The application of computerised tomography to orbital diagnosis was first evaluated by Ambrose *et al.* (1974) and by Gawler *et al.* (1974) using the original 80×80 matrix system, and subsequently the 160×160 matrix. Since that date, numerous publications have appeared detailing the technique for orbital scanning and recording the findings in specific pathological conditions such as tumours, inflammatory processes and dysthyroid exophthalmos. The presence of fat in the intraconal space, acting as a natural contrast medium, has made CT a very rewarding exercise in orbital diagnosis. It is now the principal method of investigation of patients presenting with unilateral exophthalmos, and suspected intra-orbital space-occupying lesions, after plain x-ray examination of the skull. Other modalities – ultrasound, orbital venography, carotid angiography – are ancillary to it.

The present apparatus used by the author is an EMI General Purpose Scanner (CT5005) which has been adapted for head and neck scanning and which incorporates a high-resolution facility. The latter system uses only the central 5 in of the scanning aperture, and with a 5 mm collimated slice thickness has produced the optimal orbital scans to date (figures 16.1, 16.2 and 16.3). Bone detail is particularly well shown with the high-resolution method. A general-purpose scanner is better than a dedicated brain scanner for orbital diagnosis because the larger scanning aperture means that scans are not limited to the axial plane. Coronal, oblique and even sagittal sections can be obtained.

TECHNIQUE OF EXAMINATION

Positioning of the Patient

For axial scans of the orbit, the prone position is preferred when there is an overcouch gantry and tube mounting. In this way, the incident beam of x-rays is directed for the most part through the back of the skull, reducing the radiation dose received by the lens and cornea to less than one-sixth of that received when the patient is supine. The attitude of the patient's head is most important, so that the optimum scanning plane can be obtained through the orbits. Satisfactory scans should include the globes, showing the lens, optic nerve, lateral and medial rectus muscles on the same cut. To do this, the position of the head should be adjusted so that the scanning plane forms an angle of 16° caudally from the orbito-meatal line. This line should be marked out on the skin prior to scanning. Optimum axial scans will be obtained if the posterior clinoids are shown on scans which also include the optic nerves and clearly show the globes on both sides.

For coronal scans, the patient lies prone with the

chin elevated so that the radiation port is again principally through the skull vault. A similar position can be obtained by placing the patient supine with the head hyperextended, but this incurs an unacceptable level of radiation to the lens and cornea and is therefore not recommended.

Contrast Medium

The injection of contrast medium for orbital CT scanning is no longer a routine procedure. If possible, postcontrast scans to show tissue enhancement are to be avoided since the injection of contrast converts what is essentially a non-invasive procedure into one which carries a similar morbidity and mortality to intravenous urography. Initial studies (Lloyd and Ambrose, 1977) showed that the behaviour of attenuation values pre- and postcontrast injection are unlikely, in most circumstances, to facilitate tissue characterisation. Thus, for orbital scanning, contrast medium should be used to show up doubtful space-occupying lesions in better detail and when intracranial spread is suspected. If a clearly defined lesion is shown on the unenhanced scans, injection is usually unnecessary.

ABNORMALITIES OF THE ORBIT

Primary Orbital Disease

Space-occupying lesions arising in the orbit may be divided according to their location into *intraconal* and *extraconal masses*.

Intraconal Lesions

Within the rectus muscle cone, some differentiation of intraconal lesions is possible on the basis of their shape and density (CT morphology) and of their site of origin. For example, optic nerve tumours are usually identified if there is obvious optic nerve expansion. Benign encapsulated tumours can also be readily identified by their shape and homogeneous density. The commonest in this group is a cavernous haemangioma (figure 16.1). This gives a rounded

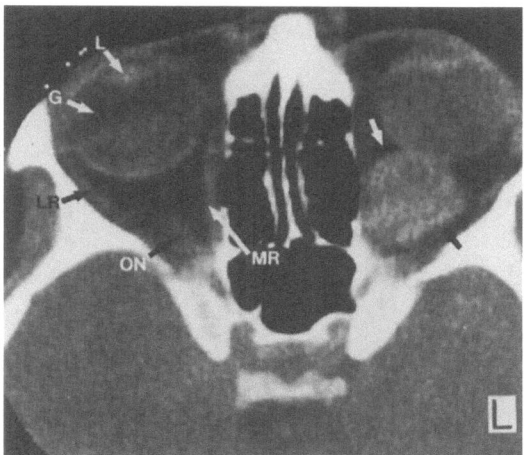

Figure 16.1   Rounded, clearly demarcated tumour mass in the left orbit, typical of a cavernous haemangioma (arrowed). Normal anatomy of the orbit is shown on the right. Globe (G), lens (L), optic nerve (ON), medial rectus (MR), lateral rectus (LR)

contour sometimes almost circular in outline and is almost invariably intraconal in location. Neurilemmoma is another intraconal tumour. It may be indistinguishable on CT from a cavernous haemangioma. In general, neurilemmomas are larger than the cavernous haemangiomata but it is not usually necessary to differentiate between the two tumours since the treatment is the same in either case, namely, excision by lateral orbitotomy. A similar appearance (i.e. a rounded clearly defined mass) is also seen with an extradural meningioma, that is, a primary meningioma arising in the orbit but not derived from the optic nerve sheath. When encapsulated tumours grow to a large size, they may fill almost the whole of the intraconal space, but even the largest will invariably leave some translucence on the scan at the orbital apex, a point of differentiation from infiltrative processes in the muscle cone. The commonest of these is a granuloma (pseudotumour) (figure 16.2). They may be distinguished from the clearly defined tumours described above by their ill-defined edge and heterogeneous density. Lymphomas may also give a similar appearance and when they occur intraconally are indistinguishable from pseudotumours.

Pseudotumours may extend both inside and

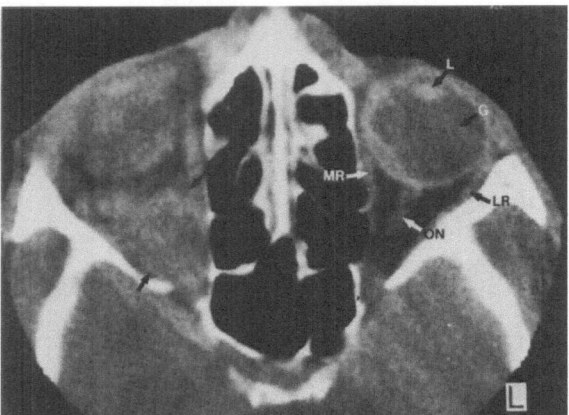

Figure 16.2 Diffuse irregular mass in the intraconal space in the right orbit due to a granuloma (arrowed). Normal anatomy is shown on the left. Globe (G), lens (L), optic nerve (ON), medial rectus (MR), lateral rectus (LR)

outside the muscle cone and may involve the lacrimal gland. They are sometimes bilateral and they may cause local muscle enlargement. Another feature of a pseudotumour or granuloma is an apparent thickening of the posterior coats of the globe – probably the result of inflammatory tissue being contiguous with the posterior surface of the sclera. In some instances, the abnormal tissue may fill the whole of the intraconal space, obliterating the outline of normal structures by an isodense mass.

Vascular Lesions

The superior ophthalmic vein is often visible crossing the optic nerve in normal scans of the upper part of the orbit and in conditions in which it becomes enlarged, for example a carotico-cavernous fistula, this may be demonstrated and the correct diagnosis deduced. However, in these patients, angiography is needed for verification of the diagnosis and remains the definitive investigation. Venous malformations may also be demonstrated on CT, although again orbital venography is needed to show their true aetiology. Negative CT scans in patients with known orbital varices have been recorded. Venous malformations present a wide spectrum of abnormality in the orbit on CT, sometimes mimicking a diffuse infiltrative process and on other occasions appearing

as a well defined mass (figure 16.3). Orbital venography should, therefore, be considered when there is a mass present which is not easily classified into the two predominant types of pathology, i.e. diffuse infiltrations or encapsulated tumours. Arteriovenous malformations in the orbit may be more readily diagnosable than venous malformations; they may give a typical worm-like appearance due to large afferent and efferent vessels (figure 16.4).

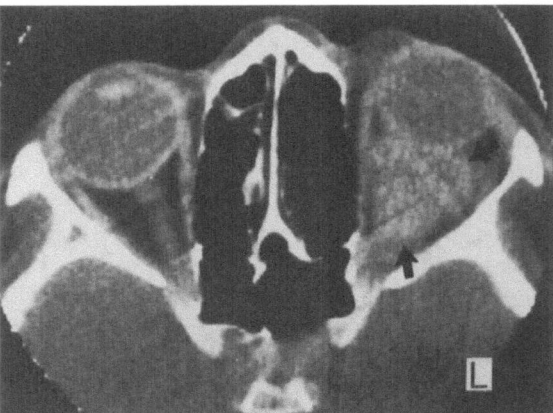

Figure 16.3 Well demarcated, somewhat rounded mass in the left orbit which was shown at surgery to be due to a venous malformation (arrowed)

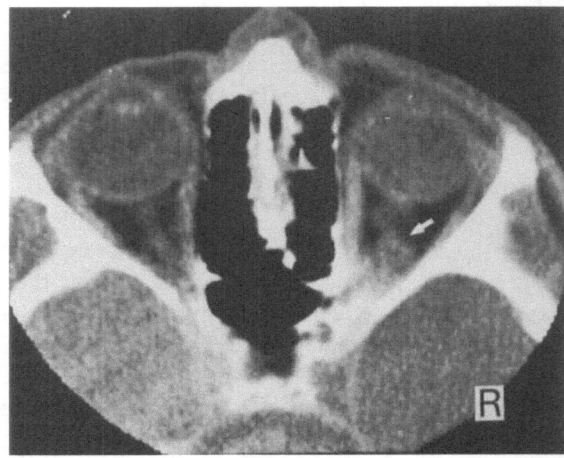

Figure 16.4 Irregular worm-like lesion in the left orbit due to an arteriovenous malformation (arrowed)

Extraconal Lesions

Tumours lying outside the muscle cone but taking their origin within the orbit can be readily demonstrated by CT. The commonest primary extraconal tumour is a lacrimal gland neoplasm. In addition to a soft-tissue mass, pressure erosion or invasion of the overlying bone of the lacrimal fossa may be demonstrated, particularly if high-resolution CT is used. Some differentiation between benign mixed lacrimal gland tumours and the carcinomata may also be possible. In general, the more widespread the tumour and less well defined, the more likely it is to be malignant. The demonstration of calcification in the tumour, either by conventional radiography or on CT, is also a sign of likely malignancy (figure 16.5). Other extraconal tumours of primary orbital

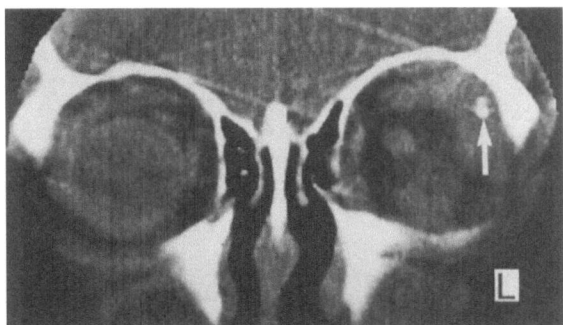

Figure 16.5   Coronal section showing soft-tissue mass of a lacrimal gland carcinoma. Note small area of calcification (arrowed)

origin include lymphomata which typically occur in the forward part of the orbit and tend to encompass the globe. A cavernous haemangioma may also rarely present as an extraconal mass, and a pseudotumour or granuloma may sometimes be confined to the extraconal space. Another important lesion in this situation is a metastasis. These frequently involve bone and will then lie extraconally in association with an area of bone destruction visible on both plain radiograph and on CT. Dermoid cysts occur extraconally, most often in the roof of the orbit. They may show areas of low attenuation due to the presence of oil or fat (figure 16.6).

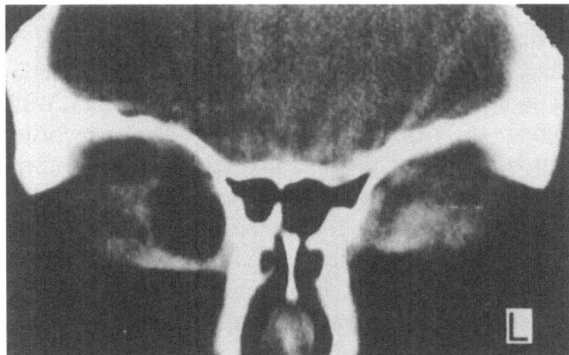

Figure 16.6   Coronal CT scan showing well circumscribed area of low attenuation in the right orbit due to a dermoid cyst

Dysthyroid Exophthalmos

Enlargement of the extra-ocular muscles which occurs in this condition may be clearly demonstrated by CT scanning. In addition to muscle enlargement, the intraconal space may appear to be enlarged, presumably due to polysaccharide infiltration in the intraconal fat. In dysthyroid patients, the degree of muscle swelling, as depicted on CT, may be uneven; in some instances, it may be entirely unilateral or there may be selective enlargement of

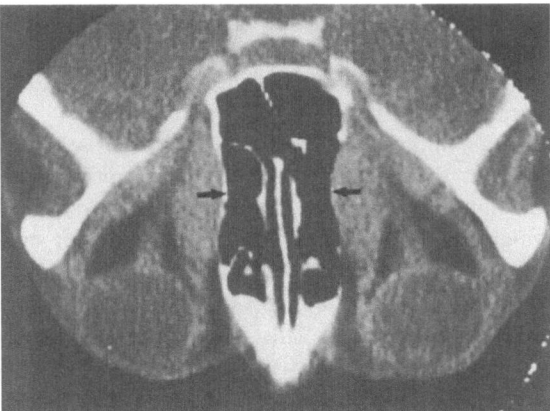

Figure 16.7   Typical appearance of dysthyroid disease showing generalised enlargement of the rectus muscles with bilateral indentation of the ethmoid labyrinth (arrowed) caused by the muscle enlargement

individual or groups of muscles. Enlargement of the medial rectus muscles may also cause a characteristic 'waisting' of the ethmoid labyrinth due to symmetrical pressure on the medial orbital walls (figure 16.7). Brismar *et al.* (1976) have recorded that bunching of the enlarged rectus muscles in the apex of the orbit may simulate tumour formation. This is an obvious pitfall in the differential diagnosis of endocrine exophthalmos and is explained by the tomographic section intersecting obliquely one or several enlarged muscles (usually the inferior rectus muscle), thus producing a false tumour-like structure. The problem has largely been overcome by the use of routine coronal sections which will identify the enlarged rectus muscles.

Secondary Orbital Disease

Tumours and other lesions arising intracranially or within the paranasal sinuses may involve the orbit secondarily. Middle fossa lesions invading the orbit and causing proptosis may be clearly demonstrated by CT. Meningiomata are the commonest tumours to extend into the orbit causing proptosis, and the majority are clearly demonstrated on both axial and coronal scans. Other middle fossa lesions such as infraclinoid aneurysms or carotico-cavernous fistulae may be demonstrated by CT, although, of course, the definitive investigation in these patients is angiography. The delineation of the herniation of the temporal lobe through a posterior encephalocele may be shown in patients with neurofibromatosis (figure 16.8).

In the majority of patients, primary pathology arising in the paranasal sinuses is diagnosable by plain films aided, where necessary, by conventional tomography. CT may act as a substitute for conventional tomography, particularly in the axial plane, and is a useful adjunct to show the soft-tissue extent of the lesion. This also applies to nasopharyngeal lesions which may extend to the orbit causing exophthalmos. Neoplasms and other expanding processes arising in the frontal sinuses and ethmoids are optimally demonstrated in their extent and spread by CT. Invasion of the anterior fossa is clearly defined by coronal CT scanning

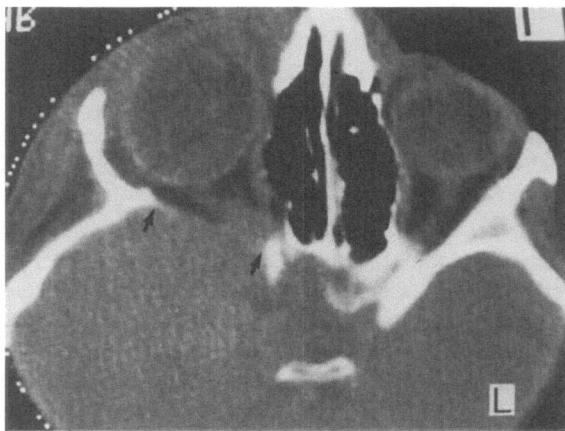

Figure 16.8 **Neurofibromatosis showing bone defect in the greater wing of the sphenoid (arrowed), enlargement of the middle fossa and buphthalmos**

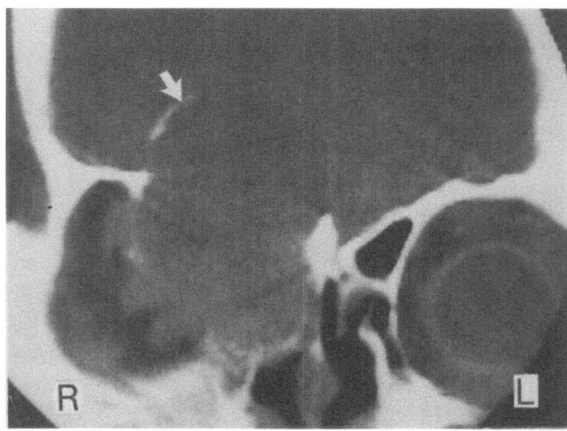

Figure 16.9 **Large fronto-ethmoidal mucocele demonstrated on coronal CT scan. The orbital invasion is demonstrated and there is upward expansion into the anterior fossa (arrowed)**

(figure 16.9). Frontal sinus pathology cannot be adequately demonstrated on axial scans alone. Coronal scans are also important to show antral or intranasal pathology invading the orbit.

USE OF COMPUTED TOMOGRAPHY IN ORBITAL DIAGNOSIS

Conventional radiology and CT are now the dominant radiological investigations of the orbit, and the majority of patients presenting with exophthalmos can be totally evaluated by these techniques without further study.

Plain x-ray examination remains the first investigation of these patients and should never be neglected. In a series of 1070 patients investigated for unilateral exophthalmos by the author, no less than 33% showed abnormality on plain films and in 21% the features were totally diagnostic without further investigation. In a high proportion of these positive cases, the pathology originated either in the middle fossa of the skull or in the paranasal sinuses. Plain x-ray investigation is concerned with bone imaging, and in some patients additional information may be required which can only be furnished by hypocycloidal tomography. This technique is used if fine bone detail is required, particularly at the apex of the orbit and optic canal. Even this technique is less necessary with the introduction of high-resolution CT, which in most instances is an adequate substitute for conventional hypocycloidal tomography. The other non-invasive technique showing the orbital soft tissues (i.e. ultrasound) has largely been superseded by CT scanning for extra-ocular orbital diagnosis.

Angiography now plays a minor role in orbital investigation. As indicated above, venography is needed principally when a venous malformation is suspected in the orbit. The introduction of CT scanning has made orbital arteriography seldom necessary for the routine investigation of exophthalmos. CT has largely taken over the previous role of carotid angiography in the exclusion of intracranial lesions causing proptosis. The technique has also made intra-orbital diagnosis far more exact preoperatively, so that in most patients the appropriate surgical approach is clearly indicated and can be safely undertaken without the risk of the morbidity which attends carotid puncture. This latter investigation should therefore only be carried out on selected patients, principally those who are clinically suspected of having a carotico-cavernous fistula or other intracranial vascular anomaly. Carotid angiography is also required in patients with a very vascular tumour in the orbit in which it is important to identify the feeding vessels prior to surgery.

REFERENCES

Ambrose, J. A. E., Lloyd, G. A. S. and Wright, J. E. (1974). A preliminary evaluation of fine matrix computerized axial tomography (EMI Scan) in the diagnosis of orbital space occupying lesions. *British Journal of Radiology*, **47**, 747

Brismar, J., Davis, K. R., Dallow, R. C. and Brismar, G. (1976). Unilateral endocrine exophthalmos. Diagnostic problems in association with computed tomography. *Neuroradiology*, **12**, 21

Gawler, J., Sanders, M. D., Bull, J. W., du Boulay, G. and Marshall, J. (1974). Computer assisted tomography in orbital disease. *British Journal of Ophthalmology*, **58**, 571

Lloyd, G. A. S. and Ambrose, J. A. E. (1977). An evaluation of C.A.T. in the diagnosis of orbital space occupying lesions. In *The First European Seminar on Computerized Axial Tomography in Clinical Practice*, eds G. du Boulay and I. F. Moseley, Berlin, Springer, p. 154

17

Computed Tomography in Oncology

CT has a major role in the diagnosis and management of malignant disease because of its ability to delineate masses. Not only can it be used for the primary diagnosis and staging of the disease but it is also ideally suited for measuring response to treatment, for detecting relapse and for radiotherapy treatment planning.

PRIMARY DIAGNOSIS

The ability of CT to demonstrate disease in individual sites in the body has been discussed in previous chapters. In general, CT will be used when simpler techniques have failed to establish the diagnosis. However, in some areas, notably the brain, the adrenal glands, the retroperitoneum and the mediastinum, CT is likely to be used early in the diagnostic sequence because these are sites in which tumours may be difficult or impossible to demonstrate by other techniques. In a series of 243 consecutive patients referred to St Bartholomew's Hospital for body scans with a possible diagnosis of malignancy, a mass was demonstrated by CT in 87 (35%). Thirty-five of these patients had no evidence of a mass on investigations carried out before the CT scan, and in half of these the masses were malignant (table 17.1). Thus, CT made a unique contribution to the detection of malignant disease in 7% of the patients.

Patients with known malignant disease in whom

Table 17.1 Thirty-five patients with masses on CT previously undiagnosed

Abdominal nodes	10	Follow up available
Pancreas	9	30 patients
Adrenals	8	
Other retroperitoneal lesions	3	17 malignant
Mediastinum	2	No false positives
Kidney, stomach, lung	1 each	

the site of the primary tumour is not established present a particular problem to the clinician, and CT scanning is not uncommonly requested in the hope of demonstrating the hidden tumour. In the authors' experience, this is rarely a rewarding exercise unless there is fairly strong clinical evidence to implicate a particular organ or site.

Patients are also sometimes referred for CT scanning in whom there is a relatively low suspicion of malignancy in order to exclude a tumour of a particular region, such as the pancreas. Clearly, the degree of confidence in reporting a negative examination depends on the area examined, the patient's build and the general quality of the CT examination. The accuracy of the technique in relation to individual organs is discussed elsewhere in this book but, in general, a good-quality CT examination in a patient with an adequate amount of body fat is an acceptable method of excluding masses more than 2 to 3 cm in diameter.

STAGING

The objective of tumour staging is to define the extent of tumour in local tissues (T-staging), in regional lymph nodes (N-staging) and distant sites (M-staging). Staging is essential for defining optimum treatment regimes, for providing a prognosis and for avoiding ineffective therapy.

The impact of CT depends not only on its ability to demonstrate tumour spread but also on the ease with which the same information can be obtained by other techniques. Assessment of the accuracy of CT in tumour staging requires correlation between CT findings and histopathology, and in many tumour types these data are still lacking. However, in broad terms, it is possible to indicate those situations where CT is making a significant contribution to staging.

Local Spread of Primary Tumour (T-stage)

Conventional radiological methods of staging frequently fail to demonstrate the complete extent of the primary tumour. Thus, the superficial or accessible growth is seen but there is no indication as to the depth of tumour infiltration within the primary organ or whether the tumour has spread into adjacent structures. Since CT distinguishes soft-tissue tumour from surrounding structures which have a significantly different density (e.g. fat), it not only demonstrates the total tumour mass but also shows tumour spread beyond the primary organ.

The role of CT in assessing the local extent of disease in individual organs has been discussed in previous chapters. In general, the clarity of definition of the primary tumour and its spread depends on the density of the tumour compared with the normal tissue of the primary organ, the density of surrounding normal tissue and the ability to define the normal anatomy in the vicinity of the tumour. It follows that local spread is more easily detected in some tumours than in others. Thus, tumours of the paranasal sinuses are relatively easy to define with CT because air and bone provide sufficient contrast to determine tumour limits and the amount of bone involvement (*see* chapter 15). Conversely, tumours of the prostate are difficult to assess because the tumour cannot be distinguished from the normal gland, and assessment of extracapsular tumour spread is difficult because there is usually only a thin layer of fat between the lateral margins of the prostate and the levator ani (*see* chapter 11).

CT is well suited to defining the local extent of disease in tumours in the nasopharynx, paranasal sinuses, the retroperitoneum (particularly the kidney) and in the bladder. The technique is less well suited for detecting early spread in tumours of the cervix and body of the uterus and prostate. The extent of primary lung tumours can also be difficult to evaluate because they are frequently associated with collapse and/or consolidation of the surrounding lung which has a similar density to tumour tissue.

Lymph Node Metastases (N-stage)

The capabilities and limitations of CT in lymph node disease of the mediastinum have been discussed in chapter 4 and of the abdomen and pelvis in chapter 10. Briefly, the detection of lymph node metastases with CT depends on the size of the involved nodes and on the site of involvement. Unlike lymphography, CT cannot detect metastases unless the nodes are enlarged Enlarged nodes are most easily observed in the retroperitoneal space and can be detected even when there is only minimal enlargement, so that CT provides an accurate method of staging patients with lymphomas and those with carcinomas which have spread to the para-aortic nodes. Lymph node enlargement in the pelvis is much more difficult to assess and, for this reason, CT is a relatively inaccurate method of estimating local spread to nodes from pelvic cancers.

At present, the conditions in which CT appears to have most impact on the detection of lymph node involvement are testicular teratomas (Husband *et al.*, 1981a), bronchogenic carcinoma (Dunnick *et al.*, 1979; Underwood *et al.*, 1979) and retroperitoneal tumours, such as carcinoma of the kidney and pancreas.

Distant Metastases (M-stage)

Blood-borne metastases from a primary tumour can occur in almost any organ, but the commonest sites are the brain, lungs, liver and bone. CT can detect metastases in all these organs with a varying degree of accuracy. Its ability to demonstrate metastases in the brain is well recognised. In the lungs, it is more sensitive than conventional radiology for the detection of pulmonary metastases (*see* chapter 4), but limited scanning time confines the use of CT to those patients in whom a major clinical decision is determined by the result. The most important of these are patients with osteogenic sarcomas, soft-tissue sarcomas and testicular teratomas.

The detection of liver metastases using CT has been discussed in detail in chapter 7. In summary,

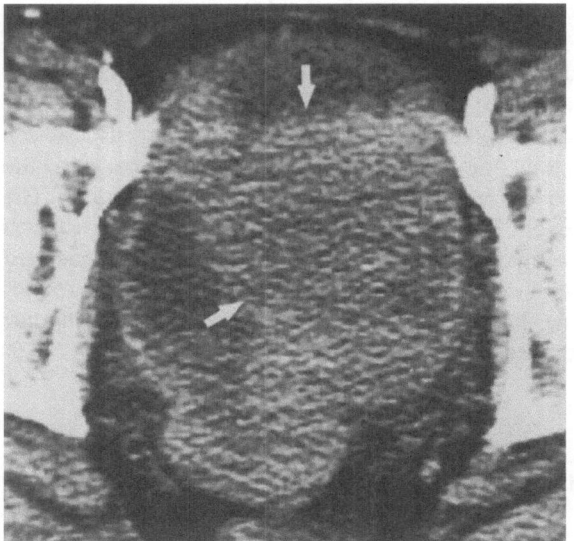

Figure 17.1(a)

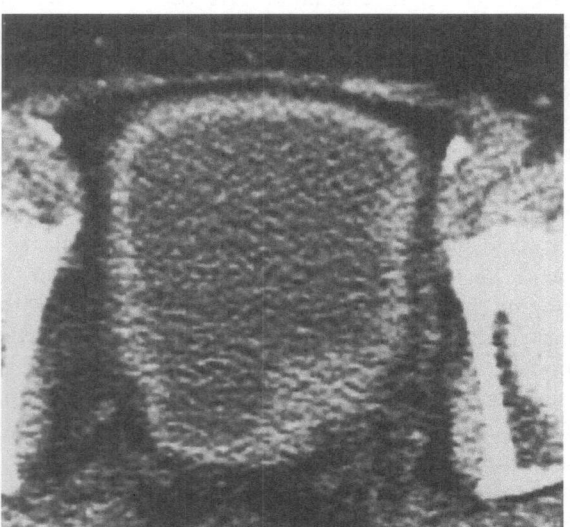

Figure 17.1(b)

Figure 17.1 Monitoring progress – carcinoma of the bladder. (a) Scan before treatment showing large tumour (arrowed). (b) Follow-up scan three months later in the same patient after a six-week course of radiotherapy. There has been marked tumour regression

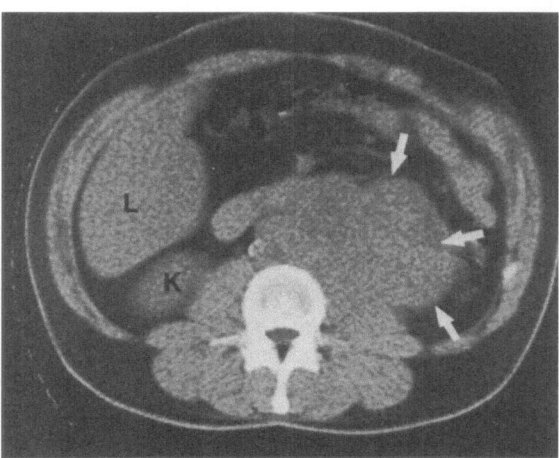

Figure 17.2(a)

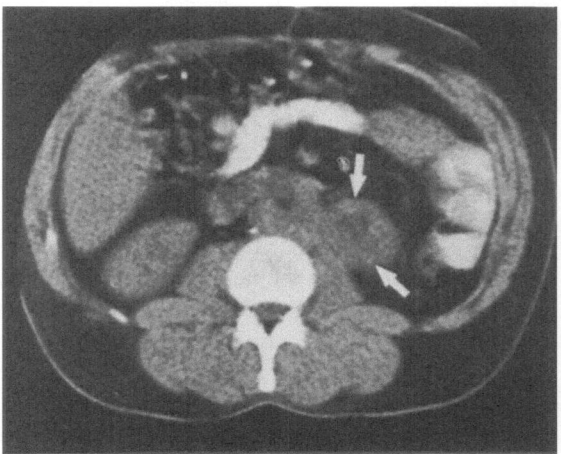

Figure 17.2(b)

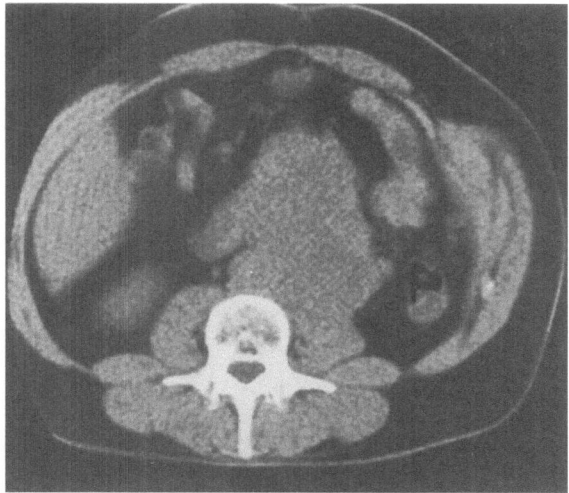

Figure 17.2(c)

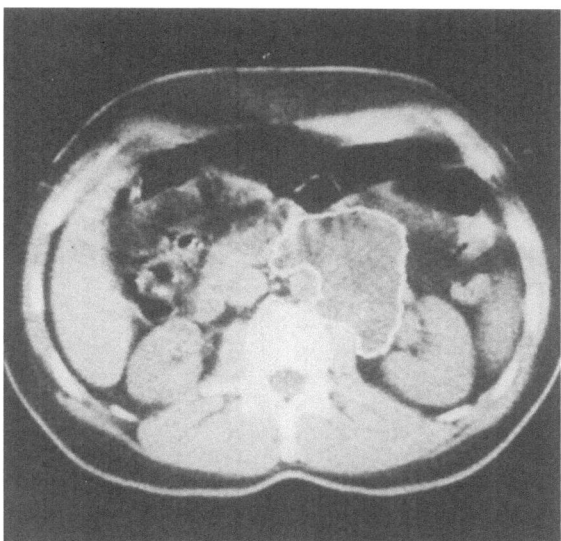

Figure 17.2 Monitoring progress – abdominal nodal metastases from testicular teratoma. (a) Large nodal mass (arrowed) on the left. Liver (L), lower pole of right kidney (K). (b) Follow-up scan in the same patient after treatment with chemotherapy for six months. The tumour is much smaller, but there is still a residual mass (arrowed). (c) The same patient five months later, showing significant regrowth of tumour. At the time of this scan, the patient complained of backache, but there were no other clinical features to suggest relapse

Figure 17.3 Tumour volume estimation. A precision touch-sensitive light pen is used to outline the tumour on each CT section throughout the tumour length

CT provides a useful alternative method to isotope scanning and to ultrasound, and in some cases can identify metastases not demonstrated by these other techniques.

CT has only a limited role in the detection of bone metastases because this is more effectively carried out by conventional skeletal surveys and radioisotope techniques. Unsuspected bony metastases can sometimes be identified during scans carried out to examine other structures.

MONITORING RESPONSE TO TREATMENT

One of the major uses of CT in oncology is to monitor changes in size of the tumour in response to therapy. Thus, a tumour which is difficult or impossible to visualise by conventional techniques can be assessed initially to provide a baseline of its size and extent and then scanned at regular intervals during treatment. An estimation of significant tumour shrinkage or growth can be made visually with CT by comparing sequential examinations (figures 17.1 and 17.2). Such information can be important to the oncologist and radiotherapist. For example, patients with various tumour types are frequently treated first with chemotherapy to reduce tumour bulk and then with radiotherapy. In such patients, CT can demonstrate the degree of tumour regression with chemotherapy, helping the clinician to decide when to introduce radiotherapy. In the same way, significant tumour growth can be appreciated, indicating failure of a particular treatment regime (figure 17.2c). Monitoring the response to treatment forms a large part of the workload of a scanner in an oncology centre; at the Royal Marsden Hospital, approximately one-third of the CT examinations are repeat scans carried out for this purpose.

Estimations of tumour volume are usually qualitative, but in centres where research facilities are available CT has opened the way to a quantitative approach. Tumour volume calculations using CT are made from the area of tumour shown on successive CT slices throughout the tumour length. Details

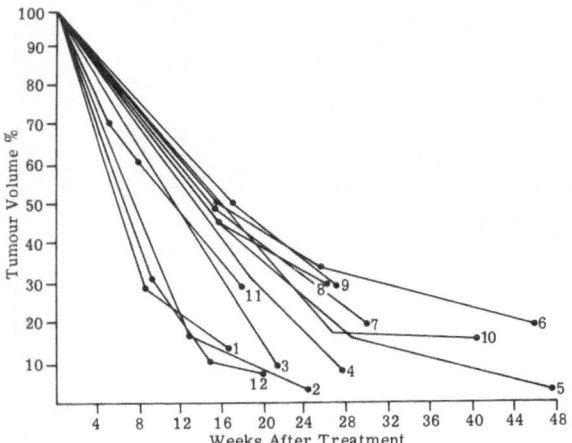

Figure 17.4 Tumour volume regression in 12 patients with abdominal nodal metastases from testicular teratoma who were treated with chemotherapy. Tumour volume is expressed as percentage of initial tumour volume for reasons of clarity

Table 17.2 Comparison of visual and quantitative estimations of tumour volume

	No. of patients	Increase	Decrease	No change
Visual report	22	—	13	9
Quantitative report	22	5	17	—

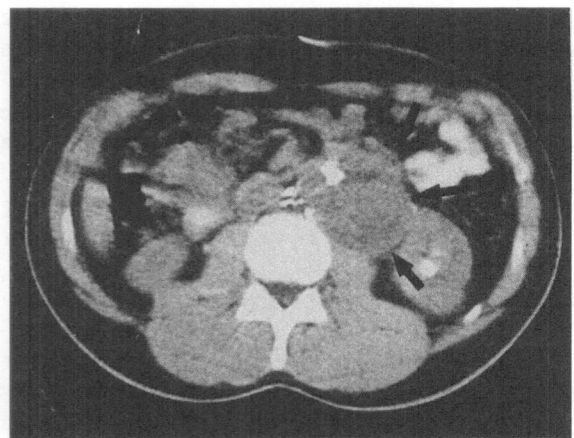

Figure 17.5(a)

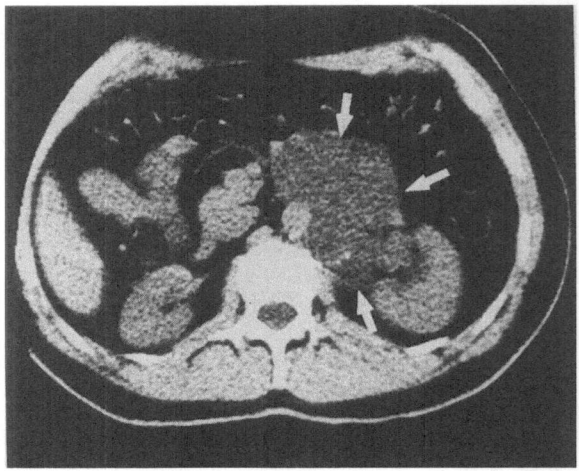

Figure 17.5(b)

Figure 17.5 Monitoring progress — cystic change in abdominal nodal mass due to testicular teratoma. (a) Large mass on the left side of the abdomen (arrowed), +18 EMI units. (b) Follow-up scan in the same patient after chemotherapy. The mass is larger but the tumour has become 'cystic', +6 EMI units. This 'cystic' mass was subsequently excised and histological examination showed no evidence of malignancy

of the technique will vary with the facilities available. At the Royal Marsden Hospital, CT images are displayed on the EMIPLAN 7000 Radiotherapy Planning System (Husband *et al.*, 1981c). A precision light pen is used to outline the tumour on the television monitor (figure 17.3). The area of tumour of each slice is calculated from the number and size of the picture elements within the outline. Possible sources of error include the algorithm used, the pixel size and the observer's ability to achieve reproducible results. Investigations using phantoms have indicated that the error of the method is considerably less than 5%. The errors incurred when attempting to measure human tumours are more difficult to assess, but initial results correlating CT volumes of human tumours with the volume of the excised specimens indicate that the method is highly accurate in selected cases. The major source of error is the difficulty in delineating precise tumour margins; this varies with tumour site and size as well as the patient's build.

Figure 17.4 illustrates tumour regression in response to chemotherapy in 12 patients with abdominal nodal metastases from testicular teratoma. Assessment of small changes in tumour volume may be impossible by visual CT reporting and precise measurement of tumour volume is then the only method of detecting tumour response or growth. Table 17.2 shows a comparison between visual CT reporting and quantitative reporting in the assessment of therapeutic response. In nine out of 22 patients, change in tumour volume was not appreciated by visual reporting although apparent when quantitative estimations were made.

Changes in composition of a tumour may also be detected with CT in patients with abdominal nodal metastases from testicular teratoma (Husband *et al.*, 1981b). In general, these tumours become less dense in response to chemotherapy, and occasionally the attenuation values change from that of a solid lesion to that of a cyst (figure 17.5).

RADIOTHERAPY TREATMENT PLANNING

The objective of radiotherapy is to administer a tumorcidal dose of x-radiation to the tumour site while ensuring that the dose received by normal structures within the radiation field is minimal. Accurate radiotherapy planning thus requires a precise knowledge of tumour site, its anatomical relation to normal structures and correct delineation of the patient's body contour. This information enables the radiotherapist and physicist to produce a treatment plan in the cross-sectional plane through the centre of the target volume. The target volume includes the macroscopic tumour and local sites of microscopic spread. The completed plan shows the position of the external radiation beams and the isodose curves superimposed on the tumour and vital normal structures. Inaccurate information regarding tumour localisation, the position of normal structures and the body contour can result in significant errors in radiotherapy treatment planning, so that the tumour may not be completely encompassed in the target volume. This means that the tumour receives a lower dose than is indicated on the treatment plan and adjacent normal structures receive a higher dose.

The cross-sectional anatomical display produced by CT has obvious application to radiotherapy treatment planning. CT can demonstrate the size of the tumour in each dimension, its position and relation to neighbouring normal structures, such as kidneys and spinal cord. If required, this information can be transferred to the scanogram film so that the clinician can visualise the tumour and the neighbouring structures in three dimensions (figure 17.6). It is important to obtain accurate measurements of the tumour on contiguous slices throughout its length in order to achieve an accurate representation. Apart from radiotherapy treatment planning, a 'map' of this kind can be a help to the surgeon when planning the operation.

The scan data can only be of use for precise radiotherapy treatment planning if the scan is obtained under conditions simulating those under which therapy is given. Hence, patients must be scanned on a flat couch rather than the usual dish-shaped couch because this alters the body contour and internal anatomy (Hobday *et al.*, 1979). Planning scans have to be obtained with the patient breathing to simulate the conditions during treatment. Such scans are likely to be of poor diagnostic

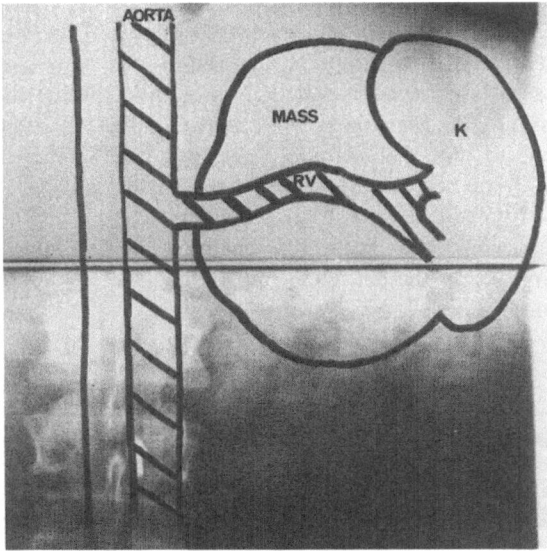

Figure 17.6   Scanogram film showing size and site of an abdominal mass and its relationship to the left renal vein (RV) and left kidney (K)

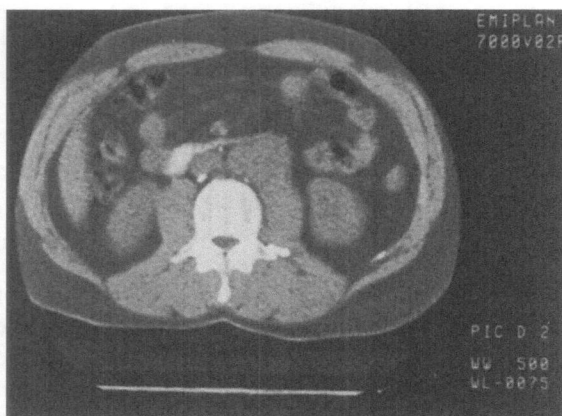

Figure 17.7(a)

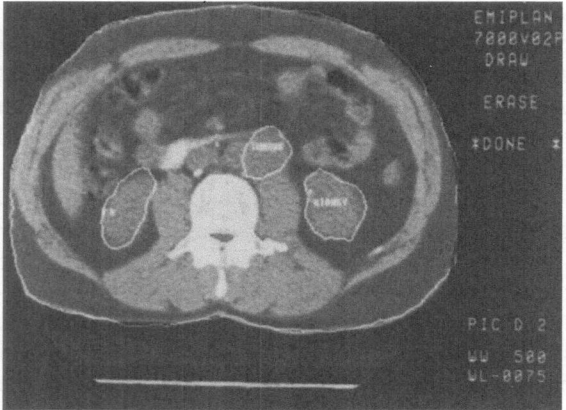

Figure 17.7(b)

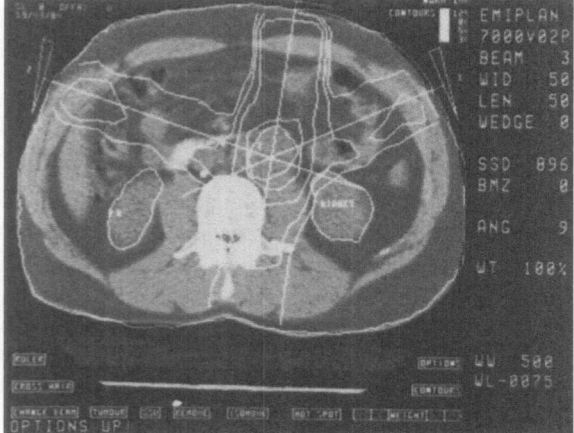

Figure 17.7(c)

quality and it is, therefore, essential to obtain high-quality scans (during suspended respiration) to diagnose the site and extent of local tumour spread before the planning scan is carried out. In this way, any significant difference in body contour or internal anatomy between the non-breathing and breathing scans can be taken into account when producing the final plan.

In order to produce accurate results, the CT information must also be obtained in the proposed treatment position. Techniques to improve the reproducibility of patient positioning include the use of skin markers such as barium paste or radiopaque plastic. Even so, correct patient positioning is one of the major difficulties of using CT for radiotherapy treatment planning. For certain tumours, the optimum position for radiotherapy is such that scanning in the treatment position is impossible. If CT data are to be used in this situation, then the treatment position must be modified.

A life-size CT image is required for radiotherapy treatment planning. There are basically two ways of achieving this. First, a hard copy of the chosen CT slice (either Polaroid print or x-ray film) can be enlarged. The tumour, normal structures and body outline are then traced from the CT image onto paper on which the final plan is produced. Secondly, CT scan data can be transferred directly from the scanner to a radiotherapy planning computer system. A precision light pen is used to outline the tumour, the relevant normal anatomy and the body contour (figure 17.7a and b). (Using the EMIPLAN 7000, the body contour is traced automatically.)

The radiotherapy treatment plan is produced by displaying the radiation beams directly superimposed on the CT image (figure 17.7c). The computed isodose levels are also shown. One of the main

Figure 17.7 Radiotherapy treatment planning. (a) Testicular teratoma showing a nodal mass at the level of the fourth lumbar vertebra. (b) The tumour, kidneys and spinal cord have been outlined using a precision touch-sensitive light pen. (c) Radiotherapy treatment plan superimposed directly on to the CT image on the EMIPLAN 7000 System. The radiation beams and computed isodose levels are shown

advantages of this integrated CT–radiotherapy planning system over other methods is that quantitative information from the CT numbers of surrounding structures through which the radiation beam passes is used in dose calculations. This facility is more important for planning radiotherapy to tumours of the lung than in other sites because significant alterations in absorbed dose result from the beam passing through low-density lung tissue.

Several studies have already indicated that CT-interfaced radiotherapy planning is more accurate than conventional methods, but the improved accuracy varies according to tumour site and size of the radiation field used by the radiotherapist (Geise and McCullough, 1977; Van Dyk *et al.*, 1980). At the Royal Marsden Hospital, a study has been carried out to compare the results of conventional tumour localisation with localisation using CT information. The final treatment plans were changed as a result of CT in 84 out of 290 patients (29%) (table 17.3). Deep-seated intra-abdominal tumours are difficult to localise by conventional methods and the information gain using CT is high; in the Royal Marsden Hospital series, changes were made to the final treatment plans in 61% of such cases.

The value of CT in radiotherapy treatment planning is influenced by the size of the radiation fields. For example, in certain sites, such as the pelvis, the practice of wide-field irradiation reduces the chance of a geographical 'miss' using conventional methods of tumour localisation and reduces the potential benefit of localisation with CT. However, improved tumour localisation should enable radiotherapists to adopt an individual approach to planning and permit higher doses of radiation to be given to smaller volumes of tissue.

Ultimately, the role of CT in radiotherapy treatment planning, and indeed in oncology as a whole, must be assessed by its effect on local tumour control and the final outcome of disease, which will take several years to evaluate. Only time will tell.

Table 17.3 Comparison of conventional methods of localisation with CT: summary of results

	Cases	Total changes
Pelvis	130	29 (22%)
Abdomen	38	23 (61%)
Thorax	94	27 (29%)
Head and neck	28	5 (18%)
Total	290	84 (29%)

REFERENCES

Dunnick, N. R., Ihde, D. C. and Johnston-Early, A. (1979). Abdominal CT in the evaluation of small cell carcinoma of the lung. *American Journal of Roentgenology*, **133**, 1085–1088

Geise, R. A. and McCullough, E. C. (1977). The use of CT scanners in megavoltage photon-beam therapy planning. *Radiology*, **124**, 133–141

Hobday, P., Hodson, N. J., Husband, J., Parker, R. P. and Macdonald, J. S. (1979). Computed tomography applied to radiotherapy treatment planning: techniques and results. *Radiology*, **133**, 477–482

Husband, J. E., Barrett, A. and Peckham, M. J. (1981a). The evaluation of the role of CT in the management of testicular teratoma. *British Journal of Urology*, **53**, 179–183

Husband, J., Hobday, P. and Cassell, K. J. (1981b). Quantitation of therapeutic response. In *Computerised Axial Tomography in Oncology*, eds. J. E. Husband and P. A. Hobday, Churchill Livingstone, Edinburgh, pp. 176–186

Husband, J. E., Peckham, M. J., Cassell, K. and Macdonald, J. S. (1981c). The role of computed tomography in the assessment of tumour volume in patients with malignant testicular teratoma. *Proceedings of the Workshop on Computerised Tomographic Scanners in Radiotherapy in Europe*, Geneva 1979. *British Institute of Radiology Special Report Series* (in press)

Underwood, G. H., Hooper, R. G., Alexander, S. P. and Goodwin, D. W. (1979). Computed tomographic scanning of the thorax in the staging of bronchogenic carcinoma. *New England Journal of Medicine*, **300**, 777–778

Van Dyk, J., Battista, J. J., Cunningham, J. R., Rider, W. D. and Sontag, M. R. (1980). On the impact of CT scanning on radiotherapy planning. *Computerised Tomography*, **4**, 55–65

Index

Abscess
  hepatic 89
  intra-abdominal 125
  pancreas 105–106
  perirenal 67
  psoas 120–121
  renal 62–63
  retroperitoneal 119
Adrenal gland
  calcification 75, 77
  cysts 75
  hyperplasia 77
  tumours, calcification in 75,
    77
    Conn's syndrome 77, 79
    cortical 73
    Cushing's syndrome 77–79
    differential diagnosis 75–77
    metastatic 75
    phaeochromocytoma 73, 75,
      77, 78–79
Aneurysm
  abdominal 123
    dissection of 123–124
  thoracic 35, 38–39
    dissection of 35
Angiomyolipoma of kidney 64
Anthropomorphic baseline 189
Aorta, abdominal 113–114
  aneurysm of 123, 125
    dissection of 123–124
  'floating' 135
Aorta, thoracic 23
  aneurysm of 35, 38–39
    dissection of 35
Aortic-pulmonary window 23
Artefacts, causes of 7, 10–12, 32
  bone 175
  circular 3

spinal canal 184
vessels at lung base 42
Arteries
  coeliac 116
  hepatic 82
  iliac, internal and external 151
  internal mammary 42
  pulmonary 23
  renal 116
  superior mesenteric 98, 99, 116
Asbestosis 53
Ascites 122–123
  in Morison's pouch 83, 122
Azygo-oesophageal recess 25
Azygos fissure 43
Azygos vein 23

Bile duct, common
  dilated 84, 91–92, 94, 107–108
  normal 84
Bile ducts, intrahepatic
  air in 93
  dilated 84, 91–92, 94, 107–108
  normal 84
  versus metastases 86
  versus portal vessels 86
Biopsy 128–130
  indications for 129–130
  technique of 128–129
Bladder
  normal 149–150
  tumours 151–154
    calcification in 152
    effect of radiotherapy on 154,
      162
    extravesical spread 152
Bone, tumours of 171–178
  primary 171–173

secondary 175–176
use of CT in 177–178
Bone islands 166, 175

Calcification in
  adrenal glands 77
  adrenal tumours 75
  aneurysm, thoracic 35
  bladder tumours 152
  corpus uteri 158
  lacrimal gland 207
  liver tumours 86
  lung nodules 47
  mediastinal masses 27
  ovaries 159
  pancreas 106
  pleura 51
  prostate 159
  renal tumours 61
  spleen 127
Calculi in
  gall-bladder 91
  kidney 66
Cavernous haemangioma
  of liver 87
  of orbit 205, 207
Cerebellar tonsils, herniation of 185
Cervix uteri
  normal 150
  tumours of 157
    staging of 162
Cholecystitis 92–93
Cirrhosis of liver 90
Congenital anomalies
  kidney,
    horseshoe 64
    pelvic 64
    polycystic 64

Congenital anomalies (*contd.*)
  skeleton,
    face 194
    hip 181
    spine 181
  thoracic, vascular 36
Conn's syndrome 77, 79
Contrast media
  bladder, demonstration of 146–148
  bowel opacification 10, 97, 146
  spinal cord 187–188
  tissue opacification 14
    dynamic CT 15
    vascular 14–15
  use of, in
    adrenals 71, 75
    biliary tract 81, 84, 93
    bone and soft-tissue tumours
      172
    inferior vena cava 124–125
    kidney 55, 58, 62, 64
    larynx 198
    liver 81, 85–87
    mediastinum 27–28, 35, 39
    orbits 205
    pancreas 98
    paranasal sinuses 189, 194
    parotid gland 201, 203
    pharynx 195
    retroperitoneal abscess 119
    retroperitoneum 137
    spinal cord 184, 185
    submandibular salivary gland
      197
    urinary tract 147
Coronary artery bypass graft 36, 39
Corpus uteri
  normal 150
  tumours of 157–158
    staging of 162
Cushing's syndrome 77–78
Cystadenocarcinoma of pancreas 105
Cysts
  adrenal glands 75
  dermoid 27, 32, 159
  kidney 58–60, 62
  liver 87–88, 93
  ovary 158–159
  pericardium 31
  spleen 126

Dermoid cyst
  mediastinum 27, 32
  orbit 107
  pelvis 159

Diaphragm, crura 27
Dissecting aneurysm
  abdominal 123–124
  thoracic 35

Exophthalmos
  dysthyroid 207
  unilateral 208–209

Fascia
  Gerota's 113
  lateroconal 113
  renal, anterior and posterior 58
Fatty infiltration of liver 89, 90

Gall-bladder
  anatomy 83–84
  cholecystitis 92–93
  dilated 91
Gallstones 91

Haematoma of
  kidney 62, 64
  perirenal space 67
  retroperitoneum 118–119
  spleen 127
Haemochromatosis 90–91
Heart 27, 36
  coronary artery bypass graft 36
Hepatoma 86
Hydatid cyst
  kidney 58
  liver 88

Inferior vena cava
  abdominal 113–115, 124–125
  thrombus of 124
  tumour of 62, 125
Internal mammary arteries 42
Ischiorectal fossa, anatomy of 149

Jaundice 94–95

Kidney
  calculi 66
  congenital anomalies 62, 64
  foetal lobulation 64
  hydronephrosis 64–65
  masses

abscess 62–63
angiomyolipoma 64
cysts
  hydatid 58
  parapelvic 59
  simple 58
fibrolipomatosis 64
haematoma 62, 64
  perinephric 67
tumours 61
  benign versus malignant 62,
    68
  recurrence 70
  staging 62
  xanthogranulomatous
    pyelonephritis 63, 64
'non-functioning', 70
pseudotumour 64
scarred 64
transplant 67
trauma 67

Lacrimal gland, tumour of 207
Larynx
  thyroid cartilage 200–201
  tumours
    aryepiglottic folds 200
    epiglottis 200
    vocal cords 200–201
Lipomatosis, of pelvis 161
Liver
  artefacts 81, 93
  diffuse disease 89–90
    cirrhosis 90
    fatty infiltration 89–90
    haemochromatosis 90–91, 94
    use of CT 93–94
  focal disease 85–89
    abscess 89, 93
    cysts
      hydatid 88
      simple 87–88
    tumours
      benign versus malignant 87
      calcification in 86
      cavernous haemangioma 87
      primary 85
      secondary 86
    use of CT 93
  trauma 89
Lung
  fissures 42–43
  nodules 44
    benign versus malignant 45, 52
    calcification in 47

Lung (*contd.*)
solitary 47
use of CT 52–53
parenchymal changes
asbestosis 53
consolidation 47
emphysematous bullae 47, 53
fibrosis 47
interstitial fibrosis 53
primary tumours
carcinoma of bronchus, staging 52–53
vessels 41–42
apical lower lobe 42
artefacts at base 42
gravity effect 41–42
normal anatomy 41
Lymph nodes, anatomy of 132–134
Lymphadenopathy
accuracy of CT 140–142
anatomical sites
coeliac 137–138
internal jugular chain 197
internal mammary chain 51
mediastinum 28, 36–37
mesentery 137–138
para-aortic 134–135
pelvis 139, 141, 144
porta hepatis 137–138
renal hilar 138–139
retrocrural 135–137
retropharyngeal 196–197
splenic hilar 138
reactive hyperplasia 135
Lymphoma
accuracy and use of abdominal CT 140–145
of orbit 205, 207

Mediastinum
masses 27–36
benign versus malignant 32
calcification in 27
cyst
dermoid 27, 32
pericardial 32
fat pad 31
lymphadenopathy 28
thymoma 27
use of CT 36
Meningioma
of orbits 205, 208
of spinal cord 185–186
Mesothelioma 51
Metastases, in

adrenal gland 75
bone 175
liver 86, 93
lung 44–47
lymph nodes 28, 36–37, 51, 132–145, 197
orbit 207
soft tissues 176
Morison's pouch 83
Muscles
gluteus maximus 148–149, 170, 171
iliacus 151
obturator internus 148
psoas 151, 170
pterygoid 190–191
pyrifomis 151, 170
sartorius 171
tensa fascia lata 171
Myelography, metrizamide 187–188

Neurilemmoma of orbit 205
Neurofibroma, spine 186
Noise 8

Oesophagus, carcinoma 34
Orbits
dythyroid exophthalmos 207–208
masses
cavernous haemangioma 205, 207
dermoid cyst 207
lymphoma 205, 207
metastasis 207
neurilemmoma 205
optic nerve tumour 205
pseudotumour 205–206, 207
venous malformation 206
tumour extension into 196, 208–209
vascular lesions 206
Ovaries
cysts 158–159
normal 150–151
tumours 159
staging of 163

Pancreas
atrophy 107, 109
masses
abscess 105, 106
carcinoma 102
cystadenocarcinoma 105

islet cell tumours 109
normal 99–101
use of CT 109–111
Pancreatitis 102, 107, 109
calcification in 106, 108
dilatation of pancreatic duct 107
pseudocyst 105, 108
Paranasal sinuses
congenital abnormalities 194
inflammatory disease 194
trauma 194
tumours 191–194
Partial volume effect 6–7
kidneys 62
ribs 43–44
spinal cord 184
vocal cords 198
Pelvis
anatomy
bone and muscles 170–171
soft tissues 148–151
frozen 162, 163
trauma of 179
Pericardium
cyst 31
effusion 36
fat pad 31
normal 27
Perirenal space
abscess 67
haematoma 67
Peritoneum, spaces 116–117
Phaeochromocytoma 73, 75, 77–79
Pharynx
tumours
nasopharynx 196
oropharynx 197
Pixel 3
Pleura 49
calcification in 51
effusion 49
thickening 49
tumour 49–51
Polycystic liver 85
Porta hepatis 82
Prostate
calcification in 159
hypertrophy of 159, 161
normal 149
tumours 159–161
staging of 163
Pseudocyst of pancreas 105, 108
Pseudotumour (granuloma)
of orbit 205–206, 207
Psoas muscle
abscess 120–121

Radiation dose 7
Radiotherapy treatment planning
    technique 215
    use of CT in 215
Rectum
    normal 148–149
    tumours
        differential diagnosis 154–155
        primary 154, 162
        recurrent 154–156
Reidel's lobe 82
Resolution 6, 8
Retroperitoneum
    abscess 119–120
    fibrosis 121, 134–135
    spaces of
        anterior pararenal 113
        perirenal 113
        posterior pararenal 113
    tumours of
        benign versus
            lymphadenopathy 118
        benign versus malignant
            117–118
        primary 117–118

Salivary gle ds
    normal
        parotid 201
        submandibular 203
    tumours
        parotid 202
Sarcoidosis, pulmonary, 53
Scanogram 13–14
Schmorl's nodes 175
Soft tissues, tumours of 174–176
Spinal cord
    metrizamide, use of 176, 187–188
    syringomyelia 185
    tumours
        extramedullary 185–187
        intramedullary 185

Spine
    congenital anomalies 181
    degenerative disease 181
    disc prolapse 183
    normal anatomy 166–168
    stenosis of 181, 188
    trauma
Spleen 126
    calcification in 127
    cyst 126
    haematoma 127
    Hodgkin's disease 127
    trauma 127
Staging of tumours 211
    bladder 162
    bronchus 38, 52
    kidney 62
    lymphomas 140–141
    oesophagus 38
    pelvis 162
    testicular tumours 37, 52,
        141–142
Superior vena cava 23
    compression of 38
Syringomyelia 185, 188

Testicular teratoma
    lymphadenopathy
        mediastinum 37
        para-aortic 135, 139, 141–142,
            144
    metastases, lung 52
Therapeutic response
    changes in composition 215
    changes in volume 213
Thrombus
    inferior vena cava 62, 124–125
    renal vein 62, 123–125
    thoracic aneurysm 35
Tymus 23–25
    normal 23
    tumours 27, 36–37

Trauma
    kidney 67
    liver 89
    skeletal system 178–180, 194
    spleen 127

Ultrasound versus CT
    adrenal glands 77, 79
    intra-abdominal masses 124–126
    kidney 68–70
    liver 94–95
    pancreas 110
Ureter
    dilatation of 66
    displacement of 68

Vagina, normal 148, 150
Veins
    azygos 23
    innominate 23–24, 27
    orbital malformations 206
    portal
        intrahepatic 82, 84
        main 82, 84, 98
        versus intrahepatic bile ducts 85
        versus metastasis 86
    pulmonary 23
    renal
        left 56, 62
        right 56, 62, 116
    splenic 99
Vesicles, seminal
    normal 149
Voxel 3

Window
    level 4–5, 82
    width 4–5, 81

Xanthogranulomatous pyelonephritis
    63